Essentials of Non-Alcoholic Fatty Liver Disease

Anca Trifan · Carol Stanciu
Cristina Muzica

Editors

Essentials of Non-Alcoholic Fatty Liver Disease

Complications and Extrahepatic Manifestations

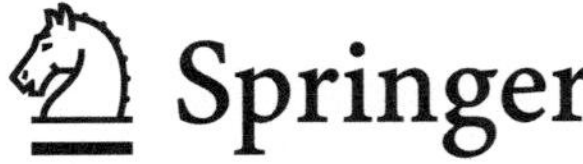

Editors
Anca Trifan
Department of Gastroenterology and
Hepatology
Grigore T. Popa University of Medicine and
Pharmacy
Iasi, Romania

Carol Stanciu
Department of Gastroenterology and
Hepatology
Grigore T. Popa University of Medicine and
Pharmacy
Iasi, Romania

Cristina Muzica
Department of Gastroenterology and
Hepatology
Grigore T. Popa University of Medicine and
Pharmacy
Iasi, Romania

ISBN 978-3-031-33550-1   ISBN 978-3-031-33548-8   (eBook)
https://doi.org/10.1007/978-3-031-33548-8

This Springer imprint is published by the registered company Springer Nature Switzerland AG
The registered company address is: Gewerbestrasse 11, 6330 Cham, Switzerland

Preface

The hepatology community recognized and drew attention in the last years to poor provision of services for liver diseases worldwide and the only focus on end-stage liver disease and its complications—cirrhosis and cancer, neglecting any preventive measures. It was emphasized that a change of paradigm is urgently needed to focus on the identification of those with progressive liver fibrosis and to find strategies to prevent chronic liver diseases. Nowadays, viral hepatitis could easily be treated if timely diagnosed by screening programs. Liver fibrosis could be assessed by simple, noninvasive methods, available for any physician. However, the burden of chronic liver disease is increasing due to a lack of effective measures for limiting inappropriate alcohol consumption and preventing obesity. Non-alcoholic fatty liver disease (NAFLD), obesity, and diabetes mellitus seem to be twenty-first century silent epidemics that require energetic policy action to limit them.

Our book tries to synthetize the latest developments in understanding the NAFLD spectrum and to offer medical practitioner of any specialty the necessary knowledge to understand the disease, to diagnose and manage patients, and more importantly enough information to engage every reader in the twenty-first century fight to prevent end-stage liver disease due to fatty liver.

We hope that we succeeded in guiding the readership to learn about NAFLD, then to understand the complexity of the problem, and ultimately to prepare for action in daily practice and in the community.

Iasi, Romania
Iasi, Romania
Iasi, Romania
December 2022

Anca Trifan
Cristina Muzica
Carol Stanciu

Contents

About the Editors

Anca Trifan MD, PhD, FEBGH, FRCP (London), Professor of Gastroenterology and Internal Medicine, and Director of the Department of Internal Medicine of the "Grigore T. Popa" University of Medicine and Pharmacy, Iasi, Romania, Head of the Institute of Gastroenterology and Hepatology, Iasi, Romania. Her research interests include viral hepatitis, liver cirrhosis, liver transplant, acute-on-chronic liver failure, noninvasive assessment of liver fibrosis, inflammatory bowel disease, biliary tract disorders, and *Clostridium difficile* infection. She has published numerous original papers, books, and chapters of books and has been actively involved in the peer-review process of many high-impact factor journals. She has been involved in medical teaching from the beginning of her career. She received many prizes form scientific organization (e.g., Rising Stars in Gastroenterology awarded by UEG). She is past president of the Romanian Society of Gastroenterology and Hepatology, member of the Academy of Medical Sciences, member of the European Board of Gastroenterology, AGA fellow, and member of the American Association for the Study of Liver Diseases.

Carol Stanciu MD, PhD, FRCP (London), Professor of Gastroenterology and Internal Medicine, University of Medicine and Pharmacy "Gr. T. Popa," Iasi, Fellow of Academy of Medical Sciences, and Fellow of Romanian Academy. Dr. Carol Stanciu (born May 17, 1937; Hasdat, Hunedoara, Romania) is one of the main founders of gastroenterology, diagnostic and therapeutic endoscopy in Romania. He graduated from the Faculty of Medicine, University of Medicine and Pharmacy "Gr. T. Popa" Iasi (1963) where he also received PhD and DSc, and served as Assistant, Associate Professor, and Professor of the Dept of Internal Medicine and Gastroenterology. He is former Rector of the University of Medicine and Pharmacy "Gr. T. Popa" Iasi (1992–2004), Dean of Faculty of Medicine (2004–2008), President of Romanian Society of Endoscopy (1996–2000), President of Romanian Society of Gastroenterology and Hepatology (2000–2008), and Chairman of the Ethics Committee of the World Organization of Gastroenterology (1994–2002). He has always been involved in all areas of academic life: medical training, especially therapeutic endoscopy, patient care, administrative work, and mentorship. His research interests include gastrointestinal motility, viral hepatitis, liver cirrhosis, liver transplant, acute-on-chronic liver failure, noninvasive assessment of liver fibrosis, inflammatory bowel disease, biliary tract disorders, and *Clostridium diffi-*

cile infection. He has published numerous original papers, books, and chapters of books and has been actively involved in the peer-review process of prestigious high-impact factor journals. He received many awards from Romanian Presidency, French Presidency, WGO, Romanian Society of Gastroenterology and Hepatology, and many universities.

Cristina Muzica MD, PhD, Assistant Professor of Gastroenterology and Internal Medicine, University of Medicine and Pharmacy "Gr. T. Popa," Iasi. Her primary research interests are in the field of hepatology and consist of hepatocellular carcinoma, viral hepatitis, non-alcoholic fatty liver disease, and alcoholic liver diseases. During her career she published several papers including book chapters about the aforementioned themes. She is a member of the Romanian Society of Gastroenterology, European Association for the Study of the Liver, United European Gastroenterology, and Romanian Society of Neurogastroenterology.

Abbreviations

5mc	5-methylcytosine
AASLD	American Association for the Study of Liver Diseases
ACLD	Advanced chronic liver disease
ACLY	ATP citrate lyase
ACTH	Adrenocorticotropic hormone
ADMA	Asymmetric dimethyl arginine
ADPN	Adiponutrin
AE	Adverse effect
AGEs	Advanced glycosylation end products
AIH	Autoimmune hepatitis
ALD	Alcoholic liver disease/alcohol-related liver disease
ALP	Alkaline phosphatase
ALT	Alanine transaminase
ANA	Antinuclear antibodies
apoB	Apolipoprotein B
APRI	AST-platelet ratio index
ARFI	Acoustic radiation force impulse
ASA	American society of anesthesiologists
ASH	Alcoholic steatohepatitis
AST	Aspartate aminotransferase
AUROC	Area under receiver-operating characteristics curve
BAFF	B cell activating factor
BAFLD	Both alcohol and metabolic associated fatty liver disease
BAs	Bile acids
BCLC	Barcelona clinic for liver cancer
BMI	Body mass index
C22orf20	Chromosome 22 open reading frame 20
cACLD	Compensated advanced chronic liver disease
CAP	Controlled attenuation parameter
CD	Celiac disease
CEUS	Contrast-enhanced ultrasonography
ChREBP	Carbohydrate response element-binding protein
CHB	Chronic hepatitis B
CHC	Chronic hepatitis C

CI	Confidence interval
CKD	Chronic kidney disease
CLD	Chronic liver disease
CPT	Complete portal tract
CRC	Colorectal cancer
CREBH	Cyclic AMP-responsive element-binding protein 3-like 3
CT	Computed tomography
CV	Cardiovascular
CVD	Cardiovascular disease
DAMPs	Damage-associated molecular patterns
DC	Dendritic cell
DDP-4i	Dipeptidyl dipeptidase-4 inhibitors
DIFLD	Drug-induced fatty liver disease
DILI	Drug-induced liver disease
DISH	Drug-induced steatohepatitis
DNA	Deoxyribonucleic acid
DNL	De novo lipogenesis
DNMTs	DNA methyltransferases
E8SJM	Exon 8 splice junction mutation
EASL	European association for the study of the liver
EGD	Esophagogastroduodenoscopy
eGFR	Estimated glomerular filtration rate
ER	Endoplasmic reticulum
ERLIN1	ER lipid raft associated 1
EUS	Endoscopic ultrasound
EV	Esophageal varices
FA	Fatty acids
FBS	Fasting blood sugar
FFA	Free fatty acid
FIB-4	Fibrosis 4
FNA	Fine-needle aspiration
FNB	Fine-needle biopsy
FPG	Fasting plasma glucose
FSH	Follicle-stimulating hormone
GALNTL4	Putative polypeptide N-acetylgalactosaminyl-transferase-like protein 4
GBD	Global burden of disease
GCKR	Glucokinase regulatory protein
GFD	Gluten-free diet
GGT	Gamma-glutamyl transferase
GLP-1 RA	Glucagon-like peptide-1 receptor agonists
GRID1	Glutamate receptor delta-1
GWAS	Genome-wide association study
HbA1c	Hemoglobin A1c
HBV	Hepatitis B virus

HCADS	Hepatitis C-associated dysmetabolic syndrome
HCC	Hepatocellular carcinoma
HCV	Hepatitis C virus
HDL	High-density lipoprotein
HIV	Human immunodeficiency virus
HOMA	Homeostasis model assessment
HOMA-IR	Homeostasis model assessment for insulin resistance
HSC	Hepatic stellate cells
hs-CRP	High-sensitivity C-reactive protein
HSD17B13	Hydroxysteroid 17-dehydrogenase
HVPG	Hepatic venous pressure gradient
ICC	Intraclass correlation coefficient
ICU	Intensive care unit
IFN	Interferon
IFN-γ	Interferon gamma
IGF1	Insulin-like growth factor 1
IGFBP2	Insulin-like growth factor binding protein 2
IL	Interleukin
IP6K3	Inositol hexaphosphate kinase 3
IPLA2epsilon	Calcium-independent phospholipase A2-epsilon
IQR	Interquartile range
IQR/M	Interquartile range-to-median ratio
IR	Insulin resistance
IRS-1	Insulin receptor substrate-1
KC	Kupffer cell
KDIGO	Kidney disease improving global outcome
LB	Liver biopsy
LDL	Low-density lipoproteins
LFT	Liver function test
LH	Luteinizing hormone
LT	Liver transplantation
MAFLD	Metabolic-associated fatty liver disease
MBOAT1	Membrane bound O-acyltransferase domain containing 1
MBOAT7	Membrane bound O-acyltransferase domain containing 7
MCP-1	Monocyte chemoattractant protein-1
MDB	Mallory-Denk bodie
MetS	Metabolic syndrome
miR	Micro RNA
miRNA	Micro RNA
MRE	Magnetic resonance elastography
MRI	Magnetic resonance imaging
MRI PDFF	Magnetic resonance imaging proton density fat fraction
MTTP	Microsomal triglyceride transfer protein
NAFL	Nonalcoholic fatty liver
NAFLD	Nonalcoholic fatty liver disease

NAS	NAFLD activity score
NASH	Nonalcoholic steatohepatitis
NASH CRN	The NASH Clinical Research Network
NCAN	Neurocan
NHANES III	Third National Health and Nutrition Examination Survey
NK	Natural killer
NLR	Nucleotide oligomerization domain-like receptor
NO	Nitric oxide
NOS	Nitric oxide synthase
NPV	Negative predictive value
NRTI	Nucleoside reverse transcriptase inhibitor
OR	Odds ratio
PAI-1	Plasminogen activator inhibitor-1
PAMPs	Pathogen-associated molecular patterns
PC	Pyruvate carboxylase
PCOS	Polycystic ovarian syndrome
PCP	Primary care practitioner
PEMT	Phosphatidylethanolamine N-methyltransferase
PET	Positron emission tomography
PLCG1	Phospholipase C-gamma-1
PNPLA3	Patting-like phospholipase domain containing 3
PPARA	Peroxisome proliferator-activated receptor alpha
PPAR-γ	Peroxisome proliferator-activated receptor-γ
PPP1R3B	Protein phosphatase 1 regulatory subunit 3B
PPV	Positive predictive value
PRKCE	Protein kinase C epsilon
PRRs	Pattern recognition receptors
PST	Performance status test
RAE	Radioembolization
RCT	Randomized controlled trial
RNA	Ribonucleic acid
ROS	Reactive oxygen species
RR	Relative risk
RT	Radiation therapy
SAM	S-adenyl methionine
SBRT	Stereotactic body radiation therapy
SEER	Surveillance, epidemiology and end results
SGLT2i	Sodium-glucose-co-transporter-2 inhibitors
SH-HCC	Steatohepatitis hepatocellular carcinoma
sLDL	Small low-density lipoprotein
SNP	Single-nucleotide polymorphism
SOD	Superoxide dismutase
SOD2	Superoxide dismutase 2
Sp	Associated specificities
SPPARMs	Selective peroxisome proliferator-activated receptor-γ modulators

SREBP1c	Sterol regulating element binding protein 1c
Ss	Observed sensitivities
T2DM	Type 2 diabetes mellitus
TACE	Transarterial chemoembolization
TARE	Transarterial radioembolization
TF	Nuclear transcription factor
TGs	Triglycerides
Th	T-helper
TJLB	Transjugular liver biopsy
TLR	Toll-like receptor
TM6SF2	Transmembrane 6 superfamily member 2
TNF-A	Tumor necrosis factor alpha
TRIB1	Tribbles pseudokinase 1
UACR	Urinary albumin to creatinine ratio
UCP2	Uncoupling protein 2
UK	United Kingdom
UPR	Unfolded protein response
US	Ultrasonography
USA	United States of America
VAFLD	Virus-associated fatty liver disease
VCTE	Vibration-controlled transient elastography
VLDL	Very low-density lipoprotein
WD	Wilson disease
XO	Xanthine oxidase

The Nomenclature and Definition of Nonalcoholic Fatty Liver Disease

1

Anca Trifan and Carol Stanciu

1.1 Introduction

The term "nonalcoholic fatty liver disease" (NAFLD) is currently used to refer to a broad and heterogeneous range of clinic and pathological entities that have one thing in common: they are all characterized by the absence of significant alcohol consumption or other causes of liver damage like steatogenic drugs, viral hepatitis, or hereditary disorders, but at least 5% of their hepatocytes show signs of steatosis (the presence of lipid droplets) [1]. The following are the most frequent concurrent diseases that must be ruled out: hemochromatosis, autoimmune hepatitis, celiac disease, Wilson's disease, a/hypobetalipoproteinemia lipoatrophy, drug-induced fatty liver disease, HCV-associated fatty liver disease (GT3), and alcoholic fatty liver disease. Inborn metabolic abnormalities, hypopituitarism, hypothyroidism, starvation, parenteral nutrition, and Wolman disease (lysosomal acid lipase deficiency) [2].

The NAFLD spectrum includes the following:

1. **Nonalcoholic fatty liver (NAFL)** which includes *pure steatosis* without any inflammation and *steatosis without significant inflammation* or signs of hepatocyte injury (no ballooning), with some *lobular inflammation* being possible [3].
2. **Nonalcoholic steatohepatitis (NASH)** is the most aggressive form of NAFLD characterized by the presence of steatosis plus significant inflammation ("which developed to remove the fat") and signs of hepatocyte's injury as ballooning. Fibrosis is the histological feature which is considered the most important pre-

A. Trifan (✉) · C. Stanciu
Gastroenterology Department, Grigore T. Popa University of Medicine and Pharmacy, Iasi, Romania

St. Spiridon Emergency Hospital, Institute of Gastroenterology and Hepatology, Iasi, Romania

A. Trifan et al. (eds.), *Essentials of Non-Alcoholic Fatty Liver Disease*, https://doi.org/10.1007/978-3-031-33548-8_1

dictor for clinical outcome. The European Association for Study of the Liver (EASL) subclassified NASH depending on the degree of fibrosis in:
(a) *Early NASH* (no or mild fibrosis)
(b) *Fibrotic NASH* (significant/advanced fibrosis)
(c) *NASH cirrhosis* is defined by stage 4 of fibrosis and presence of regeneration nodules, drastic change in normal lobular architecture associated with residual signs of steatosis, and NASH [4]

Another term which should be defined is *cryptogenic cirrhosis*, which means features of cirrhosis with no obvious etiology. In patients with cryptogenic cirrhosis, metabolic risk factors such as obesity and other metabolic syndrome (MetS) components could be frequently recognized. It is largely accepted that cryptogenic cirrhosis is part of NAFLD [5].

1.2 Hepatocellular Carcinoma (HCC)

Hepatocellular carcinoma has been suggested to be included as part of NAFLD spectrum, and the risk of NAFLD-associated HCC is increased in cirrhosis and pre-cirrhotic stages, especially when *PNPLA3* rs738409 C > G polymorphism is present [6].

The nomenclature of NAFLD includes a negation *nonalcoholic*, which should also be defined. It is considered nonalcoholic when a significant alcohol consumption is not ongoing or was not present in the past (previous 2 years). The significant alcohol consumption is inhomogeneously defined in different regions and by different scientific bodies [7].

A *standard drink*, according to the National Institute on Alcohol Abuse and Alcoholism (NIAAA), contains 14 g of pure alcohol. This value is used by the American Association for Study of the Liver (AASLD) in their consensus. The World Health Organization (WHO) and the EASL define a standard drink as any form of alcohol which contains 10 g of pure alcohol [8]. A significant alcohol consumption is defined by the AASLD and the EASL as three or more standard drinks per day (or >21 drinks per week) for men and two or more standard drinks per day (>14 drinks per week) for women. Because of the different definitions of a standard drink, the actual alcohol quantity which defines significant consumption differs between the USA and Europe (42 g daily in the USA/30 g daily in Europe for men and 28 g daily in the USA and 20 g daily in Europe for women), which can produce some inconsistencies [9].

1.3 Metabolic Syndrome

Metabolic syndrome is defined by a cluster of five features of metabolic type, in close relation with insulin resistance used to identify individuals at increased risk of atherosclerotic cardiovascular disease and vascular and neurological complications such as a cerebrovascular accident. More recently, MetS has been considered to be a risk for NAFLD and fatty liver as the early sign of insulin resistance [10]. The presence of MetS is confirmed when three of the following five features are present: (1) waist circumference more than 94 cm in men and 88 cm in women; (2) elevated triglycerides 150 mg/dL or greater; (3) reduced high-density lipoprotein cholesterol (HDL) less than 40 mg/dL in men or less than 50 mg/dL in women; (4) elevated fasting glucose of 100 mg/dL or greater; and (5) blood pressure values of systolic 130 mmHg or higher and/or diastolic 85 mmHg or higher [11].

1.4   Impaired Glucose Tolerance

Between normal glucose homeostasis and diabetes, there are intermediate stages of aberrant glucose control represented by impaired fasting glucose and impaired glucose tolerance [12]. An increased fasting plasma glucose (FPG) concentration (between 100 and 126 mg/dL) is now used to identify impaired fasting glucose. A high 2-h plasma glucose concentration (between 140 and 200 mg/dL) after a 75 g glucose load on the oral glucose tolerance test (OGTT) in the context of an FPG concentration of less than 126 mg/dL indicates impaired glucose tolerance [13].

1.5   Insulin Resistance

A major factor thought to be implicated in the pathophysiology of NAFLD is insulin resistance, which is defined as a decreased physiologic response to insulin stimulation of target tissues, primarily the liver, muscle, and adipose tissue. Hyperinsulinemia and an increase in beta-cell insulin synthesis occur as a result of impaired glucose elimination brought on by insulin resistance. It most frequently happens in connection with obesity, but there are many other underlying causes as well, including obesity-related stress (caused by an excess of the hormones that regulate stress, such as cortisol, growth hormone, catecholamines, and glucagon), medicine (such as glucocorticoids, human immunodeficiency virus antiretrovirals, oral contraceptives), pregnancy (placental lactogen), lipodystrophy associated, insulin antibodies, genetic defects in insulin-signaling pathways (type A insulin resistance), and blocking autoantibodies against the insulin receptor (type B insulin resistance) [14, 15].

When a patient exhibits the characteristics of MetS, including hyperglycemia, dyslipidemia, abdominal obesity, and hypertension, insulin resistance is presumed to be the cause. It would be helpful to measure insulin resistance in obese patients in a clinical context because they are most likely to develop type 2 diabetes mellitus and its consequences, cardiovascular disease, and several cancers linked to obesity and insulin resistance (e.g., colon, breast, and endometrial cancers) [16]. But there is not a reliable test available right now to assess insulin resistance in a clinical context. The hyperinsulinemic-euglycemic glucose clamp method is the gold standard for determining insulin resistance. Although this study method has limited clinical relevance, there are a number of insulin resistance surrogate measures that can be used in clinical settings, such as homeostasis model assessment-estimated insulin resistance (HOMA-IR) and quantitative insulin sensitivity check index (QUICKI) [17].

1.6   Obesity

The accumulation of excessive bodily fat, which is harmful to health, is what defines obesity. It is regarded as a condition with many complications that is difficult. BMI is a quick, cheap, and widely used assessment that enables an early diagnosis of obesity. It is frequently employed as a measure of relative weight. BMI is calculated by multiplying a person's weight in kilograms by the square of his or her height in meters (kg/m^2). When it falls between 18.5 and 24.9 kg/m^2, BMI is regarded as normal. When a person's BMI is between 25 and 29.9 kg/m^2 and above 30, they are termed overweight. Contrarily, when BMI is less than 18.5 kg/m^2, thinness is taken into account [18, 19].

Central obesity is characterized as an excessive buildup of abdominal fat, primarily from visceral fat. Waist circumference, a useful anthropometric parameter to assess visceral fat in adults, is the simplest technique to measure visceral fat. The top of the iliac crest (NHANES III, NCEP ATP III), the narrowest waist (ASM), the level of the navel, and the approximate halfway between the lower edge of the last palpable rib and the top of the iliac crest are all considered to represent the waist level [20]. Different cutoffs have been suggested as metabolic syndrome criteria. For different racial and gender groupings, recommended cutoffs (equal or higher) for WC are different. For European population, the cutoff measurements are 94 cm for men and 80 cm for women. On the other hand, the American standard for central obesity is 102 cm for men and 88 cm for women. Cutoffs for men and women that have been proven to be effective in a number of studies are 90 cm for South Asians, 80 cm for Chinese, and 80 cm for Japanese [21].

1.7   Lean NAFLD

Lean NAFLD defines the spectrum of NAFLD which is encountered in individuals with BMI <25 kg/m^2 in Western countries and <23 kg/m^2 in Asian population with no significant alcohol consumption and no concurrent causes of steatosis. NAFLD in lean patients, unlike conventional NAFLD, is a special subtype that develops without obesity and is linked to a lower metabolic burden [22]. These illnesses are thought to have a separate etiology, with metabolic and gut microbiota characteristics that differ from NAFLD in obese individuals [23]. Lean individuals with NAFLD may also experience more severe outcomes, including an increased risk of advanced fibrosis, cardiovascular problems, and liver-related death. Additionally, it was reported that patients with lean NAFLD have considerably higher overall mortality rates than those with non-lean NAFLD [24].

The concurrent diseases which should be meticulously excluded in lean individuals before a definitive diagnosis of NAFLD are (a) general/nutritional diseases: acute starvation, protein malnutrition, total parenteral nutrition, Mauriac syndrome, and hepatitis C; (b) metabolic: cystic fibrosis, Wilson's disease, alpha-1-antitrypsin deficiency, galactosemia, fructosemia, Wolman disease, glycogen storage disease, mitochondrial and peroxisomal defects of fatty acid oxidation, lipodystrophies, abetalipoproteinemia, and Weber-Christian disease; and (c) drug toxicity: amiodarone, methotrexate, prednisolone, L-asparaginase methotrexate, vitamin A, valproate, tamoxifen, zidovudine, and ecstasy [25, 26].

The obvious relationship in most cases between metabolic disturbances and fatty liver disease, the fact that NAFLD is an exclusion diagnosis (elimination of significant alcohol intake and concurrent causes of liver diseases), and the word alcohol (even preceded by "non") which could bring some stigmatization for patients were considered strong arguments for searching for a new nomenclature and new definition which could solve these shortcomings, which allows a positive diagnosis and could include patients with concomitant liver diseases [26, 27].

The term **metabolic dysfunction-associated fatty liver disease (MAFLD)** was coined and defined as hepatic steatosis (proved by any of the following: histology, imaging, or blood biomarker) in addition to one of the following three criteria, namely *overweight/obesity, type 2 diabetes mellitus* (T2DM), or evidence of *metabolic dysregulation* [28].

At least two metabolic risk abnormalities are required to establish metabolic dysregulation: waist measurements of Caucasian men and women of 102/88 cm or Asian men and women of 90/80 cm; blood pressure measurements of 130/85 mmHg or use of a particular medication; plasma triglycerides less than 150 mg/dL (1.70 mmol/L) or using a particular medication; prediabetes, which is defined as fasting plasma glucose of 5.6–6.9 mmol/L, or HOMA-IR of 2.5; plasma HDL cholesterol 1.0 mmol/L for males and 2 mg/L for women; or lipid-lowering medication treatment [29].

There are many discussions and an international debate going on in order to find out if MAFLD could replace the term NAFLD, if these distinct nomenclatures are naming the same disease or a new disease is born. Until a straight conclusion is reached, we choose to use the old good term of NAFLD.

References

1. Chalasani N, Younossi Z, Lavine JE, Diehl AM, Brunt EM, Cusi K, Charlton M, Sanyal AJ. The diagnosis and management of non-alcoholic fatty liver disease: practice guideline by the American Association for the Study of Liver Diseases, American College of Gastroenterology, and the American Gastroenterological Association. Hepatology. 2012;55(6):2005–23.
2. Ahadi M, Molooghi K, Masoudifar N, Namdar AB, Vossoughinia H, Farzanehfar M. A review of non-alcoholic fatty liver disease in non-obese and lean individuals. J Gastroenterol Hepatol. 2021;36(6):1497–507.
3. Puri P, Sanyal AJ. Nonalcoholic fatty liver disease: definitions, risk factors, and workup. Clin Liver Dis. 2012;1:99–103.

4. Fingas CD, Best J, Sowa J-P, Canbay A. Epidemiology of nonalcoholic steatohepatitis and hepatocellular carcinoma. Clin Liver Dis. 2016;8:119–22.
5. Mercado-Irizarry A, Torres EA. Cryptogenic cirrhosis: current knowledge and future directions. Clin Liver Dis, vol. 7; 2016. p. 69.
6. Shah PA, Patil R, Harrison SA. NAFLD-related hepatocellular carcinoma: the growing challenge. Hepatology. 2022;00:1–17.
7. Hajifathalian K, Torabi Sagvand B, McCullough AJ. Effect of alcohol consumption on survival in nonalcoholic fatty liver disease: a national prospective cohort study. Hepatology. 2019;70:511–21.
8. What is a standard drink? National Institute on Alcohol Abuse and Alcoholism (NIAAA) Alcohol & Your Health website. https://www.niaaa.nih.gov/alcohol-health/overview-alcohol-consumption/what-standard-drink. Accessed 1 Nov 2022.
9. Mukamal KJ. A safe level of alcohol consumption: the right answer demands the right question. J Intern Med. 2020;288(5):550–9.
10. Marchesini G, Bugianesi E, Forlani G, Cerrelli F, Lenzi M, Manini R, Natale S, Vanni E, Villanova N, Melchionda N, Rizzetto M. Nonalcoholic fatty liver, steatohepatitis, and the metabolic syndrome. Hepatology. 2003;37:917–23.
11. Day C. Metabolic syndrome, or what you will: definitions and epidemiology. Diabetes Vasc Dis Res. 2007;4(1):32–8.
12. Nathan DM, Davidson MB, DeFronzo RA, Heine RJ, Henry RR, Pratley R, Zinman B, American Diabetes Association. Impaired fasting glucose and impaired glucose tolerance: implications for care. Diabetes Care. 2007;30(3):753–9.
13. Freeman AM, Pennings N. Insulin resistance. [updated 2022 Jul 4]. In: StatPearls [Internet]. Treasure Island (FL): StatPearls Publishing; 2022.
14. Ascaso JF, Pardo S, Real JT, Lorente RI, Priego A, Carmena R. Diagnosing insulin resistance by simple quantitative methods in subjects with normal glucose metabolism. Diabetes Care. 2003;26(12):3320–5.
15. Gołacki J, Matuszek M, Matyjaszek-Matuszek B. Link between insulin resistance and obesity-from diagnosis to treatment. Diagnostics (Basel). 2022;12(7):1681. Published 2022 Jul 10.
16. Avgerinos KI, Spyrou N, Mantzoros CS, Dalamaga M. Obesity and cancer risk: emerging biological mechanisms and perspectives. Metabolism. 2019;92:121–35. https://doi.org/10.1016/j.metabol.2018.11.001. Epub 2018 Nov 13.
17. Rössner SM, Neovius M, Mattsson A, Marcus C, Norgren S. HOMA-IR and QUICKI: decide on a general standard instead of making further comparisons. Acta Paediatr. 2010;99(11):1735–40.
18. Jensen MD, Ryan DH, Apovian CM, et al. 2013 AHA/ACC/TOS guideline for the management of overweight and obesity in adults: a report of the American College of Cardiology/American Heart Association task force on practice guidelines and the Obesity Society. Circulation. 2014;129:S102.
19. Bray GA, Frühbeck G, Ryan DH, Wilding JP. Management of obesity. Lancet. 2016;387:1947.
20. Turkbey EB, McClelland RL, Kronmal RA, Burke GL, Bild DE, Tracy RP, Arai AE, Lima JA, Bluemke DA. The impact of obesity on the left ventricle: the multi-ethnic study of atherosclerosis (MESA). JACC Cardiovasc Imaging. 2010;3(3):266–74.
21. Dansinger ML, Gleason JA, Griffith JL, et al. Comparison of the Atkins, Ornish, Weight Watchers, and Zone diets for weight loss and heart disease risk reduction: a randomized trial. JAMA. 2005;293:43.
22. Younossi ZM, Stepanova M, Negro F, et al. Nonalcoholic fatty liver disease in lean individuals in the United States. Medicine (Baltimore). 2012;91:319–27.
23. Eslam M, Sanyal AJ, George J. International consensus panel. MAFLD: a consensus-driven proposed nomenclature for metabolic associated fatty liver disease. Gastroenterology. 2020;158:1999–2014.e1.
24. Younes R, Govaere O, Petta S, et al. Caucasian lean subjects with non-alcoholic fatty liver disease share long-term prognosis of non-lean: time for reappraisal of BMI-driven approach? Gut. 2022;71:382–90.

25. Cruz ACD, Bugianesi E, George J, et al. Characteristics and long-term prognosis of lean patients with nonalcoholic fatty liver disease. Gastroenterology. 2014;5:S909.
26. Loomis AK, Kabadi S, Preiss D, Hyde C, Bonato V, St Louis M, Desai J, Gill JM, Welsh P, Waterworth D, Sattar N. Body mass index and risk of nonalcoholic fatty liver disease: two electronic health record prospective studies. J Clin Endocrinol Metab. 2016;101(3):945–52.
27. WHO Expert Consultation. Appropriate body-mass index for Asian populations and its implications for policy and intervention strategies. Lancet. 2004;363(9403):157–63.
28. Younossi ZM, Rinella ME, Sanyal AJ, Harrison SA, Brunt EM, Goodman Z, Cohen DE, Loomba R. From NAFLD to MAFLD: implications of a premature change in terminology. Hepatology. 2021;73:1194–8.
29. van Kleef LA, de Knegt RJ. The transition from NAFLD to MAFLD: one size still does not fit all—time for a tailored approach? Hepatology. 2022;76:1243–5.

Nonalcoholic Fatty Liver Disease Versus Metabolic Associated Fatty Liver Disease

Sebastian Zenovia and Irina Girleanu

2.1 Introduction

In the last century, the burden of obesity, type 2 diabetes mellitus (T2DM), metabolic syndrome (MS), as well as its components has been rising [1]. The impact of these diseases is also reflected in the structure of liver parenchyma, by overloading the hepatocytes with fat leading to a high proportion of patients with liver fibrosis. Nonalcoholic fatty liver disease (NAFLD) has become one of the few pandemics that increase the risk of chronic liver disease by its subtypes, including nonalcoholic steatohepatitis (NASH) [2].

As a short history, fatty liver generally known as steatosis has been described since 1845 due to the work of Addison, who identified alcohol-induced liver histological abnormalities [3]. Lately, after one century, Connor identified the possibility for alcoholic or diabetic fatty liver disease to evolve into liver cirrhosis, while in 1964, Dianzani elucidated the etiology of steatosis [4, 5]. The words NASH and NAFLD were not coined until the 1980s by Ludwig et al. and Shaffner and Thaler, respectively [6, 7]. After several decades of study in this area, it is now common knowledge that NAFLD and NASH are caused by different pathogens, are ubiquitous in the overall population worldwide, impose substantial direct and indirect expenses, and lack a safe and efficient pharmacological therapy [8].

A panel of worldwide experts established an agreement in 2020 to reconsider the present concept of fatty liver disease, including renaming it as metabolic dysfunction-associated fatty liver disease (MAFLD) and establishing a simplified set of "positive" diagnostic criteria for both adults and children [9, 10]. MAFLD is diagnosed when a

S. Zenovia (✉) · I. Girleanu
Gastroenterology Department, Grigore T. Popa University of Medicine and Pharmacy, Iasi, Romania

St. Spiridon Emergency Hospital, Institute of Gastroenterology and Hepatology, Iasi, Romania

© The Author(s), under exclusive license to Springer Nature Switzerland AG 2023
A. Trifan et al. (eds.), *Essentials of Non-Alcoholic Fatty Liver Disease*, https://doi.org/10.1007/978-3-031-33548-8_2

patient has hepatic steatosis, is overweight or obese, and has T2DM or two or more of the following: ethnicity-specific waist circumference cutoffs for central obesity; blood pressure ≥135/85 mmHg; plasma triglycerides ≥150 mg/dL; plasma HDL cholesterol <40 mg/dL for men and <50 mg/dL for women; fasting plasma glucose ≥100 mg/dL, 2-h post-load glucose ≥140 mg/dL, or hemoglobin A1c ≥5.7%; homeostasis model assessment of insulin resistance ≥2.5 and plasma high-sensitivity C-reactive protein >2 mg/L (Fig. 2.1, Table 2.1); or a specific drug treatment to counterbalance these metabolic disorders. This request garnered strong support from hepatologists throughout the world, hepatology scientific organizations, nursing and allied health leaders, pharmaceutical and regulatory science specialists, and patient associations. Notwithstanding, the new terminology has also generated criticism, emphasizing the necessity for a redefinition of NAFLD based on consensus [11].

The incidence of MAFLD is growing, even among nonobese persons, and affects 50% of the world's overweight and obese adult population. This rise is found worldwide, mostly in low- and low-middle-income nations in Africa, Asia, and South America, and it constitutes a significant worldwide burden on healthcare expenses [12, 13]. Lifestyle modifications and a balanced diet remain the mainstay of the therapeutic management of these individuals, as there are no currently authorized drugs [12]. The majority of patients with fatty liver disease are previously identified and then managed in clinical settings by primary care physicians (PCPs). There is unambiguous evidence of the health-promoting effects of primary care and its involvement in sickness and mortality prevention [14]. In addition, in contrast to specialty care, the provision of primary care as a healthcare service for all populations is more egalitarian. In this setting, primary care is crucial and may thus aid or hinder the delivery of effective treatment for chronic diseases. To offer effective and high-quality treatment, PCPs must include new information, abilities, and positive attitudes toward care that emphasize system transformation and participatory patient and primary care team connections.

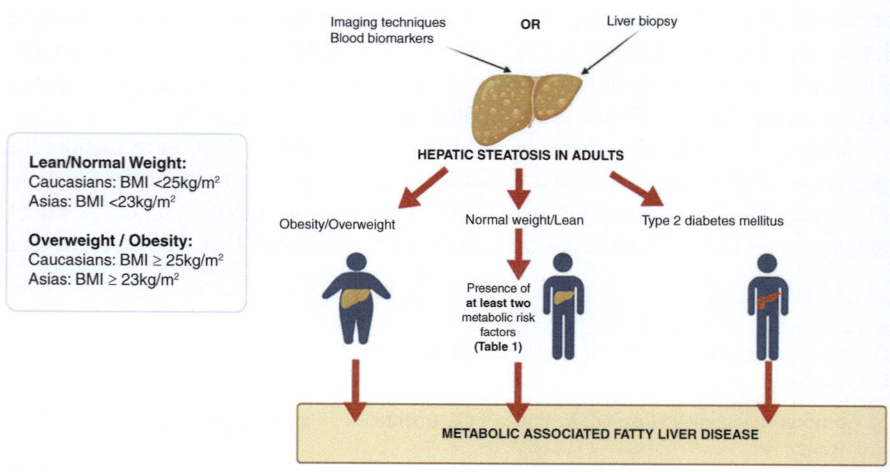

Fig. 2.1 A flowchart with the proposed diagnostic criteria for MAFLD

Table 2.1 Metabolic risk factors

Waist circumference ≥102/88 cm in Caucasian men and women (or ≥90/80 cm in Asian men and women)
Blood pressure ≥130/85 mmHg or specific drug treatment
Plasma triglycerides/150 mg/dL (≥1.70 mmol/L) or specific drug treatment
Plasma HDL cholesterol <40 mg/dL (<1.0 mmol/L) for men and <50 mg/dL (<1.3 mmol/L) for women or specific drug treatment
Prediabetes (i.e., fasting glucose levels 100–125 mg/dL (5.6–6.9 mmol/L), or 2-h post-load glucose levels 140–199 mg/dL (7.8–11.0 mmol), or HbA1c 5.7–6.4% (39–47 mmol/mol))
Homeostasis model assessment (HOMA)-insulin resistance score ≥2.5
Plasma high-sensitivity C-reactive protein (hs-CRP) level >2 mg/L

2.2 NAFLD Roadblocks

NAFLD, which includes the complete range of alcohol-like liver disorders present in nonalcoholics, was originally regarded as "the hepatic manifestation of the MS" [15]. However, this outmoded notion is at best unsatisfactory, and accumulating data suggests that the relationship between NAFLD and MS is complementary and bidirectional [1]. In the absence of competing causes of (steatogenic) liver disease, NAFLD is diagnosed noninvasively (through biomarkers and/or imaging modalities). Compared to these highly sensitive and specific biomarkers, conventional ultrasonography (US) retains a significant role since it is inexpensive, repeatable, widely available, and cost-efficient for excluding focal liver disease, with a semi-quantitative assessment of liver structure changes including steatogenic and focal lesion diagnosing [16].

However, liver biopsy (LB) is the gold standard for diagnosis providing a definitive characterization of the fundamental histological lesions: steatosis, ballooning, inflammation, and fibrosis, allowing differentiation between the more indolent, uncomplicated steatosis and the more rapidly progressive NASH forms [17]. According to the categorization, NAFLD is considered "primary" when it is coupled with MS or is seen as a precursor to its occurrence. "Secondary" types of NAFLD are many and include, among others, illnesses resulting from dietary abnormalities, consequences of abdominal surgery, drug use, occupational exposure to chemical solvents, and (rarely) metabolic disorders [18–21]. In addition, NAFLD is frequently caused by common viral infections (viral associated fatty liver disease—VAFLD) and recurrent endocrine problems. These secondary types of NAFLD must be recognized from the main NAFLD because, for example, VAFLD caused by HIV infection has a poorer prognosis than primary NAFLD and NAFLD caused by hypothyroidism has a particular pathophysiology that, in theory, may be entirely reversed by thyroid replacement treatment [22].

NAFLD is notoriously underdiagnosed in primary care, data from current literature derived mostly from US studies indicating a prevalence of 2% and 5%, respectively, well below the anticipated population prevalence of 25–30% [23, 24]. NAFLD is not detected even in the presence of MS comorbidities and US or imaging testing findings of hepatic steatosis. The reasons for these "missed" diagnostics are complicated, with survey research indicating that NAFLD is not a priority in primary care and that there is a significant knowledge gap in NAFLD diagnosis and therapy [25]. These occurrences result in a significant gap between existing standards and actual clinical practice. However, the problems that led to a change in nomenclature to eliminate the confusing factor are the following: (1) in routine primary care settings, adherence to NAFLD clinical practice recommendations appears to be problematic for reasons other than a lack of understanding; (2) the intricacy of the diagnostic criteria for NAFLD poses a considerable hurdle for PCPs to initiate screening or active case diagnosis; (3) simplifying the diagnostic criteria for fatty liver disease acceptable for a busy primary care setting is essential for expanding therapy into primary care settings; and (4) with the time necessary to collect a complete and accurate alcohol history, patient care may be misdirected as a result of this dichotomization into alcoholic and nonalcoholic [26]. In addition, the limited availability and use of sensitive direct alcohol markers in primary, secondary, and tertiary care settings in various regions of the world render interviews or questionnaires the only method for distinguishing between alcoholic and nonalcoholic fatty liver disease.

2.3   NAFLD and the Metabolic Syndrome: Common Pathophysiology Pathway and Bidirectional Interplay

Insulin resistance is the shared pathophysiological common denominator between NAFLD and MS, as previously stated. In the medical literature, the "chicken-and-egg" issue regarding the temporal relationship of NAFLD and MS was finally resolved by recent evidence demonstrating that NAFLD is both the cause and the result of MS [27, 28]. Nonetheless, it became evident immediately that tackling the major pathogenic causes of NASH would not necessarily improve disease outcomes. Insulin sensitizers did not restore or even exacerbate mitochondrial defects in NASH, but pharmaceutical treatments, such as vitamin E, acting via pathways other than insulin sensitization led to histological improvement in at least some individuals [29]. Therefore, in blatant contradiction to pathogenesis studies, there are a few questions that arise. Firstly, is the treatment of insulin resistance never adequate to successfully cure NASH in the vast majority of patients? This is likely the outcome of a variety of pathogenic pathways that interact to cause varying degrees of liver damage in particular patients. Based on this premise, therapy should be individualized for each patient. However, it is not clear how this may be achieved. Determining the role of each pathophysiological process in the development of NAFLD/NASH in an individual patient remains a scientific and clinical practice obstacle. Second, should people with NAFLD who do not have MS and those with lean NAFLD be treated similarly to those who are obese? In the absence of supporting data, should men and women be treated equally? Regardless of whether NAFLD is the cause or outcome of MS (which is both, as we now know), it is essential to recognize that these two conditions are synergistic HCC risk factors [29, 30]. HCC is the most prevalent primary liver cancer and the fourth leading cause of cancer-related death [31].

In their landmark publication, Bellentani et al. correctly noted the limits of a "negative" definition of NAFLD and NASH as opposed to a "positive" one, i.e., "metabolic," raising concerns from an established pipeline of prior investigations [32]. In accord, Fouad et al. identified that the reference to alcohol in the phrase "nonalcoholic" posed concerns of trivialization, stigmatization, and disregard by health authorities [33]. Recently, the factors that can influence clinical trials regarding NASH have been debated, for example their differentiation according to the fibrotic status of the patient (cirrhotic or non-cirrhotic), the differentiation between clinical and preclinical studies, but also the homogeneity of the studies regarding the histological diagnosis of NASH by LB, not emphasizing the extrahepatic manifestations or rather the patient's comorbidities [34]. Recent studies emphasize a rapid progression of the degree of liver fibrosis in patients with NASH in patients with metabolic comorbidities, who are at a high risk of developing cirrhosis. Therefore, a change in nomenclature is necessary to establish the risk of individual mortality and morbidity.

2.4 NAFLD-MAFLD: A Debate Near the End

An expert group from as many as 22 nations developed the word MAFLD in an effort to combine ideas about the inaccuracy and potential detrimental implications of using the term "NAFLD" that had gathered over the previous few decades [9–12]. This idea has quickly garnered support across Latin America, North Africa, and the Middle East, suggesting a consensus that the justifications for discarding the existing nomenclature exceed those for preserving it [35, 36]. The diagnostic criteria for MAFLD exceed the inconveniences that were previously encountered for the diagnosis of NAFLD; for example, NAFLD in diabetic patients will follow the same path as in metabolically healthy obese patients. Similarly, it is unknown whether persons with altered metabolic derangements would be susceptible to the same risk of developing hepatic and extrahepatic problems as are usually associated with overt diabetes [9]. NAFLD and its subtypes nonalcoholic fatty liver (NAFL) and NASH were more thoroughly characterized than MAFLD from a histological standpoint, and characterizing liver histology remains a milestone in our ability to predict the clinical consequences of illness. Nevertheless, physicians and patients will welcome the option of noninvasively identifying MAFLD, considering the numerous critiques that may be linked to LB [27, 37]. Experts developed a set of diagnostic criteria to establish the diagnosis of MAFLD-associated cirrhosis, hence removing the phrase cryptogenic cirrhosis among dysmetabolic individuals. Considering that fatty changes could disappear over time, the committee proposed that patients with existing cirrhosis, despite the absence of histopathologic proof of steatohepatitis, should then be deemed to have MAFLD-related cirrhosis if at least one of the following requirements is met: past or present evidence of dysmetabolic features that meet the criteria for the diagnosis of MAFLD (as described above) that have at least one of the following criteria in their medical history: prior histopathology-proven MAFLD or confirmation of liver steatosis using imaging modalities [9–12]. In this light, it is essential to note the 1999 pivotal research in which Caldwell, based on his series of 70 cases, was the first to argue that "NASH plays an under-recognized role in many patients with cryptogenic cirrhosis, the majority of whom are older, T2DM-positive, and obese females" [38]. MAFLD takes a step further to accurately describe NAFLD individuals; however, it is unlikely to be the ultimate answer to all unmet clinical requirements. In addition, the unique concept of MAFLD integrates the insights acquired on the alarming interplay between NAFLD and MS, a relationship that impairs liver histology, accelerates fibrosis advancement, raises the chance of developing HCC, and diminishes the life expectancy of NAFLD patients.

2.5 Pro Arguments for MAFLD: Improve Disease Awareness

Decades of effort have been expended to raise the knowledge of NAFLD; nevertheless, a recent study demonstrates that switching from NAFLD to MAFLD boosted awareness of the illness among primary care providers and physicians of other specialties. Two further investigations have demonstrated that the new label MAFLD has increased patient awareness [35, 39]. Despite moderate acceptance, this illustrates the efficacy of the MAFLD criteria in the context of ordinary clinical care and suggests that the results are generalizable. Utilizing the MAFLD criteria more broadly could result in even larger gains in the care of MAFLD patients if this momentum is capitalized on [40] (Fig. 2.2).

The existing MAFLD care strategy can be reduced based on a transformational shift from NAFLD to MAFLD: better allocation of resources to diagnose more patients (expanding access and coverage), improved identification of patients at risk of disease progression and accelerated treatment initiation (linkage to care),

Fig. 2.2 Implications for redefining fatty liver disease from a primary care perspective

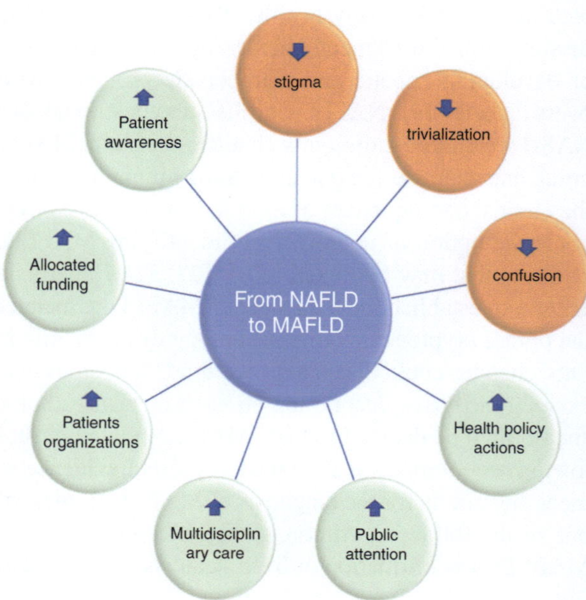

reduction in complications among high-risk populations, and reduction in the long-term medical costs of complications, such as those associated with advanced liver disease, extrahepatic cholestasis, and extrahepatic cholestasis (optimizing referral pathway).

Unfortunately, the fact that current NAFLD diagnosis is centered on the rejection of other liver diseases poses a substantial barrier to the holistic management of patients with liver diseases, as well as the advancement of research into the interplay among fatty liver disease and other liver diseases. This may result in misclassification, underreporting, and suboptimal care for these patients, particularly in light of increasing evidence that patients with MAFLD and other consequent liver diseases, such as chronic viral hepatitis, alcohol intake, or autoimmune hepatitis, have a more severe liver injury than those with each disease alone [41–43]. An international committee of experts has emphasized the need of including MAFLD in the hepatitis C eradication campaign. Notably, numerous recent studies have indicated that in patients with simultaneous chronic hepatitis B or chronic hepatitis C, the MAFLD criteria are superior to the previous NAFLD criteria for detecting individuals with more severe liver damage, such as steatosis, fibrosis, and increased liver enzymes. On the other hand, the transition to MAFLD will permit the establishment of a multidisciplinary clinic with contributions from primary care, hepatology, endocrinology, and cardiology to improve both liver-related and cardiometabolic health [44].

2.6 Conclusion

The MAFLD definition's revolutionary simplification of the diagnosis and evaluation may facilitate the implementation of effective fatty liver disease management, prevent overdiagnosis and overtreatment, and reduce underdiagnosis by PCPs. Thereby, this modification will enable PCPs to continue contributing to the health and well-being of patients in the community, based on accessibility, equity, and respect for the patient's individuality, with a possible decrease in morbidity and mortality due to fatty liver worldwide.

References

1. Muzica CM, Sfarti C, Trifan A, Zenovia S, Cuciureanu T, Nastasa R, Huiban L, Cojocariu C, Singeap AM, Girleanu I, Chiriac S, Stanciu C. Nonalcoholic fatty liver disease and type 2 diabetes mellitus: a bidirectional relationship. Can J Gastroenterol Hepatol. 2020;28:6638306. https://doi.org/10.1155/2020/6638306.
2. Younossi ZM, Koenig AB, Abdelatif D, Fazel Y, Henry L, Wymer M. Global epidemiology of nonalcoholic fatty liver disease-meta-analytic assessment of prevalence, incidence, and outcomes. Hepatology. 2016;64(1):73–84. https://doi.org/10.1002/hep.28431. Epub 2016 Feb 22.
3. Addison T. Observations on fatty degeneration of the liver. Guys Hosp Rep. 1836;1:485.
4. Connor CL. Fatty infiltration of the liver and the development of cirrhosis in diabetes and chronic alcoholism. Am J Pathol. 1938;14(3):347–364.9.

 5. Dianzani MU. Sulla patogenesi dell'accumulo del grasso nella steatosi epatica. Rass Med Sarda. 1964;66:67–90. Italian.
 6. Ludwig J, Viggiano TR, McGill DB, Oh BJ. Nonalcoholic steatohepatitis: Mayo Clinic experiences with a hitherto unnamed disease. Mayo Clin Proc. 1980;55:434–8.
 7. Schaffner F, Thaler H. Nonalcoholic fatty liver disease. Prog Liver Dis. 1986;8:283–98.
 8. Younossi Z, Anstee QM, Marietti M, Hardy T, Henry L, Eslam M, George J, Bugianesi E. Global burden of NAFLD and NASH: trends, predictions, risk factors and prevention. Nat Rev Gastroenterol Hepatol. 2018;15(1):11–20. https://doi.org/10.1038/nrgastro.2017.109. Epub 2017 Sep 20.
 9. Eslam M, Newsome PN, Sarin SK, et al. A new definition for metabolic dysfunction-associated fatty liver disease: an international expert consensus statement. J Hepatol. 2020;73(1):202–9.
10. Eslam M, Alkhouri N, Vajro P, et al. Defining paediatric metabolic (dysfunction)-associated fatty liver disease: an international expert consensus statement. Lancet Gastroenterol Hepatol. 2021;6:864–73.
11. Younossi ZM, Rinella ME, Sanyal A, et al. From NAFLD to MAFLD: implications of a premature change in terminology. Hepatology. 2020;73(3):1194–8. https://doi.org/10.1002/hep.31420.
12. Eslam M, Fan J-G, Mendez-Sanchez N. Non-alcoholic fatty liver disease in non-obese individuals: the impact of metabolic health. Lancet Gastroenterol Hepatol. 2020;5:713–5.
13. Ye Q, Zou B, Yeo YH, et al. Global prevalence, incidence, and outcomes of non-obese or lean non-alcoholic fatty liver disease: a systematic review and meta-analysis. Lancet Gastroenterol Hepatol. 2020;5:739–52.
14. Starfield B, Shi L, Macinko J. Contribution of primary care to health systems and health. Milbank Q. 2005;83(3):457–502.
15. Diehl AM, Goodman Z, Ishak KG. Alcohol-like liver disease in nonalcoholics. A clinical and histologic comparison with alcohol-induced liver injury. Gastroenterology. 1988;95:1056–62.
16. Zenovia S, Stanciu C, Sfarti C, Singeap A-M, Cojocariu C, Girleanu I, Dimache M, Chiriac S, Muzica CM, Nastasa R, Huiban L, Cuciureanu T, Trifan A. Vibration-controlled transient elastography and controlled attenuation parameter for the diagnosis of liver steatosis and fibrosis in patients with nonalcoholic fatty liver disease. Diagnostics. 2021;11:787. https://doi.org/10.3390/diagnostics11050787.
17. Ratziu V, Charlotte F, Heurtier A, Gombert S, Giral P, Bruckert E, Grimaldi A, Capron F, Poynard T. Sampling variability of liver biopsy in nonalcoholic fatty liver disease. Gastroenterology. 2005;128:1898–906.
18. Lonardo A, Ballestri S, Marchesini G, Angulo P, Loria P. Nonalcoholic fatty liver disease: a precursor of the metabolic syndrome. Dig Liver Dis. 2015;47:181–90.
19. Ballestri S, Zona S, Targher G, Romagnoli D, Baldelli E, Nascimbeni F, Roverato A, Guaraldi G, Lonardo A. Nonalcoholic fatty liver disease is associated with an almost twofold increased risk of incident type 2 diabetes and metabolic syndrome. Evidence from a systematic review and meta-analysis. J Gastroenterol Hepatol. 2016;31:936–44.
20. Guaraldi G, Lonardo A, Ballestri S, Zona S, Stentarelli C, Orlando G, Carli F, Carulli L, Roverato A, Loria P. Human immunodeficiency virus is the major determinant of steatosis and hepatitis C virus of insulin resistance in virus-associated fatty liver disease. Arch Med Res. 2011;42:690–7.
21. Lonardo A, Mantovani A, Lugari S, Targher G. NAFLD in some common endocrine diseases: prevalence, pathophysiology, and principles of diagnosis and management. Int J Mol Sci. 2019;20:2841.
22. Vodkin I, Valasek MA, Bettencourt R, Cachay E, Loomba R. Clinical, biochemical and histological differences between HIV-associated NAFLD and primary NAFLD: a case-control study. Aliment Pharmacol Ther. 2015;41:368–78.
23. Alexander M, Loomis AK, Fairburn-Beech J, et al. Real-world data reveal a diagnostic gap in non-alcoholic fatty liver disease. BMC Med. 2018;16(1):130.
24. Loomba R, Wong R, Fraysse J, et al. Nonalcoholic fatty liver disease progression rates to cirrhosis and progression of cirrhosis to decompensation and mortality: a real world analysis of Medicare data. Aliment Pharmacol Ther. 2020;51:1149–59.

25. Standing HC, Jarvis H, Orr J, et al. GPs' experiences and perceptions of early detection of liver disease: a qualitative study in primary care. Br J Gen Pract. 2018;68(676):e743–9.
26. Eslam M, Sanyal AJ, George J. Toward more accurate nomenclature for fatty liver diseases. Gastroenterology. 2019;157(3):590–3.
27. Lonardo A, Carani C, Carulli N, Loria P. Chicken or egg turned into head or belly. J Hepatol. 2006;45:454–6.
28. Lonardo A. Renaming NAFLD to MAFLD: could the LDE system assist in this transition? J Clin Med. 2021;10(3):492. https://doi.org/10.3390/jcm10030492.
29. Lonardo A, Bellentani S, Ratziu V, Loria P. Insulin resistance in nonalcoholic steatohepatitis: necessary but not sufficient—death of a dogma from analysis of therapeutic studies? Expert Rev Gastroenterol Hepatol. 2011;5:279–89.
30. Wainwright P, Byrne CD. Bidirectional relationships and disconnects between NAFLD and features of the metabolic syndrome. Int J Mol Sci. 2016;17:367.
31. Lonardo A, Ballestri S, Chow PKH, Suzuki A. Sex disparity in hepatocellular carcinoma owing to NAFLD and non-NAFLD etiology. Epidemiological findings and patho-mechanisms. Hepatoma Res. 2020;6:83.
32. Bellentani S, Tiribelli C. Is it time to change NAFLD and NASH nomenclature? Lancet Gastroenterol Hepatol. 2017;2:547–8.
33. Fouad Y, Waked I, Bollipo S, Gomaa A, Ajlouni Y, Attia D. What's in a name? Renaming 'NAFLD' to 'MAFLD'. Liver Int. 2020;40:1254–61.
34. Ratziu V, Friedman SL. Why do so many NASH trials fail? Gastroenterology. 2020;18:S0016-5085(20)30680-6.
35. Mendez-Sanchez N, Arrese M, Gadano A, Oliveira CP, Fassio E, Arab JP, Chávez-Tapia NC, Dirchwolf M, Torre A, Ridruejo E, et al. The Latin American association for the study of the liver (ALEH) position statement on the redefinition of fatty liver disease. Lancet Gastroenterol Hepatol. 2021;6:65–72.
36. Shiha G, Alswat K, Al Khatry M, Sharara AI, Örmeci N, Waked I, Benazzouz M, Al-Ali F, Hamed AE, Hamoudi W, et al. Nomenclature and definition of metabolic-associated fatty liver disease: a consensus from the Middle East and north Africa. Lancet Gastroenterol Hepatol. 2021;6:57–64.
37. Polyzos SA, Kang ES, Tsochatzis EA, Kechagias S, Ekstedt M, Xanthakos S, Lonardo A, Mantovani A, Tilg H, Côté I, et al. Commentary: nonalcoholic or metabolic dysfunction-associated fatty liver disease? The epidemic of the 21st century in search of the most appropriate name. Metabolism. 2020;113:154413.
38. Caldwell SH, Oelsner DH, Iezzoni JC, Hespenheide EE, Battle EH, Driscoll CJ. Cryptogenic cirrhosis: clinical characterization and risk factors for underlying disease. Hepatology. 1999;29:664–9.
39. Abdel Alem SGY, AbdAlla M, Said E, Fouad Y. Capturing patient experience: a qualitative study of change from NAFLD to MAFLD real-time feedback. J Hepatol. 2021;74(5):1261–2.
40. Eslam M, George J. MAFLD: now is the time to capitalize on the momentum. J Hepatol. 2020;74(5):1262–3.
41. Fouad Y, Saad Z, Raheem EA, et al. Clinical validity of the diagnostic criteria for metabolic-associated fatty liver disease: a real-world experience. medRxiv. 2020;8(20):20176214. https://doi.org/10.1101/2020.08.20.20176214.
42. Gaber Y, AbdAllah M, Salama A, Sayed M, Abdel Alem S, Nafady S. Metabolic-associated fatty liver disease and autoimmune hepatitis: an overlooked interaction. Expert Rev Gastroent. 2021;15:1–9.
43. Choi HS, Brouwer WP, Zanjir WM, et al. Nonalcoholic steatohepatitis is associated with liver-related outcomes and all-cause mortality in chronic hepatitis B. Hepatology. 2020;71(2):539–48.
44. Eslam M, Ahmed A, Després J-P, et al. Incorporating fatty liver disease in multidisciplinary care and novel clinical trial designs for patients with metabolic diseases. Lancet Gastroenterol Hepatol. 2021;9(6):P743–53. https://doi.org/10.1016/S2468-1253(21)00132-1.

Natural History of Nonalcoholic Fatty Liver Disease

3

Abdulrahman Ismaiel, Piero Portincasa, and Dan L. Dumitrascu

3.1 Introduction

Nonalcoholic fatty liver disease (NAFLD) encompasses a spectrum of hepatic histopathological changes and is defined by the excessive ($\geq 5\%$) deposition of fat in the hepatocytes, in the absence of secondary causes of hepatic steatosis such as significant alcohol consumption, viral infection, or drugs. The term NAFLD includes simple steatosis, known as nonalcoholic fatty liver (NAFL), that might progress to steatosis with necro-inflammatory changes, known as nonalcoholic steatohepatitis (NASH), and subsequently advanced fibrosis, liver cirrhosis, and even HCC [1, 2].

NAFLD is currently the most frequent cause of chronic liver disease (CLD) in the USA and in other industrialized nations [3]. It is estimated that NAFLD will soon become the most frequent cause of end-stage liver disease, leading to liver cirrhosis and hepatocellular carcinoma (HCC), and as a result becoming the most frequent indication for liver transplantation (LT) [4, 5]. The increasing prevalence of metabolic syndrome (MetS), overweight, and obesity worldwide over the past 30 years [6] are closely related to the rising trends of NAFLD. Hence, the clinical burden of NAFLD is significant and is expected to increase as the obesity and type 2 diabetes mellitus (T2DM) epidemics expand [4]. This combination poses the most

A. Ismaiel · D. L. Dumitrascu (✉)
2nd Department of Internal Medicine, "Iuliu Hatieganu" University of Medicine and Pharmacy, Cluj-Napoca, Romania
e-mail: ddumitrascu@umfcluj.ro

P. Portincasa
Department of Biomedical Sciences and Human Oncology, Clinica Medica "A. Murri", University of Bari "Aldo Moro" Medical School, Bari, Italy
e-mail: piero.portincasa@uniba.it

A. Trifan et al. (eds.), *Essentials of Non-Alcoholic Fatty Liver Disease*, https://doi.org/10.1007/978-3-031-33548-8_3

serious burden and health risk due to its multisystemic effects, which include rising rates of cardiovascular, oncologic, and liver-related morbidity and mortality [7–9].

Research conducted in the late 1980s and early 1990s showed the potential of progression to liver cirrhosis and HCC, which led to the link between NASH and several cases of cryptogenic cirrhosis [10–13]. The recognition of NAFLD subtypes provided a rationale for these opposing perspectives [14]. The spectrum of NAFLD is defined in Table 3.1 according to the American Association for the Study of Liver Diseases [15]. Moreover, Fig. 3.1 summarizes the recently published diagnosis criteria for the recently proposed term, metabolic dysfunction-associated fatty liver disease (MAFLD) [16–18].

NAFLD is becoming more widely acknowledged as a clinically significant disease, and like any disease, the clinical significance depends on the prevalence and natural history of the condition [19]. The natural history of NAFLD is similarly significant in terms of therapeutic relevance, yet there is still a lot of uncertainty and controversy around this topic. The consensus is that NAFLD is not a completely benign disorder, as a limited number of patients progress to significant liver fibrosis or develop related morbidity and mortality [20]. In fact, as new evidence emerges over time, our knowledge of the natural history of NAFLD constantly changes.

A variety of factors, including genetic, environmental, and lifestyle factors, interact and contribute to the dynamic natural history of NAFLD. Understanding the natural history of NAFLD, which was crucial to comprehending the clinical characteristics of the condition, has significantly improved over the past 20 years [21]. With the aim of reducing or preventing hepatic and extrahepatic complications, this in turn allowed for more accurate risk assessment and establishment of appropriate diagnostic strategies [22].

Table 3.1 The spectrum of NAFLD

NAFLD spectrum	Definition
NAFLD	Encompasses the whole spectrum of fatty liver disease in subjects without secondary causes of hepatic steatosis, ranging from fatty liver to steatohepatitis, and subsequently liver cirrhosis
NAFL	Lack of hepatocellular injury, as demonstrated by ballooning of the hepatocytes, or fibrosis in the presence of $\geq 5\%$ hepatic steatosis. The risk of progressing to liver cirrhosis and hepatic failure is regarded as minimal
NASH	The presence of $\geq 5\%$ hepatic steatosis with hepatocellular ballooning and inflammation, in the presence or absence of liver fibrosis. Progression can lead to cirrhosis, hepatic failure, and seldomly liver cancer
NASH cirrhosis	Liver cirrhosis in association with previous or actual histopathological confirmation of hepatic steatosis or steatohepatitis
Cryptogenic cirrhosis	The presence of cirrhosis without a clear etiology. Metabolic risk factors like obesity and MetS are greatly higher in patients with cryptogenic cirrhosis

From the American Association for the Study of Liver Diseases [15]

Abbreviations: *MetS* Metabolic syndrome, *NAFL* Nonalcoholic fatty liver, *NAFLD* Nonalcoholic fatty liver disease, *NASH* Nonalcoholic steatohepatitis

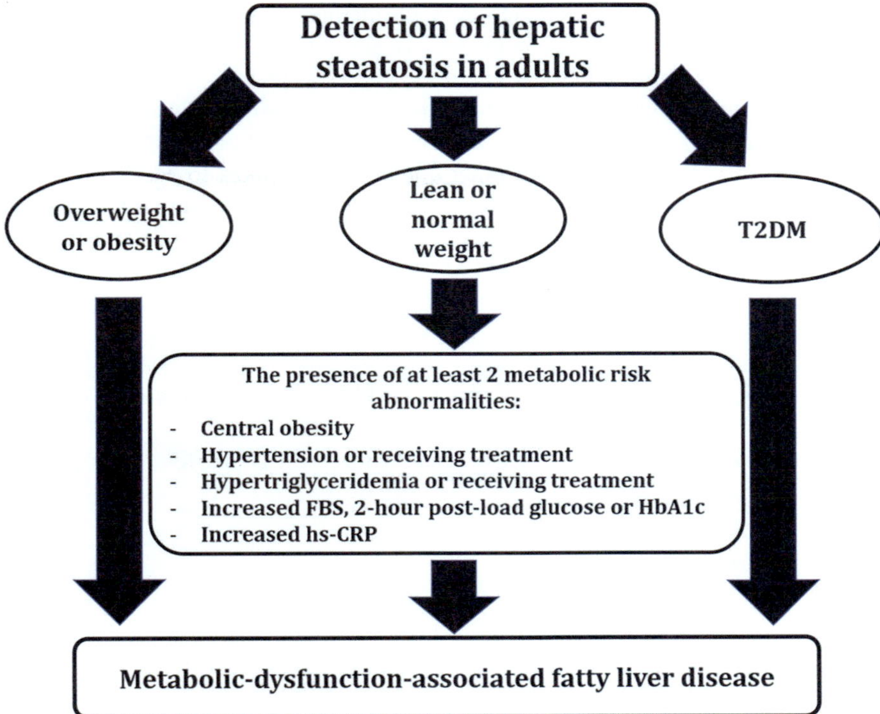

Fig. 3.1 The proposed "positive" diagnosis criteria for diagnosing MAFLD. *Abbreviations: FBS* Fasting blood sugar, *HbA1c* Glycated hemoglobin, *hs-CRP* High-sensitivity C-reactive protein, *T2DM* Type 2 diabetes mellitus

Understanding the natural history of NAFLD is crucial for determining the clinical relevance of NAFLD, defining long-term outcomes, and risk-stratifying patients for complications and mortality. In addition, to balance the risks and advantages of various therapies more accurately, it is crucial to understand the natural history and consequences of any disease [23]. This is certainly relevant in NAFLD, given the vast spectrum range of associated comorbidities [24, 25].

In this chapter, we present the latest evidence regarding the natural history of NAFLD and its implications for a more rational and personalized approach to this disease that presents characteristics of a global epidemic.

3.2   Rationale for Understanding the Natural History of NAFLD

Diet and exercise carry minimal risk in comparison to their potential advantages and are therefore generally encouraged. On the contrary, in individuals with active steatohepatitis and red flags of progressive advancing fibrosis, pharmacological interventions should be taken into consideration [23]. However, unless they are very well targeted at the patient subset, such therapies are probably going to be associated with high costs and considerable side effects, possibly outweighing their benefit.

Furthermore, the majority of patients with NAFLD also have insulin resistance or MetS [23, 26]. Therefore, there is an even greater need to understand the spectrum of NAFLD in the context of other comorbidities linked to MetS, given the strong relationship of NAFLD with, for instance, cardiovascular disease (CVD) [9, 27, 28]. NAFLD patients present an increased mortality rate due to CVD, being the most common cause of death in NAFLD patients, as well as cirrhosis and hepatic and extrahepatic cancers [29–32].

3.3   Risk Factors and Predictors for NAFLD Progression

Numerous risk factors appear to be associated with NAFLD progression (Fig. 3.2).

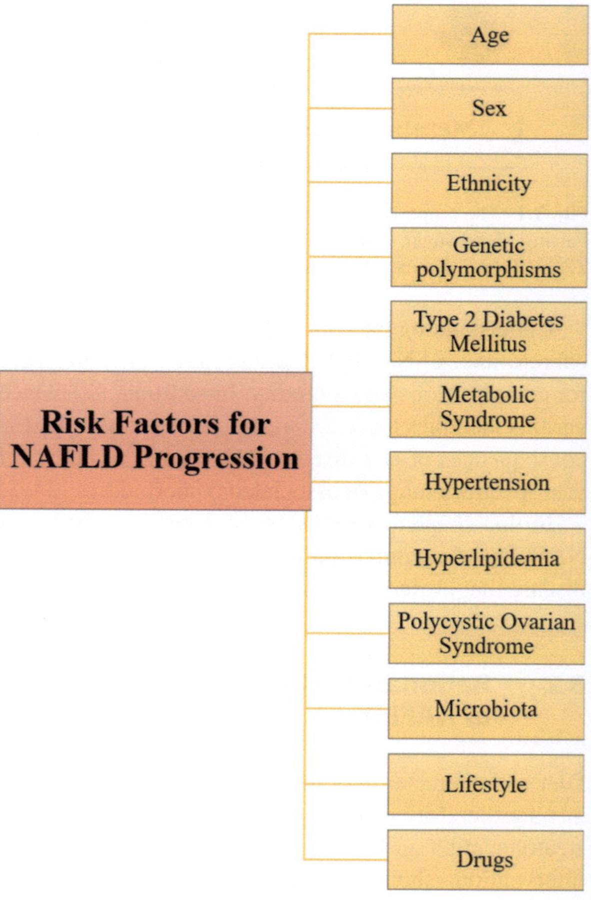

Fig. 3.2 Risk factors and predictors for NAFLD progression. *Abbreviations: NAFLD* Nonalcoholic fatty liver disease

3.3.1 Age

The prevalence of NAFLD and NAFLD-related fibrosis increases with age, even though NAFLD has been characterized in individuals of all ages [33–36]. Along with the correlation between age and NAFLD prevalence, NAFLD patients of older age also present an increased risk of disease progression or mortality [37–39].

Because older patients frequently also have significantly higher rates of other risk factors including MetS, T2DM, and obesity, it might be challenging to determine whether age *per se* is indeed an independent risk factor. Although this may be due to the accumulation of metabolic exposures over time and the prolonged duration of NAFLD in these populations, cross-sectional studies have consistently shown an association between aging and more severe fibrosis in NASH patients [40, 41]. The likelihood of associated conditions such as severe liver fibrosis, HCC, and T2DM also rises with age [42–44]. These risk factors are undoubtedly more prevalent in older age populations. On the other hand, longitudinal studies have not consistently shown how age affects the quick progression of fibrosis [45].

It is noteworthy that NAFLD prevalence is rising in all age groups, including in the youth [46]. Comprehensive research is required in this area, even if age seems to be a plausible risk factor for NAFLD and NASH. It is unclear whether age is an independent risk factor for the progression of NAFLD and liver fibrosis. Notably, the relationship between age and increased prevalence of NAFLD, advanced liver fibrosis, and cirrhosis in NAFLD may be attributed to the duration or to the preponderance of other risk factors in older patients, presenting stronger associations with NAFLD and a higher rate of progression to NASH and fibrosis than to age itself.

3.3.2 Sex

The published data regarding sex as an independent risk factor for NAFLD are contradictory. NAFLD was once believed to affect females more frequently, although more recent studies report male sex being a risk factor for NAFLD [33, 46–49]. According to studies assessing the prevalence of NASH in Western populations, females make up between 60% and 83% of NASH diagnoses [50]. On the other hand, prospective studies reported that males present with NAFLD more frequently than females [51, 52]. NAFLD was shown to be prevalent in 16% of females and 31% of males in a study involving 26,527 Asian subjects who received medical health examinations [53]. The occurrence of histological NASH, hepatic fibrosis, and increased aminotransferase levels and overall mortality in NAFLD patients were also found to be associated with male sex [37, 54, 55]. However, limited research proposed a link between female sex with NAFLD and liver fibrosis [38, 56], while one study found that female patients with MetS presented an independent risk factor for NASH [57]. Given these differences, it is likely that males and females develop NAFLD and its progression in distinct manners. Whether such gender-related differences are partly related to the hormonal profile is still a matter of discussion. More research is needed on this topic to clarify the current gaps in evidence.

3.3.3 Race and Ethnicity

Recent research demonstrated that racial and ethnic differences influence the prevalence of NAFLD. Nevertheless, their impact as a risk factor for NAFLD remains unclear. The prevalence of NAFLD, hepatic steatosis, and increased aminotransferase levels is highest among Hispanics and then non-Hispanic Whites, with African Americans having the lowest prevalence [54, 58, 59].

Although it was suggested that instead of being a real risk factor, ethnicity and race most likely correlate with the incidence of obesity and the underlying MetS, it was reported that several indicators of NAFLD, like the degree of visceral adiposity, are consistent across racial and ethnic groups [46, 59]. When compared to Caucasians, Hispanic patients were shown to have a higher prevalence of NAFLD, without any difference in the severity of liver damage between the two ethnic groups [54, 60]. African American patients may have less severe histology than Asian patients, though this difference may be confounded by factors including diet [61, 62]. Asian patients may also be more prone to more severe histological changes, such as ballooning. While serum adiponectin levels are only related with NAFLD in African Americans, other correlates (such as age, triglycerides, and plasminogen activator inhibitor-1 [PAI-1]) are only associated with NAFLD in Hispanics [59]. These apparent racial and familial disparities might be an indication of an underlying genetic predisposition or environmental variables.

3.3.4 Genetic Polymorphisms

The often-recorded familial clustering of NAFLD raises the question of whether genetic variants play a pathogenic role [63, 64]. Several genetic polymorphisms have been linked to NAFLD, as outlined in Fig. 3.3 [65, 66]. After adjusting for age, sex, and metabolic factors, a study including over 1000 participants with biopsy-proven NAFLD reported that patatin-like phospholipase-3 (*PNPLA3*) and transmembrane 6 superfamily member 2 (*TM6SF2*) polymorphisms were linked to a 40–88% higher risk for advanced fibrosis [67].

According to genotyping data related to the epidemiology of NAFLD, a polymorphism in *PNPLA3*, which encodes the I148M protein variant, is probably the most significant genetic determinant of hepatic steatosis and serum ALT levels [68]. The mechanisms known as lipogenesis and lipolysis were believed to play a role in the ability of *PNPLA3* to regulate adipocyte formation as well as the production and breakdown of fats in hepatocytes and adipocytes [69]. The ethnicity most at risk for NAFLD, Hispanics, had the highest frequency of this allele (0.49), while Caucasians (0.23) and African Americans have lower frequencies (0.17) [46]. This polymorphism also predisposes subjects without hepatic steatosis to approximately 28% elevations in ALT levels [70]. Furthermore, I148M homozygotes are more likely to develop NASH (OR 3.488) [70]. This is thought to be caused by *PNPLA3* interfering with triglyceride hydrolysis in hepatocytes, which predisposes to NAFLD [71].

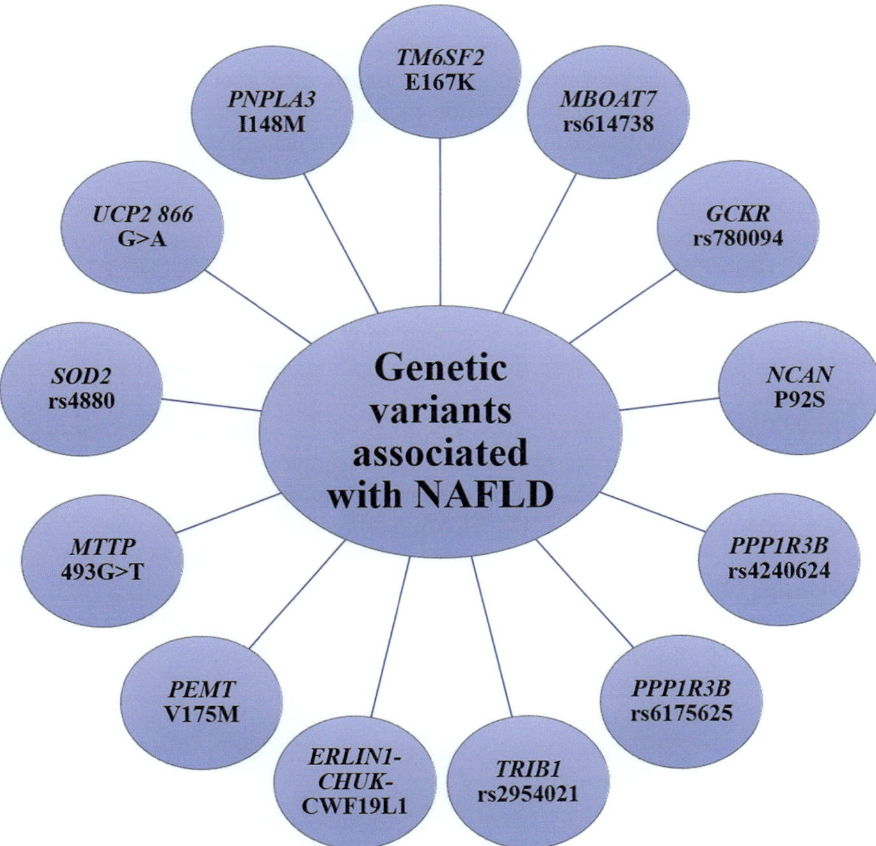

Fig. 3.3 Genetic variants associated with NAFLD. *Abbreviations: ERLIN1* ER lipid raft associated 1, *GCKR* Glucokinase regulator, *MBOAT7* Membrane-bound O-acyltransferase domain-containing 7, *MTTP* Microsomal triglyceride transfer protein, *NAFLD* Nonalcoholic fatty liver disease, *NCAN* Neurocan, *PEMT* Phosphatidylethanolamine N-methyltransferase, *PNPLA3* Patatin-like phospholipase domain-containing protein 3, *PPP1R3B* Protein phosphatase 1 regulatory subunit 3B, *SOD2* Superoxide dismutase 2, *TM6SF2* Transmembrane 6 superfamily member 2, *TRIB1* Tribbles pseudokinase 1, *UCP2* Uncoupling protein 2

Additionally, another common genetic polymorphism in the general population is the *TM6SF2* [67]. Genome-wide association studies have found that the rs738409 and rs58542926 single nucleotide polymorphisms (SNPs) of these respective genes are linked to an elevated risk of NAFLD as well as the development of more severe liver histology [67, 68, 72]. The role of *TM6SF2* in promoting triglyceride and cholesterol retention in the liver may predispose to NAFLD and liver fibrosis. With this mutation, unexpectedly, a cardioprotective role described as the "Catch-22" paradigm has been observed because of decreased levels of VLDL production and improved blood triglyceride levels with unmodified insulin sensitivity [73].

Furthermore, membrane-bound O-acyltransferase domain containing 7 (*MBOAT7*) rs647138 polymorphism was also evaluated in NAFLD patients. Irrespective of genetic background, downregulation of *MBOAT7* is a maladaptive response to hyperinsulinemia that promotes intracellular hepatic fat deposition due to impaired arachidonoyl-phosphatidylinositol, which increases lipogenesis by promoting the conversion of saturated lysophosphatidylinositol to triglycerides, potentially increasing the risk of hepatic steatosis, NASH, and hepatic fibrosis [74]. Several studies including systematic reviews and meta-analyses reported that *MBOAT7* rs641738C>T is associated with increased hepatic fat, NAFLD severity, susceptibility to develop NASH, advanced fibrosis, and HCC in adults from Caucasian, Hispanic, and African American ethnicities, as well as elevated ALT levels in children [75, 76]. Nevertheless, these findings were inconclusive in Asian populations.

An SNP in the *IFNL4* gene, which was found to be related to interferon-based treatment response in chronic hepatitis C, was also reported to be associated with liver fibrosis in NAFLD [72, 77]. Additionally, significant NAFLD contributors include genetic variations in *NCAN*, *GCKR*, and *LYPLAL1* [78]. Moreover, *GCKR* has been independently found to be a genetic determinant for NAFLD in Chinese individuals [79].

Numerous additional genetic variants have also been linked to NAFLD or NASH risk and may be responsible for the racial and ethnic differences in populations. Further studies are being done on this field.

3.3.5 Metabolic Conditions

In comparison to the general population, cohorts of patients with preexisting metabolic disorders had higher rates of NAFLD. Particularly close associations exist between T2DM and obesity in NAFLD. An increase or decrease in body mass index (BMI) over time has also been linked to liver fibrosis improvement or worsening in NAFLD patients. Despite conflicting results between hypertension as a risk factor for the progression of liver fibrosis, a recent meta-analysis considered hypertension to be a risk factor for fibrosis progression [45, 58].

An essential component of the MetS is T2DM, while T2DM and fatty liver disease have long been known to be closely related. The development of T2DM was found to parallel liver fibrosis progression, while better glycemic control was found to be associated with liver fibrosis resolution [80–82]. A total of 69% of individuals with T2DM were found to have ultrasound-diagnosed NAFLD [83]. It is essential to remember that advanced fibrosis and NASH are frequently seen in diabetic patients who are clinically asymptomatic and, in some situations, have normal liver enzymes. The risk of developing hepatic steatosis is also increased in diabetic patients due to their susceptibility to obesity and hypertriglyceridemia. Evidence also suggests that diabetic NAFLD patients present with increased mortality, cirrhosis, and progression rates than nondiabetic NAFLD patients. According to the analysis conducted by Stepanova et al. including the NHANES III (1988–1994) data, T2DM was an independent predictor of mortality as well as a substantial risk factor for liver-related mortality [84].

Obesity has long been recognized as a risk factor for NAFLD. It is important to highlight that other risk factors that predispose to hepatic steatosis can be additive to obesity. For instance, obesity doubles the risk of steatosis in heavy drinkers [85]. Due to the obesity pandemic, bariatric surgery is one of the procedures with the fastest growth in the USA. Since intraoperative liver biopsies during bariatric surgery have become commonplace during the past 10 years, numerous studies have been conducted on morbidly obese patients, who have a high prevalence of NAFLD and NASH [44, 56, 86–88]. These findings provide significant support for the hypothesis that obesity is a major risk factor for NAFLD and NASH, with bariatric surgery patients also showing advanced fibrosis [56]. The likelihood of developing fibrosis in obese individuals varies depending on the fibrosis type. Although 67% of patients undergoing gastric bypass surgery exhibited portal fibrosis, perisinusoidal fibrosis was found in approximately 4% [86, 89–91]. Interestingly, NAFLD rates in obese nondiabetic patients range from 57 to 98% [89, 92, 93]. Moreover, a study reported that central obesity rather than an increased BMI was found to be a risk factor for NAFLD [94]. According to experts, central obesity, as measured by the waist-to-hip ratio, is significantly linked to insulin resistance.

Another crucial component of the MetS is elevated cholesterol, or more precisely hypertriglyceridemia, which is usually linked to both obesity and T2DM [46]. Dyslipidemia is acknowledged as a known risk factor for NAFLD development.

Furthermore, it was recently suggested that polycystic ovarian syndrome (PCOS) is the ovarian manifestation of the MetS [95]. In one study, it was observed that hepatic steatosis and elevated HOMA-IR values were present in 55% of PCOS patients [96]. According to hepatic steatosis and elevated ALT levels, 41% of PCOS patients had concurrent NAFLD [97]. Additionally, several research have revealed that obese PCOS patients had even greater rates of being diagnosed and a higher likelihood to develop NAFLD or NASH [98].

3.4 Natural History of Nonalcoholic Fatty Liver Disease

3.4.1 Evolution of Simple Steatosis

A comprehensive understanding of NAFLD progression is summarized in Fig. 3.4. Whereas previous research suggested that NAFL/simple steatosis had a benign natural history [99], later research has shown that even NAFL has the potential for progression [100]. Notably, while progression from NAFL to NASH and severe fibrosis is possible in a subgroup of individuals, regression from NASH to NAFL under certain circumstances can also occur over time. Therefore, although patients with NAFL may have the smallest progression risk, the presence of NAFL or NASH on a baseline histological assessment offers minimal overall prognostic value. According to current theories, NAFL and NASH cycle dynamically throughout NAFLD initial phases [101].

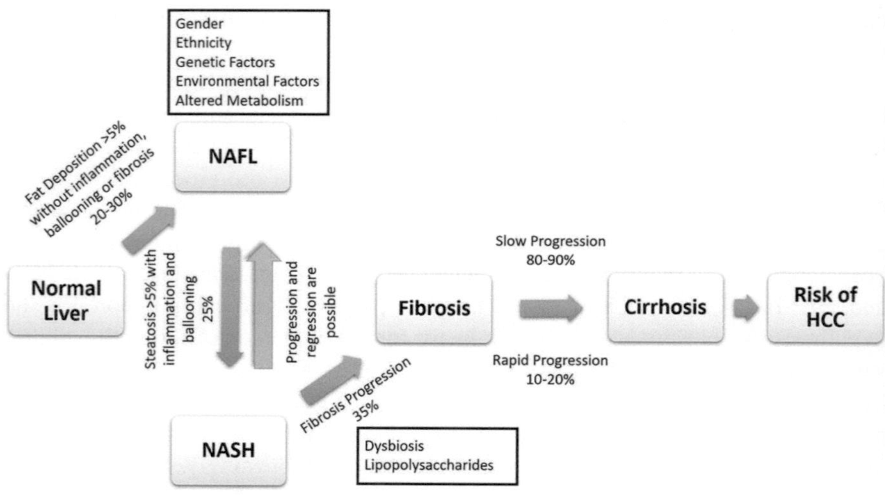

Fig. 3.4 The progression spectrum of NAFLD. *Abbreviations: HCC* Hepatocellular carcinoma, *NAFL* Nonalcoholic fatty liver, *NAFLD* Nonalcoholic fatty liver disease, *NASH-* Nonalcoholic steatohepatitis

Approximately 80% of patients who experience some liver fibrosis progress to mild stages of fibrosis (F0–F2) [101]. Nevertheless, 20% of individuals experience a substantial progression of fibrosis, leading to advanced fibrosis (F3–F4) within a couple of years. The prolonged disease duration and the fact that steatosis typically precedes NASH may help to explain the advanced fibrosis stages seen in NASH, compared with NAFL. In recent research, patients with NASH were found to be 9 years older than NAFL patients, supporting this hypothesis [102]. A total of 39% and 23% of participants with simple steatosis had advanced to borderline and definite NASH, respectively, according to a longitudinal Asian cohort study including 52 patients with biopsy-proven NAFLD who underwent repeat biopsies following 3 years [80]. In a cohort of 70 NAFLD patients with paired biopsies, of whom 25 patients had simple steatosis, Pais et al. reported that 64% of patients with simple steatosis developed progression to NASH, while 24% presented with advanced fibrosis after an average of 3.7 years [81].

Interesting insights into the dynamic evolution of the natural history of NAFLD were obtained from a systematic review and meta-analysis of paired biopsies from 11 cohort studies that included 411 patients with biopsy-proven NAFLD (150 with NAFL and 261 with NASH) and over 2145.5 person-years of follow-up [45]. Altogether, 33.6% of patients had fibrosis that progressed, compared to 43.1% who had stable fibrosis and 22.3% who had regression of the fibrosis [45]. In NAFL patients, the mean fibrosis progression rate was 0.07 stages per year, while it was 0.14 stages per year in NASH patients. Hence, this data suggests that in NAFL and NASH, hepatic fibrosis progresses by one stage every 14 and 7 years, respectively. Interestingly, 20% of patients without fibrosis at baseline proceeded quite quickly to advanced-stage (F3–F4) fibrosis, regardless of the presence of NAFL or NASH on baseline biopsy, while 80% of patients had little to no hepatic fibrosis progression [45]. In another study, 80% of NAFL patients with fibrosis progression also developed T2DM, compared to NAFL patients who did not progress, considering T2DM as a clinical indicator of a more aggressive disease [102].

The increased risk of T2DM and mortality in NAFLD was validated by a meta-analysis that included 40 studies, where NASH was linked to a greater overall and liver-related mortality when compared to NAFL, with an odds ratio of 5.7 and 1.8, respectively [103]. Nevertheless, cardiovascular mortality in NASH did not differ significantly from NAFL (OR 0.91) [103]. Even though fibrotic NASH and NASH-related cirrhosis patients are more likely to develop HCC, recent research reveals that HCC can still develop in individuals with NAFL who show no signs of fibrosis, hence leading to HCC arising from non-cirrhotic NASH [104, 105]. Accordingly, the emphasis should be on accurately and promptly identifying the small group of rapid progressors, with T2DM being an important risk factor [45].

3.4.2 NASH and Evolution of Liver Fibrosis

The prognosis of each NAFLD patient can vary greatly. In contrast to simple steatosis, the development of NASH and associated progression risk factors were extensively studied lately and are well documented in numerous studies. In patients with NASH, which is frequently defined by the NAFLD activity score (NAS score), a higher probability of progressing disease was first described [72]. The NAS score was initially created as a method for evaluating efficacy in clinical trials, but it has since been used more broadly to define NASH and evaluate histological activity. The NAS is the disproportionate sum of steatosis, ballooning, and lobular inflammation [106].

The global prevalence of NASH in NAFLD patients has been estimated to be 59% in a recent meta-analysis of biopsy-proven NAFLD patients [21]. Age, male sex, weight, insulin resistance, hypertension, total cholesterol, MetS, hyperuricemia, inflammation at index biopsy, low baseline AST to ALT, and specific genetic polymorphisms, as well as thyroid-stimulating hormone and vitamin D levels, are all predictors of histologic findings linked to the advancement of fibrosis in NASH patients [107–112].

A systematic review conducted by Argo et al. found that throughout the mean period of 5.3 years as follow-up, 37% of 221 patients with NASH developed progressive fibrosis [113]. In a more recent meta-analysis including 7 studies with 116 NASH patients, it was observed that 34.5% of the patients progressed toward fibrosis, while 38.8% remained stable, and 26.7% developed resolution or improvement of their fibrosis. Accordingly, the rate of annual fibrosis progression in NASH patients without fibrosis at baseline was 0.14 stages (95% CI 0.07–0.21 stages), indicating a progression time of 7.1 years on average [45]. The pooled mean fibrosis progression rate was estimated to be 0.09 (95% CI 0.06–0.12) in a recent meta-analysis of four studies involving biopsy-proven NASH patients. Moreover, the percentage of fibrosis progression was estimated to be 40.76% (95% CI 34.69–47.13) in a meta-analysis of six studies with histologically confirmed NASH. Nevertheless, it is worrying to highlight that one in five individuals with progression was classified as "fast progressors," patients who advanced from stage 0 fibrosis on the initial biopsy to bridging fibrosis or cirrhosis during follow-up [21]. Nevertheless, the design of the analysis prevented parameters linked to rapid progression from being identified, highlighting a critical gap in evidence of the natural history of NAFLD and associated fibrosis and necessitating more research.

To establish the importance of the NAFLD histologic features for long-term prognosis, Angulo et al. performed an international multicenter cohort research [114]. Their study revealed that the most significant histological characteristic linked to overall survival and liver-related morbidity was fibrosis stage, not NASH. Noteworthy, only those with advanced fibrosis (F3–F4) had a higher risk of liver-related complications including ascites, encephalopathy, or varices. However, even patients with mild fibrosis had a higher risk for overall mortality compared to those with no fibrosis. Ekstedt et al. evaluated a cohort of 229 patients with biopsy-proven NAFLD who were followed for an average of 26.4 years [115]. NAFLD individuals with F3–F4 fibrosis stages at baseline presented the worse outcome (HR 3.3 [95% CI 2.27–4.76, p-value <0.001]). Furthermore, NAFLD patients presented higher mortality rates compared to a matched reference sample. Patients with a high NAS (5–8) who did not have significant fibrosis, however, did not have an increase in mortality rates when compared to the reference sample.

These findings highlight the necessity of routinely evaluating fibrosis in all NAFLD patients to determine their prognosis and, consequently, the necessity of monitoring and liver-specific treatment. The identification of NAFLD patients known as quick progressors, who can rapidly progress to advanced fibrosis in a very short period of time, is concerning with significant importance [45].

3.4.3   Advanced Fibrosis and Cirrhosis

In general, we know less about the long-term effects and natural course of advanced fibrosis and cirrhosis caused by NAFLD. In approximately 10–25% of NASH patients, progressive fibrosis or cirrhosis could develop [14, 116–118]. Patients with NASH who develop cirrhosis have a poor prognosis because of the associated consequences.

A meta-analysis has estimated the global incidence of advanced fibrosis in NASH patients to be 67.95 per 1000 person-years, with fibrosis progression affecting 41% of NASH patients and an average yearly progression rate of 0.09% [21]. NAFLD patients can develop cirrhosis in up to 25% of the cases [119, 120] and end-stage liver disease in 7% [121]. In NASH patients, progressive fibrosis and cirrhosis are predicted by carotid artery disease, T2DM, and obesity [122–124]. Additionally, a systematic review including ten studies that involved 221 NASH patients found that advanced fibrosis was independently correlated with age and inflammation related to baseline liver biopsy [113].

In a cohort study of 23 patients with NASH-related cirrhosis in Australia, outcomes were contrasted to patients with chronic hepatitis C virus (HCV)-related cirrhosis [125]. A total of 39% of patients with NASH-related cirrhosis experienced liver-related complications over a 7-year follow-up period, while survival was not significantly different between the NASH and HCV-related cirrhosis groups [125]. On the contrary, another study comparing 152 NASH-related cirrhosis patients to 150 matched HCV-related cirrhosis patients found a decreased mortality rate, as well as a lower likelihood of developing ascites, hyperbilirubinemia, and HCC during a 10-year follow-up duration. Nevertheless, patients with NASH-related cirrhosis had a higher frequency of cardiovascular mortality [126]. NAFLD patients showed lower risks of liver-related complications than age- and sex-matched patients with HCV-related advanced fibrosis or cirrhosis, including HCC, in a prospective, multinational analysis of 247 patients with biopsy-proven NAFLD advanced fibrosis (grade 3) or cirrhosis. The two groups' rates of cardiovascular events and total mortality were comparable [127].

Powell et al. observed that the progression of advanced fibrosis/cirrhosis was accompanied by a decrease in steatosis and inflammatory modifications, which was highlighted as one significant finding regarding the natural history of NASH to cirrhosis [10]. Patients with NAFLD-related cirrhosis appear to experience less liver-related morbidity and mortality compared to HCV-related cirrhosis. Hui et al. compared patients with NASH-related cirrhosis and HCV-related cirrhosis, reporting that both had similar rates of liver-related complications and overall mortality, while NASH-related cirrhosis patients presented lower rates of HCC [125].

There is growing acknowledgment that NASH makes up a significant amount of what was formerly known as cryptogenic cirrhosis, the term used to describe any cirrhosis with an undetermined origin. Data on cryptogenic cirrhosis may provide indirect information regarding the natural course of NAFLD-related cirrhosis [125]. Powell's preliminary findings justify reclassifying a significant number of patients who were first diagnosed with cryptogenic cirrhosis as having burned-out NASH [10]. Many of these patients have established risk factors for MetS [11, 12], despite not presenting histological NASH features. This might be due to regression concomitantly with fibrosis progression [11, 128]. The increasing prevalence of NASH in patients who underwent liver transplants for cryptogenic cirrhosis confirms this theory [129].

The assumption that progressive NASH accounts for a considerable proportion of cryptogenic cirrhosis is further supported by the fact that these patients have a high prevalence of diseases linked to MetS and that NASH can recur after liver transplant [129]. It is also important to remember that in the USA, burned-out NASH is now thought to have been the primary cause in most subjects with cryptogenic cirrhosis. Subacute liver failure can occasionally be evident in patients with cirrhosis who had not previously been diagnosed. Uncertainty surrounds the triggering factors for such a severe deterioration. These patients have a higher chance of developing HCC.

3.4.4 Hepatocellular Carcinoma

Nearly all types of CLD, including NAFLD, carry a considerable likelihood of developing HCC [128]. The occurrence of HCC provides additional proof of the progressive character of some NAFLD subsets. HCC incidence has been rapidly rising in developed countries such as the USA and Europe, formerly thought of as having low HCC prevalence, concomitant with the NAFLD epidemic [130]. This may reflect the rising prevalence of NAFLD [131]. Patients with cirrhosis are likely to be at risk for developing HCC among the NASH cohorts. The incidence of HCC is increasing worldwide, and it is one of the six most frequent cancers in the world [131, 132]. It is also the third most common cause of cancer-related mortality.

Patients with HCC attributable to NAFLD tend to be older and of female sex than those with HCC compared to alternative CLD etiologies such as viral hepatitis, autoimmune, or metabolic liver disease that add to the overall burden of HCC [133]. Numerous studies have shown a link between MetS, T2DM, and obesity with HCC, indicating that NAFLD is significantly contributing to the increased incidence of HCC [132, 134, 135]. In the absence of cirrhosis, the possible processes linking MetS, obesity, T2DM, NAFLD, and HCC are likely connected to the etiology of the underlying condition rather than to fibrosis solely. Insulin resistance, hepatic steatosis-promoting adipose tissue-derived inflammation, adipokines, oxidative stress, lipotoxicity, activation of insulin-like growth factor, gut microbiome, nutrition, genetics, and other factors all contribute to liver carcinogenesis [134–138].

Patients with NASH cirrhosis and cryptogenic cirrhosis linked to prior NASH are two main risk groups [23]. In a cohort of 1500 US veterans with HCC identified over a 6-year period, NASH was identified to be the third most prevalent risk factor for HCC [139]. Due to insufficient surveillance, delayed diagnosis of HCC can commonly occur [140]. According to a recent study conducted using data from the Surveillance, Epidemiology, and End Results (SEER) database, individuals with NAFLD had a 2.6-fold higher risk of developing HCC, and the prevalence of NAFLD-related HCC may be rising by roughly 10% yearly [141]. With cumulative incidence rates reported to be between 2.4 and 12.8% [142], advanced fibrosis continues to be a significant risk factor for the development of HCC. In some areas, it has been reported that more than 40% of NASH-related cirrhosis patients would progress to develop HCC [143]. Although it is currently unknown if the biology of NAFLD-associated HCC exhibits special features, this can be assumed and may present distinctive therapeutic options [104]. A recently published systematic review and meta-analysis showed a pooled incidence rate of HCC being 1.25 per 1000 person-years (95% CI 1.01–1.49; $I^2 = 94.8\%$) [144]. Moreover, the incidence rate of HCC was 14.46 per 1000 person-years in NAFLD patients with advanced liver fibrosis or cirrhosis (95% CI 10.89–18.04; $I^2 = 91.3\%$) [144].

HCC is still a rare consequence of NAFLD, while liver cirrhosis plays an important influence for disease progression. A Japanese study involving 6508 ultrasound-diagnosed NAFLD patients found that after 8 years, the incidence of HCC was just 0.2%, whereas patients with advanced fibrosis as defined by the AST-platelet ratio index (APRI) had higher risk with a 25-fold [145]. Alarmingly, it has been reported that HCC developed in non-cirrhotic NAFLD patients without considerable fibrosis, pointing to the possibility that steatosis itself increases the risk of cancer [42, 142, 146]. Due to limited surveillance, HCC is commonly discovered at an advanced stage compared to individuals with viral hepatitis, hence possibly providing an explanation for the worse outcomes reported in various studies [140]. The extent of this risk has yet to be determined.

3.5 Liver Transplantation

Patients with decompensated NASH-related cirrhosis can become candidates for LT [147]. Since T2DM and cardiovascular risk factors are prevalent in this group, other underlying risk factors most likely also aggravate matters. According to published research, the outcomes of LT in NASH-related cirrhosis patients are comparable to those of patients receiving transplants for liver disorders caused by different etiologies. Recurrence occurs often in the posttransplant liver, appearing in 20–33% of cases, and periportal fibrosis is detected in 18% of patients by 18 months, with reported 5-year survival rates ranging from 71 to 75% [148, 149].

The connections between developing NASH and LT for severe cirrhosis have been concealed by a variety of factors [23]. First off, a lot of these individuals have coexisting MetS-related diseases that preclude them from being transplant candidates. In addition to diseases like CVD, a BMI >35–40 is another frequent exclusion criterion. Second, early series might not have recognized the underlying disease because the connection between NASH and cryptogenic cirrhosis has only been more apparent in the last decade. Finally, throughout time, the established terminology and nomenclature for NASH-related cirrhosis have changed. This may be seen in the UNOS databases, as cryptogenic cirrhosis has marginally decreased during this period while NASH-related cirrhosis has become more widely recognized since the early 2000s. It should come as no surprise that systemic comorbidities have a considerable impact on the outcome of LT in this group [150].

Additionally, it has been shown that individuals who have undergone LT experience recurrence of NAFLD and NASH, which is linked to the continuation of the MetS after LT and is adversely correlated with weight loss following LT [148, 151, 152]. This topic was assessed by several systematic reviews and meta-analyses. Saeed et al. conducted a meta-analysis of 17 studies, representing 2378 patients [153]. The authors reported mean incidence rates for recurrent NAFLD of 59%, 57%, and 82%; de novo NAFLD of 67%, 40%, and 78%; recurrent NASH of 53%, 57.4%, and 38%; and de novo NASH of 13%, 16%, and 17%. Moreover, multivariate analysis showed that hyperlipidemia and post-LT BMI were the most accurate outcome predictors. Using data from 12 studies and 2166 participants, Losurdo et al. conducted another meta-analysis and found that the prevalence of de novo NAFLD was 26% (95% CI 20–31%) [154]. In another recent meta-analysis, the recipient age, functional status, pre-LT hepatoma, MELD score, T2DM, pre-LT dialysis, hepatic encephalopathy, portal vein thrombosis, hospitalization/ICU at LT, and year of LT were found to be predictive variables of post-LT NASH patient survival [155].

3.6 Resolution of Nonalcoholic Fatty Liver Disease

There is scarce data in the current literature about successful NAFLD resolution. Large population-based studies with a lack of long-term follow-up and limited biopsy data further limit our knowledge regarding this topic. Studies about bariatric surgery patients have provided the most convincing data to date. Inflammation was resolved by bariatric surgery in 50% of patients (95% CI 35–64%), ballooning degeneration by 76% (95% CI 64–86%), and fibrosis by 40% (95% CI 29–51%), according to a systematic review and meta-analysis of 32 cohort studies that included 3093 liver biopsy specimens. After having bariatric surgery, patients' mean NAFLD activity scores were considerably lower (mean difference 2.39 [95% CI 1.58–3.20; *p*-value <0.001]) [156]. However, 12% of patients (95% CI 5–20%) who underwent bariatric surgery experienced new or worsening of NAFLD characteristics, such as fibrosis [156].

3.7 Conclusion and Future Perspectives

NAFLD is the most prevalent CLD worldwide, and its incidence is rising in parallel with the epidemic of obesity and MetS. Despite a small amount of disagreement in the evidence regarding the natural history of NAFLD, it appears that some subsets of NAFLD may be more susceptible than previously believed to disease progression, possibly leading to steatohepatitis, and subsequently to fibrosis and cirrhosis, as well as HCC. Metabolic risks including diabetes, obesity, and hypertension, in addition to several genetic and environmental factors, affect the severity of the underlying liver histology and are therefore likely to affect the likelihood of developing cirrhosis and HCC. With a significant clinical burden for the present and the future, NAFLD emerges as a serious disease entity.

It is necessary to continue researching NAFLD natural history and its consequences by conducting high-quality prospective research. Enhanced prevention, screening, monitoring, and treatment modalities can be established with a better understanding of the natural history of NAFLD and the factors that influence its progression and long-term effects.

References

1. Sporea I, Popescu A, Dumitraşcu D, Brisc C, Nedelcu L, Trifan A, et al. Nonalcoholic fatty liver disease: status quo. J Gastrointestin Liver Dis. 2018;27(4):439–48. https://doi.org/10.15403/jgld.2014.1121.274.quo.
2. Chalasani N, Younossi Z, Lavine JE, Diehl AM, Brunt EM, Cusi K, et al. The diagnosis and management of non-alcoholic fatty liver disease: practice guideline by the American Association for the Study of Liver Diseases, American College of Gastroenterology, and the American Gastroenterological Association. Hepatology. 2012;55(6):2005–23. https://doi.org/10.1002/hep.25762.
3. Ando Y, Jou JH. Nonalcoholic fatty liver disease and recent guideline updates. Clin Liver Dis. 2021;17(1):23–8. https://doi.org/10.1002/cld.1045.
4. Mikolasevic I, Filipec-Kanizaj T, Mijic M, Jakopcic I, Milic S, Hrstic I, et al. Nonalcoholic fatty liver disease and liver transplantation—where do we stand? World J Gastroenterol. 2018;24(14):1491–506. https://doi.org/10.3748/wjg.v24.i14.1491.
5. Younossi ZM, Marchesini G, Pinto-Cortez H, Petta S. Epidemiology of nonalcoholic fatty liver disease and nonalcoholic steatohepatitis: implications for liver Transplantation. Transplantation. 2019;103(1):22–7. https://doi.org/10.1097/tp.0000000000002484.

6. (NCD-RisC) NRFC. Trends in adult body-mass index in 200 countries from 1975 to 2014: a pooled analysis of 1698 population-based measurement studies with 19·2 million participants. Lancet. 2016;387(10026):1377–96. https://doi.org/10.1016/s0140-6736(16)30054-x.

7. Mantovani A, Petracca G, Beatrice G, Csermely A, Tilg H, Byrne CD, et al. Non-alcoholic fatty liver disease and increased risk of incident extrahepatic cancers: a meta-analysis of observational cohort studies. Gut. 2021;71(4):gutjnl-2021-324191. https://doi.org/10.1136/gutjnl-2021-324191.

8. Tan DJH, Ng CH, Lin SY, Pan XH, Tay P, Lim WH, et al. Clinical characteristics, surveillance, treatment allocation, and outcomes of non-alcoholic fatty liver disease-related hepatocellular carcinoma: a systematic review and meta-analysis. Lancet Oncol. 2022;23(4):521–30. https://doi.org/10.1016/S1470-2045(22)00078-X.

9. Ismaiel A, Dumitrascu DL. Cardiovascular risk in fatty liver disease: the liver-heart axis-literature review. Front Med (Lausanne). 2019;6:202. https://doi.org/10.3389/fmed.2019.00202.

10. Powell EE, Cooksley WG, Hanson R, Searle J, Halliday JW, Powell LW. The natural history of nonalcoholic steatohepatitis: a follow-up study of forty-two patients for up to 21 years. Hepatology. 1990;11(1):74–80.

11. Caldwell SH, Oelsner DH, Iezzoni JC, Hespenheide EE, Battle EH, Driscoll CJ. Cryptogenic cirrhosis: clinical characterization and risk factors for underlying disease. Hepatology. 1999;29(3):664–9. https://doi.org/10.1002/hep.510290347.

12. Poonawala A, Nair SP, Thuluvath PJ. Prevalence of obesity and diabetes in patients with cryptogenic cirrhosis: a case-control study. Hepatology. 2000;32(4 Pt 1):689–92. https://doi.org/10.1053/jhep.2000.17894.

13. Fazel Y, Koenig AB, Sayiner M, Goodman ZD, Younossi ZM. Epidemiology and natural history of non-alcoholic fatty liver disease. Metabolism. 2016;65(8):1017–25. https://doi.org/10.1016/j.metabol.2016.01.012.

14. Matteoni CA, Younossi ZM, Gramlich T, Boparai N, Liu YC, McCullough AJ. Nonalcoholic fatty liver disease: a spectrum of clinical and pathological severity. Gastroenterology. 1999;116(6):1413–9. https://doi.org/10.1016/s0016-5085(99)70506-8.

15. Chalasani N, Younossi Z, Lavine JE, Charlton M, Cusi K, Rinella M, et al. The diagnosis and management of nonalcoholic fatty liver disease: Practice guidance from the American Association for the Study of Liver Diseases. Hepatology. 2018;67(1):328–57. https://doi.org/10.1002/hep.29367.

16. Eslam M, Sanyal AJ, George J. MAFLD: a consensus-driven proposed nomenclature for metabolic associated fatty liver disease. Gastroenterology. 2020; https://doi.org/10.1053/j.gastro.2019.11.312.

17. Eslam M, Newsome PN, Anstee QM, Targher G, Gomez MR, Zelber-Sagi S, et al. A new definition for metabolic associated fatty liver disease: an international expert consensus statement. J Hepatol. 2020; https://doi.org/10.1016/j.jhep.2020.03.039.

18. Méndez-Sánchez N, Bugianesi E, Gish RG, Lammert F, Tilg H, Nguyen MH, et al. Global multi-stakeholder endorsement of the MAFLD definition. Lancet Gastroenterol Hepatol. 2022;7(5):388–90. https://doi.org/10.1016/S2468-1253(22)00062-0.

19. Falck-Ytter Y, Younossi ZM, Marchesini G, McCullough AJ. Clinical features and natural history of nonalcoholic steatosis syndromes. Semin Liver Dis. 2001;21(1):17–26. https://doi.org/10.1055/s-2001-12926.

20. Goh GB, McCullough AJ. Natural history of nonalcoholic fatty liver disease. Dig Dis Sci. 2016;61(5):1226–33. https://doi.org/10.1007/s10620-016-4095-4.

21. Younossi ZM, Koenig AB, Abdelatif D, Fazel Y, Henry L, Wymer M. Global epidemiology of nonalcoholic fatty liver disease-meta-analytic assessment of prevalence, incidence, and outcomes. Hepatology. 2016;64(1):73–84. https://doi.org/10.1002/hep.28431.

22. (EASL). EAftSotL, (EASD). EAftSoD, (EASO). EAftSoO. EASL–EASD–EASO Clinical Practice Guidelines for the management of non-alcoholic fatty liver disease. J Hepatol. 2016;64(6):1388–402. https://doi.org/10.1016/j.jhep.2015.11.004.

23. Caldwell S, Argo C. The natural history of non-alcoholic fatty liver disease. Dig Dis. 2010;28(1):162–8. https://doi.org/10.1159/000282081.

24. Dumitrascu DL, Neuman MG. Non-alcoholic fatty liver disease: an update on diagnosis. Clujul Med (1957). 2018;91(2):147–50. https://doi.org/10.15386/cjmed-993.

25. Filipović B, Forbes A, Tepeš B, Dumitraşcu DL. Nonalcoholic fatty liver disease. Can J Gastroenterol Hepatol. 2018;2018:2097435. https://doi.org/10.1155/2018/2097435.

26. Ismaiel A, Dumitrascu DL. How to reduce cardiovascular risk in nonalcoholic fatty liver disease. Am J Ther. 2020; Publish Ahead of Print.; https://doi.org/10.1097/mjt.0000000000001174.

27. Ismaiel A, Popa S-L, Dumitrascu DL. Acute coronary syndromes and nonalcoholic fatty liver disease: "Un Affaire de Coeur". Can J Gastroenterol Hepatol. 2020;2020:8825615. https://doi.org/10.1155/2020/8825615.

28. Ismaiel A, Colosi HA, Rusu F, Dumitrascu DL. Cardiac arrhythmias and electrocardiogram modifications in non-alcoholic fatty liver disease. a systematic review. J Gastrointestin Liver Dis. 2019;28(4):483–93. https://doi.org/10.15403/jgld-344.

29. Mantovani A, Petracca G, Beatrice G, Csermely A, Tilg H, Byrne CD, et al. Non-alcoholic fatty liver disease and increased risk of incident extrahepatic cancers: a meta-analysis of observational cohort studies. Gut. 2022;71(4):778–88. https://doi.org/10.1136/gutjnl-2021-324191.

30. Liu SS, Ma XF, Zhao J, Du SX, Zhang J, Dong MZ, et al. Association between nonalcoholic fatty liver disease and extrahepatic cancers: a systematic review and meta-analysis. Lipids Health Dis. 2020;19(1):118. https://doi.org/10.1186/s12944-020-01288-6.

31. Orci LA, Sanduzzi-Zamparelli M, Caballol B, Sapena V, Colucci N, Torres F, et al. Incidence of hepatocellular carcinoma in patients with nonalcoholic fatty liver disease: a systematic review, meta-analysis, and meta-regression. Clin Gastroenterol Hepatol. 2022;20(2):283–92. e10. https://doi.org/10.1016/j.cgh.2021.05.002.

32. Mantovani A, Csermely A, Petracca G, Beatrice G, Corey KE, Simon TG, et al. Non-alcoholic fatty liver disease and risk of fatal and non-fatal cardiovascular events: an updated systematic review and meta-analysis. Lancet Gastroenterol Hepatol. 2021;6(11):903–13. https://doi.org/10.1016/s2468-1253(21)00308-3.

33. Fan JG, Zhu J, Li XJ, Chen L, Li L, Dai F, et al. Prevalence of and risk factors for fatty liver in a general population of Shanghai, China. J Hepatol. 2005;43(3):508–14. https://doi.org/10.1016/j.jhep.2005.02.042.

34. Amarapurkar D, Kamani P, Patel N, Gupte P, Kumar P, Agal S, et al. Prevalence of non-alcoholic fatty liver disease: population based study. Ann Hepatol. 2007;6(3):161–3.

35. Li H, Wang YJ, Tan K, Zeng L, Liu L, Liu FJ, et al. Prevalence and risk factors of fatty liver disease in Chengdu, Southwest China. Hepatobiliary Pancreat Dis Int. 2009;8(4):377–82.

36. Park SH, Jeon WK, Kim SH, Kim HJ, Park DI, Cho YK, et al. Prevalence and risk factors of non-alcoholic fatty liver disease among Korean adults. J Gastroenterol Hepatol. 2006;21(1 Pt 1):138–43. https://doi.org/10.1111/j.1440-1746.2005.04086.x.

37. Ong JP, Pitts A, Younossi ZM. Increased overall mortality and liver-related mortality in non-alcoholic fatty liver disease. J Hepatol. 2008;49(4):608–12. https://doi.org/10.1016/j.jhep.2008.06.018.

38. Hashimoto E, Yatsuji S, Kaneda H, Yoshioka Y, Taniai M, Tokushige K, et al. The characteristics and natural history of Japanese patients with nonalcoholic fatty liver disease. Hepatol Res. 2005;33(2):72–6. https://doi.org/10.1016/j.hepres.2005.09.007.

39. Adams LA, Lymp JF, St Sauver J, Sanderson SO, Lindor KD, Feldstein A, et al. The natural history of nonalcoholic fatty liver disease: a population-based cohort study. Gastroenterology. 2005;129(1):113–21.

40. Hossain N, Afendy A, Stepanova M, Nader F, Srishord M, Rafiq N, et al. Independent predictors of fibrosis in patients with nonalcoholic fatty liver disease. Clin Gastroenterol Hepatol. 2009;7(11):1224-9, 9.e1-2. https://doi.org/10.1016/j.cgh.2009.06.007.

41. Tarantino G, Conca P, Riccio A, Tarantino M, Di Minno MN, Chianese D, et al. Enhanced serum concentrations of transforming growth factor-beta1 in simple fatty liver: is it really benign? J Transl Med. 2008;6:72. https://doi.org/10.1186/1479-5876-6-72.

42. Ascha MS, Hanouneh IA, Lopez R, Tamimi TA, Feldstein AF, Zein NN. The incidence and risk factors of hepatocellular carcinoma in patients with nonalcoholic steatohepatitis. Hepatology. 2010;51(6):1972–8. https://doi.org/10.1002/hep.23527.
43. Hashimoto E, Yatsuji S, Tobari M, Taniai M, Torii N, Tokushige K, et al. Hepatocellular carcinoma in patients with nonalcoholic steatohepatitis. J Gastroenterol. 2009;44(Suppl 19):89–95. https://doi.org/10.1007/s00535-008-2262-x.
44. Liew PL, Lee WJ, Wang W, Lee YC, Chen WY, Fang CL, et al. Fatty liver disease: predictors of nonalcoholic steatohepatitis and gallbladder disease in morbid obesity. Obes Surg. 2008;18(7):847–53. https://doi.org/10.1007/s11695-007-9355-0.
45. Singh S, Allen AM, Wang Z, Prokop LJ, Murad MH, Loomba R. Fibrosis progression in nonalcoholic fatty liver vs nonalcoholic steatohepatitis: a systematic review and meta-analysis of paired-biopsy studies. Clin Gastroenterol Hepatol. 2015;13(4):643–654.e1-9; quiz e39-40. https://doi.org/10.1016/j.cgh.2014.04.014.
46. Vernon G, Baranova A, Younossi ZM. Systematic review: the epidemiology and natural history of non-alcoholic fatty liver disease and non-alcoholic steatohepatitis in adults. Aliment Pharmacol Ther. 2011;34(3):274–85. https://doi.org/10.1111/j.1365-2036.2011.04724.x.
47. Singh SP, Nayak S, Swain M, Rout N, Mallik RN, Agrawal O, et al. Prevalence of nonalcoholic fatty liver disease in coastal eastern India: a preliminary ultrasonographic survey. Trop Gastroenterol. 2004;25(2):76–9.
48. Omagari K, Kadokawa Y, Masuda J, Egawa I, Sawa T, Hazama H, et al. Fatty liver in non-alcoholic non-overweight Japanese adults: incidence and clinical characteristics. J Gastroenterol Hepatol. 2002;17(10):1098–105. https://doi.org/10.1046/j.1440-1746.2002.02846.x.
49. Jamali R, Khonsari M, Merat S, Khoshnia M, Jafari E, Bahram Kalhori A, et al. Persistent alanine aminotransferase elevation among the general Iranian population: prevalence and causes. World J Gastroenterol. 2008;14(18):2867–71. https://doi.org/10.3748/wjg.14.2867.
50. Reid AE. Nonalcoholic steatohepatitis. Gastroenterology. 2001;121(3):710–23. https://doi.org/10.1053/gast.2001.27126.
51. Hamaguchi M, Kojima T, Takeda N, Nakagawa T, Taniguchi H, Fujii K, et al. The metabolic syndrome as a predictor of nonalcoholic fatty liver disease. Ann Intern Med. 2005;143(10):722–8. https://doi.org/10.7326/0003-4819-143-10-200511150-00009.
52. Hamaguchi M, Kojima T, Takeda N, Nagata C, Takeda J, Sarui H, et al. Nonalcoholic fatty liver disease is a novel predictor of cardiovascular disease. World J Gastroenterol. 2007;13(10):1579–84.
53. Chen ZW, Chen LY, Dai HL, Chen JH, Fang LZ. Relationship between alanine aminotransferase levels and metabolic syndrome in nonalcoholic fatty liver disease. J Zhejiang Univ Sci B. 2008;9(8):616–22. https://doi.org/10.1631/jzus.B0720016.
54. Kallwitz ER, Kumar M, Aggarwal R, Berger R, Layden-Almer J, Gupta N, et al. Ethnicity and nonalcoholic fatty liver disease in an obesity clinic: the impact of triglycerides. Dig Dis Sci. 2008;53(5):1358–63. https://doi.org/10.1007/s10620-008-0234-x.
55. Papatheodoridis GV, Goulis J, Christodoulou D, Manolakopoulos S, Raptopoulou M, Andrioti E, et al. High prevalence of elevated liver enzymes in blood donors: associations with male gender and central adiposity. Eur J Gastroenterol Hepatol. 2007;19(4):281–7. https://doi.org/10.1097/MEG.0b013e328011438b.
56. Ong JP, Elariny H, Collantes R, Younoszai A, Chandhoke V, Reines HD, et al. Predictors of nonalcoholic steatohepatitis and advanced fibrosis in morbidly obese patients. Obes Surg. 2005;15(3):310–5. https://doi.org/10.1381/0960892053576820.
57. Sorrentino P, Tarantino G, Conca P, Perrella A, Terracciano ML, Vecchione R, et al. Silent non-alcoholic fatty liver disease-a clinical-histological study. J Hepatol. 2004;41(5):751–7. https://doi.org/10.1016/j.jhep.2004.07.010.
58. Williams CD, Stengel J, Asike MI, Torres DM, Shaw J, Contreras M, et al. Prevalence of nonalcoholic fatty liver disease and nonalcoholic steatohepatitis among a largely middle-aged population utilizing ultrasound and liver biopsy: a prospective study. Gastroenterology. 2011;140(1):124–31. https://doi.org/10.1053/j.gastro.2010.09.038.

59. Wagenknecht LE, Scherzinger AL, Stamm ER, Hanley AJ, Norris JM, Chen YD, et al. Correlates and heritability of nonalcoholic fatty liver disease in a minority cohort. Obesity (Silver Spring, MD). 2009;17(6):1240–6. https://doi.org/10.1038/oby.2009.4.

60. Lomonaco R, Ortiz-Lopez C, Orsak B, Finch J, Webb A, Bril F, et al. Role of ethnicity in overweight and obese patients with nonalcoholic steatohepatitis. Hepatology. 2011;54(3):837–45. https://doi.org/10.1002/hep.24483.

61. Mohanty SR, Troy TN, Huo D, O'Brien BL, Jensen DM, Hart J. Influence of ethnicity on histological differences in non-alcoholic fatty liver disease. J Hepatol. 2009;50(4):797–804. https://doi.org/10.1016/j.jhep.2008.11.017.

62. Solga SF, Clark JM, Alkhuraishi AR, Torbenson M, Tabesh A, Schweitzer M, et al. Race and comorbid factors predict nonalcoholic fatty liver disease histopathology in severely obese patients. Surg Obes Relat Dis. 2005;1(1):6–11. https://doi.org/10.1016/j.soard.2004.12.006.

63. Schwimmer JB, Celedon MA, Lavine JE, Salem R, Campbell N, Schork NJ, et al. Heritability of nonalcoholic fatty liver disease. Gastroenterology. 2009;136(5):1585–92. https://doi.org/10.1053/j.gastro.2009.01.050.

64. Struben VM, Hespenheide EE, Caldwell SH. Nonalcoholic steatohepatitis and cryptogenic cirrhosis within kindreds. Am J Med. 2000;108(1):9–13. https://doi.org/10.1016/s0002-9343(99)00315-0.

65. Eslam M, George J. Genetic and epigenetic mechanisms of NASH. Hepatol Int. 2016;10(3):394–406. https://doi.org/10.1007/s12072-015-9689-y.

66. Eslam M, Valenti L, Romeo S. Genetics and epigenetics of NAFLD and NASH: clinical impact. J Hepatol. 2018;68(2):268–79. https://doi.org/10.1016/j.jhep.2017.09.003.

67. Liu YL, Reeves HL, Burt AD, Tiniakos D, McPherson S, Leathart JB, et al. TM6SF2 rs58542926 influences hepatic fibrosis progression in patients with non-alcoholic fatty liver disease. Nat Commun. 2014;5:4309. https://doi.org/10.1038/ncomms5309.

68. Romeo S, Kozlitina J, Xing C, Pertsemlidis A, Cox D, Pennacchio LA, et al. Genetic variation in PNPLA3 confers susceptibility to nonalcoholic fatty liver disease. Nat Genet. 2008;40(12):1461–5. https://doi.org/10.1038/ng.257.

69. Xiang H, Wu Z, Wang J, Wu T. Research progress, challenges and perspectives on PNPLA3 and its variants in liver diseases. J Cancer. 2021;12(19):5929–37. https://doi.org/10.7150/jca.57951.

70. Sookoian S, Pirola CJ. Meta-analysis of the influence of I148M variant of patatin-like phospholipase domain containing 3 gene (PNPLA3) on the susceptibility and histological severity of nonalcoholic fatty liver disease. Hepatology. 2011;53(6):1883–94. https://doi.org/10.1002/hep.24283.

71. He S, McPhaul C, Li JZ, Garuti R, Kinch L, Grishin NV, et al. A sequence variation (I148M) in PNPLA3 associated with nonalcoholic fatty liver disease disrupts triglyceride hydrolysis. J Biol Chem. 2010;285(9):6706–15. https://doi.org/10.1074/jbc.M109.064501.

72. Calzadilla Bertot L, Adams LA. The natural course of non-alcoholic fatty liver disease. Int J Mol Sci. 2016;17(5) https://doi.org/10.3390/ijms17050774.

73. Francque SM, van der Graaff D, Kwanten WJ. Non-alcoholic fatty liver disease and cardiovascular risk: pathophysiological mechanisms and implications. J Hepatol. 2016;65(2):425–43. https://doi.org/10.1016/j.jhep.2016.04.005.

74. Chandrasekharan K, Alazawi W. Genetics of non-alcoholic fatty liver and cardiovascular disease: implications for therapy? Front Pharmacol. 2020;10:1413. https://doi.org/10.3389/fphar.2019.01413.

75. Ismaiel A, Dumitrascu DL. Genetic predisposition in metabolic-dysfunction-associated fatty liver disease and cardiovascular outcomes-systematic review. Eur J Clin Invest. 2020;50(10):1–14. https://doi.org/10.1111/eci.13331.

76. Teo K, Abeysekera KWM, Adams L, Aigner E, Anstee QM, Banales JM, et al. rs641738C>T near MBOAT7 is associated with liver fat, ALT and fibrosis in NAFLD: a meta-analysis. J Hepatol. 2021;74(1):20–30. https://doi.org/10.1016/j.jhep.2020.08.027.

77. Neuschwander-Tetri BA, Clark JM, Bass NM, Van Natta ML, Unalp-Arida A, Tonascia J, et al. Clinical, laboratory and histological associations in adults with nonalcoholic fatty liver disease. Hepatology. 2010;52(3):913–24. https://doi.org/10.1002/hep.23784.

78. Speliotes EK, Yerges-Armstrong LM, Wu J, Hernaez R, Kim LJ, Palmer CD, et al. Genome-wide association analysis identifies variants associated with nonalcoholic fatty liver disease that have distinct effects on metabolic traits. PLoS Genet. 2011;7(3):e1001324. https://doi.org/10.1371/journal.pgen.1001324.

79. Yang Z, Wen J, Tao X, Lu B, Du Y, Wang M, et al. Genetic variation in the GCKR gene is associated with non-alcoholic fatty liver disease in Chinese people. Mol Biol Rep. 2011;38(2):1145–50. https://doi.org/10.1007/s11033-010-0212-1.

80. Wong VW, Wong GL, Choi PC, Chan AW, Li MK, Chan HY, et al. Disease progression of non-alcoholic fatty liver disease: a prospective study with paired liver biopsies at 3 years. Gut. 2010;59(7):969–74. https://doi.org/10.1136/gut.2009.205088.

81. Pais R, Charlotte F, Fedchuk L, Bedossa P, Lebray P, Poynard T, et al. A systematic review of follow-up biopsies reveals disease progression in patients with non-alcoholic fatty liver. J Hepatol. 2013;59(3):550–6. https://doi.org/10.1016/j.jhep.2013.04.027.

82. Adams LA, Sanderson S, Lindor KD, Angulo P. The histological course of nonalcoholic fatty liver disease: a longitudinal study of 103 patients with sequential liver biopsies. J Hepatol. 2005;42(1):132–8. https://doi.org/10.1016/j.jhep.2004.09.012.

83. Leite NC, Salles GF, Araujo AL, Villela-Nogueira CA, Cardoso CR. Prevalence and associated factors of non-alcoholic fatty liver disease in patients with type-2 diabetes mellitus. Liver Int. 2009;29(1):113–9. https://doi.org/10.1111/j.1478-3231.2008.01718.x.

84. Stepanova M, Rafiq N, Younossi ZM. Components of metabolic syndrome are independent predictors of mortality in patients with chronic liver disease: a population-based study. Gut. 2010;59(10):1410–5. https://doi.org/10.1136/gut.2010.213553.

85. Bellentani S, Saccoccio G, Masutti F, Crocè LS, Brandi G, Sasso F, et al. Prevalence of and risk factors for hepatic steatosis in Northern Italy. Ann Intern Med. 2000;132(2):112–7. https://doi.org/10.7326/0003-4819-132-2-200001180-00004.

86. Boza C, Riquelme A, Ibañez L, Duarte I, Norero E, Viviani P, et al. Predictors of nonalcoholic steatohepatitis (NASH) in obese patients undergoing gastric bypass. Obes Surg. 2005;15(8):1148–53. https://doi.org/10.1381/0960892055002347.

87. Abrams GA, Kunde SS, Lazenby AJ, Clements RH. Portal fibrosis and hepatic steatosis in morbidly obese subjects: a spectrum of nonalcoholic fatty liver disease. Hepatology. 2004;40(2):475–83. https://doi.org/10.1002/hep.20323.

88. Dolce CJ, Russo M, Keller JE, Buckingham J, Norton HJ, Heniford BT, et al. Does liver appearance predict histopathologic findings: prospective analysis of routine liver biopsies during bariatric surgery. Surg Obes Relat Dis. 2009;5(3):323–8. https://doi.org/10.1016/j.soard.2008.12.008.

89. Beymer C, Kowdley KV, Larson A, Edmonson P, Dellinger EP, Flum DR. Prevalence and predictors of asymptomatic liver disease in patients undergoing gastric bypass surgery. Arch Surg. 2003;138(11):1240–4. https://doi.org/10.1001/archsurg.138.11.1240.

90. Gholam PM, Flancbaum L, Machan JT, Charney DA, Kotler DP. Nonalcoholic fatty liver disease in severely obese subjects. Am J Gastroenterol. 2007;102(2):399–408. https://doi.org/10.1111/j.1572-0241.2006.01041.x.

91. Harnois F, Msika S, Sabaté JM, Mechler C, Jouet P, Barge J, et al. Prevalence and predictive factors of non-alcoholic steatohepatitis (NASH) in morbidly obese patients undergoing bariatric surgery. Obes Surg. 2006;16(2):183–8. https://doi.org/10.1381/096089206775565122.

92. Machado M, Marques-Vidal P, Cortez-Pinto H. Hepatic histology in obese patients undergoing bariatric surgery. J Hepatol. 2006;45(4):600–6. https://doi.org/10.1016/j.jhep.2006.06.013.

93. Colicchio P, Tarantino G, del Genio F, Sorrentino P, Saldalamacchia G, Finelli C, et al. Non-alcoholic fatty liver disease in young adult severely obese non-diabetic patients in South Italy. Ann Nutr Metab. 2005;49(5):289–95. https://doi.org/10.1159/000087295.

94. Farrell GC, Larter CZ. Nonalcoholic fatty liver disease: from steatosis to cirrhosis. Hepatology. 2006;43(2 Suppl 1):S99–s112. https://doi.org/10.1002/hep.20973.

95. Baranova A, Tran TP, Birerdinc A, Younossi ZM. Systematic review: association of polycystic ovary syndrome with metabolic syndrome and non-alcoholic fatty liver disease. Aliment Pharmacol Ther. 2011;33(7):801–14. https://doi.org/10.1111/j.1365-2036.2011.04579.x.

96. Romanowski MD, Parolin MB, Freitas AC, Piazza MJ, Basso J, Urbanetz AA. Prevalence of non-alcoholic fatty liver disease in women with polycystic ovary syndrome and its correlation with metabolic syndrome. Arq Gastroenterol. 2015;52(2):117–23. https://doi.org/10.1590/s0004-28032015000200008.

97. Kelley CE, Brown AJ, Diehl AM, Setji TL. Review of nonalcoholic fatty liver disease in women with polycystic ovary syndrome. World J Gastroenterol. 2014;20(39):14172–84. https://doi.org/10.3748/wjg.v20.i39.14172.

98. Hossain N, Stepanova M, Afendy A, Nader F, Younossi Y, Rafiq N, et al. Non-alcoholic steatohepatitis (NASH) in patients with polycystic ovarian syndrome (PCOS). Scand J Gastroenterol. 2011;46(4):479–84. https://doi.org/10.3109/00365521.2010.539251.

99. Teli MR, James OFW, Burt AD, Bennett MK, Day CP. The natural history of nonalcoholic fatty liver: a follow-up study. Hepatology. 1995;22(6):1714–9. https://doi.org/10.1002/hep.1840220616.

100. Adams LA, Ratziu V. Non-alcoholic fatty liver—perhaps not so benign. J Hepatol. 2015;62(5):1002–4. https://doi.org/10.1016/j.jhep.2015.02.005.

101. De A, Duseja A. Natural history of simple steatosis or nonalcoholic fatty liver. J Clin Exp Hepatol. 2020;10(3):255–62. https://doi.org/10.1016/j.jceh.2019.09.005.

102. McPherson S, Hardy T, Henderson E, Burt AD, Day CP, Anstee QM. Evidence of NAFLD progression from steatosis to fibrosing-steatohepatitis using paired biopsies: Implications for prognosis and clinical management. J Hepatol. 2015;62(5):1148–55. https://doi.org/10.1016/j.jhep.2014.11.034.

103. Musso G, Gambino R, Cassader M, Pagano G. Meta-analysis: natural history of non-alcoholic fatty liver disease (NAFLD) and diagnostic accuracy of non-invasive tests for liver disease severity. Ann Med. 2011;43(8):617–49. https://doi.org/10.3109/07853890.2010.518623.

104. Paradis V, Zalinski S, Chelbi E, Guedj N, Degos F, Vilgrain V, et al. Hepatocellular carcinomas in patients with metabolic syndrome often develop without significant liver fibrosis: a pathological analysis. Hepatology. 2009;49(3):851–9. https://doi.org/10.1002/hep.22734.

105. Kawada N, Imanaka K, Kawaguchi T, Tamai C, Ishihara R, Matsunaga T, et al. Hepatocellular carcinoma arising from non-cirrhotic nonalcoholic steatohepatitis. J Gastroenterol. 2009;44(12):1190–4. https://doi.org/10.1007/s00535-009-0112-0.

106. Angulo P, Hui JM, Marchesini G, Bugianesi E, George J, Farrell GC, et al. The NAFLD fibrosis score: a noninvasive system that identifies liver fibrosis in patients with NAFLD. Hepatology. 2007;45(4):846–54. https://doi.org/10.1002/hep.21496.

107. Ballestri S, Nascimbeni F, Romagnoli D, Lonardo A. The independent predictors of non-alcoholic steatohepatitis and its individual histological features.: Insulin resistance, serum uric acid, metabolic syndrome, alanine aminotransferase and serum total cholesterol are a clue to pathogenesis and candidate targets for treatment. Hepatol Res. 2016;46(11):1074–87. https://doi.org/10.1111/hepr.12656.

108. Dixon JB, Bhathal PS, O'Brien PE. Nonalcoholic fatty liver disease: predictors of non-alcoholic steatohepatitis and liver fibrosis in the severely obese. Gastroenterology. 2001;121(1):91–100. https://doi.org/10.1053/gast.2001.25540.

109. Carulli L, Canedi I, Rondinella S, Lombardini S, Ganazzi D, Fargion S, et al. Genetic polymorphisms in non-alcoholic fatty liver disease: interleukin-6-174G/C polymorphism is associated with non-alcoholic steatohepatitis. Dig Liver Dis. 2009;41(11):823–8. https://doi.org/10.1016/j.dld.2009.03.005.

110. Petta S, Camma C, Cabibi D, Di Marco V, Craxi A. Hyperuricemia is associated with histological liver damage in patients with non-alcoholic fatty liver disease. Aliment Pharmacol Ther. 2011;34(7):757–66. https://doi.org/10.1111/j.1365-2036.2011.04788.x.

111. Carulli L, Ballestri S, Lonardo A, Lami F, Violi E, Losi L, et al. Is nonalcoholic steatohepatitis associated with a high-though-normal thyroid stimulating hormone level and lower cholesterol levels? Intern Emerg Med. 2013;8(4):297–305. https://doi.org/10.1007/s11739-011-0609-4.

112. Dasarathy J, Periyalwar P, Allampati S, Bhinder V, Hawkins C, Brandt P, et al. Hypovitaminosis D is associated with increased whole body fat mass and greater severity of non-alcoholic fatty liver disease. Liver Int. 2014;34(6):e118–27. https://doi.org/10.1111/liv.12312.

113. Argo CK, Northup PG, Al-Osaimi AM, Caldwell SH. Systematic review of risk factors for fibrosis progression in non-alcoholic steatohepatitis. J Hepatol. 2009;51(2):371–9. https://doi.org/10.1016/j.jhep.2009.03.019.
114. Angulo P, Kleiner DE, Dam-Larsen S, Adams LA, Bjornsson ES, Charatcharoenwitthaya P, et al. Liver fibrosis, but no other histologic features, is associated with long-term outcomes of patients with nonalcoholic fatty liver disease. Gastroenterology. 2015;149(2):389–97.e10. https://doi.org/10.1053/j.gastro.2015.04.043.
115. Ekstedt M, Hagstrom H, Nasr P, Fredrikson M, Stal P, Kechagias S, et al. Fibrosis stage is the strongest predictor for disease-specific mortality in NAFLD after up to 33 years of follow-up. Hepatology. 2015;61(5):1547–54. https://doi.org/10.1002/hep.27368.
116. Portillo-Sanchez P, Bril F, Maximos M, Lomonaco R, Biernacki D, Orsak B, et al. High prevalence of nonalcoholic fatty liver disease in patients with type 2 diabetes mellitus and normal plasma aminotransferase levels. J Clin Endocrinol Metab. 2015;100(6):2231–8. https://doi.org/10.1210/jc.2015-1966.
117. Ratziu V, Cadranel JF, Serfaty L, Denis J, Renou C, Delassalle P, et al. A survey of patterns of practice and perception of NAFLD in a large sample of practicing gastroenterologists in France. J Hepatol. 2012;57(2):376–83. https://doi.org/10.1016/j.jhep.2012.03.019.
118. Younossi ZM, Henry L. Economic and quality-of-life implications of non-alcoholic fatty liver disease. Pharmacoeconomics. 2015;33(12):1245–53. https://doi.org/10.1007/s40273-015-0316-5.
119. McCullough AJ. The clinical features, diagnosis and natural history of nonalcoholic fatty liver disease. Clin Liver Dis. 2004;8(3):521–33., viii. https://doi.org/10.1016/j.cld.2004.04.004.
120. Önnerhag K, Nilsson PM, Lindgren S. Increased risk of cirrhosis and hepatocellular cancer during long-term follow-up of patients with biopsy-proven NAFLD. Scand J Gastroenterol. 2014;49(9):1111–8. https://doi.org/10.3109/00365521.2014.934911.
121. Ekstedt M, Franzen LE, Mathiesen UL, Thorelius L, Holmqvist M, Bodemar G, et al. Long-term follow-up of patients with NAFLD and elevated liver enzymes. Hepatology. 2006;44(4):865–73. https://doi.org/10.1002/hep.21327.
122. Koehler EM, Plompen EP, Schouten JN, Hansen BE, Darwish Murad S, Taimr P, et al. Presence of diabetes mellitus and steatosis is associated with liver stiffness in a general population: the Rotterdam study. Hepatology. 2016;63(1):138–47. https://doi.org/10.1002/hep.27981.
123. You SC, Kim KJ, Kim SU, Kim BK, Park JY, Kim DY, et al. Factors associated with significant liver fibrosis assessed using transient elastography in general population. World J Gastroenterol. 2015;21(4):1158–66. https://doi.org/10.3748/wjg.v21.i4.1158.
124. Roulot D, Czernichow S, Le Clésiau H, Costes JL, Vergnaud AC, Beaugrand M. Liver stiffness values in apparently healthy subjects: influence of gender and metabolic syndrome. J Hepatol. 2008;48(4):606–13. https://doi.org/10.1016/j.jhep.2007.11.020.
125. Hui JM, Kench JG, Chitturi S, Sud A, Farrell GC, Byth K, et al. Long-term outcomes of cirrhosis in nonalcoholic steatohepatitis compared with hepatitis C. Hepatology. 2003;38(2):420–7. https://doi.org/10.1053/jhep.2003.50320.
126. Sanyal AJ, Banas C, Sargeant C, Luketic VA, Sterling RK, Stravitz RT, et al. Similarities and differences in outcomes of cirrhosis due to nonalcoholic steatohepatitis and hepatitis C. Hepatology. 2006;43(4):682–9. https://doi.org/10.1002/hep.21103.
127. Bhala N, Angulo P, van der Poorten D, Lee E, Hui JM, Saracco G, et al. The natural history of nonalcoholic fatty liver disease with advanced fibrosis or cirrhosis: an international collaborative study. Hepatology. 2011;54(4):1208–16. https://doi.org/10.1002/hep.24491.
128. Bugianesi E, Leone N, Vanni E, Marchesini G, Brunello F, Carucci P, et al. Expanding the natural history of nonalcoholic steatohepatitis: from cryptogenic cirrhosis to hepatocellular carcinoma. Gastroenterology. 2002;123(1):134–40. https://doi.org/10.1053/gast.2002.34168.
129. Ong J, Younossi ZM, Reddy V, Price LL, Gramlich T, Mayes J, et al. Cryptogenic cirrhosis and posttransplantation nonalcoholic fatty liver disease. Liver Transpl. 2001;7(9):797–801. https://doi.org/10.1053/jlts.2001.24644.
130. McGlynn KA, Petrick JL, London WT. Global epidemiology of hepatocellular carcinoma: an emphasis on demographic and regional variability. Clin Liver Dis. 2015;19(2):223–38. https://doi.org/10.1016/j.cld.2015.01.001.

131. Baffy G, Brunt EM, Caldwell SH. Hepatocellular carcinoma in non-alcoholic fatty liver disease: an emerging menace. J Hepatol. 2012;56(6):1384–91. https://doi.org/10.1016/j.jhep.2011.10.027.

132. Dyson J, Jaques B, Chattopadyhay D, Lochan R, Graham J, Das D, et al. Hepatocellular cancer: the impact of obesity, type 2 diabetes and a multidisciplinary team. J Hepatol. 2014;60(1):110–7. https://doi.org/10.1016/j.jhep.2013.08.011.

133. Lindenmeyer CC, McCullough AJ. The natural history of nonalcoholic fatty liver disease—an evolving view. Clin Liver Dis. 2018;22(1):11–21. https://doi.org/10.1016/j.cld.2017.08.003.

134. Park EJ, Lee JH, Yu GY, He G, Ali SR, Holzer RG, et al. Dietary and genetic obesity promote liver inflammation and tumorigenesis by enhancing IL-6 and TNF expression. Cell. 2010;140(2):197–208. https://doi.org/10.1016/j.cell.2009.12.052.

135. Zámbó V, Simon-Szabó L, Szelényi P, Kereszturi E, Bánhegyi G, Csala M. Lipotoxicity in the liver. World J Hepatol. 2013;5(10):550–7. https://doi.org/10.4254/wjh.v5.i10.550.

136. Duan XF, Tang P, Li Q, Yu ZT. Obesity, adipokines and hepatocellular carcinoma. Int J Cancer. 2013;133(8):1776–83. https://doi.org/10.1002/ijc.28105.

137. Oliveira CP, Stefano JT. Genetic polymorphisms and oxidative stress in non-alcoholic steatohepatitis (NASH): A mini review. Clin Res Hepatol Gastroenterol. 2015;39(Suppl 1):S35–40. https://doi.org/10.1016/j.clinre.2015.05.014.

138. Henao-Mejia J, Elinav E, Jin C, Hao L, Mehal WZ, Strowig T, et al. Inflammasome-mediated dysbiosis regulates progression of NAFLD and obesity. Nature. 2012;482(7384):179–85. https://doi.org/10.1038/nature10809.

139. Mittal S, Sada YH, El-Serag HB, Kanwal F, Duan Z, Temple S, et al. Temporal trends of nonalcoholic fatty liver disease-related hepatocellular carcinoma in the veteran affairs population. Clin Gastroenterol Hepatol. 2015;13(3):594–601.e1. https://doi.org/10.1016/j.cgh.2014.08.013.

140. Giannini EG, Marabotto E, Savarino V, Trevisani F, di Nolfo MA, Del Poggio P, et al. Hepatocellular carcinoma in patients with cryptogenic cirrhosis. Clin Gastroenterol Hepatol. 2009;7(5):580–5. https://doi.org/10.1016/j.cgh.2009.01.001.

141. Younossi ZM, Otgonsuren M, Henry L, Venkatesan C, Mishra A, Erario M, et al. Association of nonalcoholic fatty liver disease (NAFLD) with hepatocellular carcinoma (HCC) in the United States from 2004 to 2009. Hepatology. 2015;62(6):1723–30. https://doi.org/10.1002/hep.28123.

142. White DL, Kanwal F, El-Serag HB. Association between nonalcoholic fatty liver disease and risk for hepatocellular cancer, based on systematic review. Clin Gastroenterol Hepatol. 2012;10(12):1342–59.e2. https://doi.org/10.1016/j.cgh.2012.10.001.

143. Yatsuji S, Hashimoto E, Tobari M, Taniai M, Tokushige K, Shiratori K. Clinical features and outcomes of cirrhosis due to non-alcoholic steatohepatitis compared with cirrhosis caused by chronic hepatitis C. J Gastroenterol Hepatol. 2009;24(2):248–54. https://doi.org/10.1111/j.1440-1746.2008.05640.x.

144. Thomas JA, Kendall BJ, Dalais C, Macdonald GA, Thrift AP. Hepatocellular and extrahepatic cancers in non-alcoholic fatty liver disease: A systematic review and meta-analysis. Eur J Cancer. 2022;173:250–62. https://doi.org/10.1016/j.ejca.2022.06.051.

145. Kawamura Y, Arase Y, Ikeda K, Seko Y, Imai N, Hosaka T, et al. Large-scale long-term follow-up study of Japanese patients with non-alcoholic fatty liver disease for the onset of hepatocellular carcinoma. Am J Gastroenterol. 2012;107(2):253–61. https://doi.org/10.1038/ajg.2011.327.

146. Ertle J, Dechêne A, Sowa JP, Penndorf V, Herzer K, Kaiser G, et al. Non-alcoholic fatty liver disease progresses to hepatocellular carcinoma in the absence of apparent cirrhosis. Int J Cancer. 2011;128(10):2436–43. https://doi.org/10.1002/ijc.25797.

147. Mishra A, Younossi ZM. Epidemiology and natural history of non-alcoholic fatty liver disease. J Clin Exp Hepatol. 2012;2(2):135–44. https://doi.org/10.1016/S0973-6883(12)60102-9.

148. Bhagat V, Mindikoglu AL, Nudo CG, Schiff ER, Tzakis A, Regev A. Outcomes of liver transplantation in patients with cirrhosis due to nonalcoholic steatohepatitis versus patients

with cirrhosis due to alcoholic liver disease. Liver Transpl. 2009;15(12):1814–20. https://doi.org/10.1002/lt.21927.

149. Yalamanchili K, Saadeh S, Klintmalm GB, Jennings LW, Davis GL. Nonalcoholic fatty liver disease after liver transplantation for cryptogenic cirrhosis or nonalcoholic fatty liver disease. Liver Transpl. 2010;16(4):431–9. https://doi.org/10.1002/lt.22004.

150. Malik SM, deVera ME, Fontes P, Shaikh O, Ahmad J. Outcome after liver transplantation for NASH cirrhosis. Am J Transplant. 2009;9(4):782–93. https://doi.org/10.1111/j.1600-6143.2009.02590.x.

151. Kim WR, Poterucha JJ, Porayko MK, Dickson ER, Steers JL, Wiesner RH. Recurrence of nonalcoholic steatohepatitis following liver transplantation. Transplantation. 1996;62(12):1802–5. https://doi.org/10.1097/00007890-199612270-00021.

152. Malik SM, Devera ME, Fontes P, Shaikh O, Sasatomi E, Ahmad J. Recurrent disease following liver transplantation for nonalcoholic steatohepatitis cirrhosis. Liver Transpl. 2009;15(12):1843–51. https://doi.org/10.1002/lt.21943.

153. Saeed N, Glass L, Sharma P, Shannon C, Sonnenday CJ, Tincopa MA. Incidence and risks for nonalcoholic fatty liver disease and steatohepatitis post-liver transplant: systematic review and meta-analysis. Transplantation. 2019;103(11):e345–e54. https://doi.org/10.1097/tp.0000000000002916.

154. Losurdo G, Castellaneta A, Rendina M, Carparelli S, Leandro G, Di Leo A. Systematic review with meta-analysis: de novo non-alcoholic fatty liver disease in liver-transplanted patients. Aliment Pharmacol Ther. 2018;47(6):704–14. https://doi.org/10.1111/apt.14521.

155. Minich A, Arisar FAQ, N-uS S, Herman L, Azhie A, Orchanian-Cheff A, et al. Predictors of patient survival following liver transplant in non-alcoholic steatohepatitis: a systematic review and meta-analysis. eClinicalMedicine. 2022:50. https://doi.org/10.1016/j.eclinm.2022.101534.

156. Lee Y, Doumouras AG, Yu J, Brar K, Banfield L, Gmora S, et al. Complete resolution of nonalcoholic fatty liver disease after bariatric surgery: a systematic review and meta-analysis. Clin Gastroenterol Hepatol. 2019;17(6):1040–60 e11. https://doi.org/10.1016/j.cgh.2018.10.017.

Hepatocellular Carcinoma in Nonalcoholic Fatty Liver Disease

4

Corina Pop and Sorina Diaconu

4.1 Epidemiology

Nonalcoholic fatty liver disease (NAFLD) is defined as hepatic fat accumulation without any other known causes of liver damage, classified as nonalcoholic fatty liver (simple steatosis) and nonalcoholic steatohepatitis (NASH), which is defined as fatty infiltration associated with necroinflammation. In the USA, NAFLD is present in one-third of the adult population. Over time, the prevalence has increased and has been attributed to the obesity epidemic, increasing with a 21% from 2015 to 2019 [1].

Rafiq et al. observed a higher mortality in those with NAFLD when compared to the general population; the percentage for liver-related deaths was 13% compared to <1% in general population, and 3% of those with NAFLD developed cirrhosis [2].

Primary liver cancer represents the sixth most common cancer and also the third cause of cancer-related death in the entire world, accounting 80% of all primary liver cancers [3].

Liver cancer encompasses a multistep process of chronic inflammation → fibrosis → cirrhosis → and hepatocellular carcinoma (HCC). The most important risk factor for HC is cirrhosis; however, 12% of patients progress in the absence of cirrhosis [3] (Fig. 4.1). An important percentage of people with NASH presents, during the entire life, an evolution to fibrosis (34–42%), and to cirrhosis also.

NAFLD is the fastest growing cause of cirrhosis and HCC in the USA [4].

Patients with NASH are more likely to develop an advanced progressive liver disease. There are a lot of studies which demonstrated that the rates of cirrhosis in patients with NASH are increased compared to those with fatty liver without NASH (25% compared with 3%). For these people, the risk of liver disease-related death is increased (11% versus 2%) [2].

C. Pop (✉) · S. Diaconu
University of Medicine and Pharmacy Carol Davila Bucharest, Bucharest, Romania

© The Author(s), under exclusive license to Springer Nature Switzerland AG 2023

A. Trifan et al. (eds.), *Essentials of Non-Alcoholic Fatty Liver Disease*,
https://doi.org/10.1007/978-3-031-33548-8_4

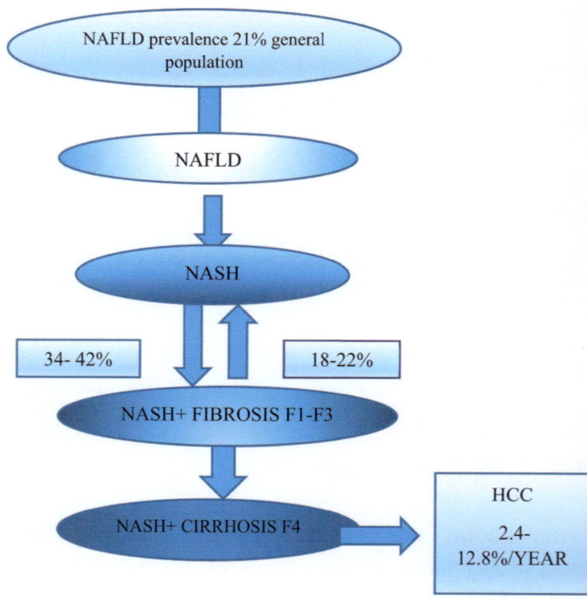

Fig. 4.1 The sequential pathophysiological states of NAFLD → HCC [7]

A meta-analysis of 19 studies published in August 2022 which included 168,517 participants determined that nonalcoholic steatohepatitis (NASH) was the most common cause of non-cirrhotic HCC patients [3].

A study published in 2019 in the USA showed a 2.6% yearly cumulative incidence of HCC and 4% in cirrhosis in NAFLD patients [5]. Diabetes and obesity were two independent risk factors for HCC, and that association with NAFLD increased the risk for HCC.

Another study published in Germany established that NAFLD is the most common etiology of HCC (24%), followed by chronic hepatitis C (23.3%), chronic hepatitis B (19.3%), and alcoholic liver disease (12.7%) [5].

The incidence of HCC has increased in the USA during the past 25 years due to increase in HCV infection, increase in immigrants from HBV-endemic countries, and, the most important, increase in nonalcoholic liver disease [5].

Over the course of 20 years between 1995–1999 and 2010–2014, the prevalence of NASH-associated HCC increased from 2.6% to 19.5%. NASH is the second most common indication for liver transplantation in the USA after chronic C hepatitis [3, 6].

The development of HCC on a NASH background was described for the first time in literature in 1990 by Powell and colleagues when they reported a 5-year follow-up study of 42 patients with NASH. In another study from the USA, the yearly cumulative incidence of HCC was 2.6% in patients with NASH-associated cirrhosis compared with 4% in HCV-related cirrhosis [7]. However, retrospective Korean study including 25,947 individuals, monitoring an average period of 7.5 years, reported a higher incidence of HCC in patients with NAFLD (23.1 versus 0.9 per 100,000 subjects) [7]. In Japanese patients, the annual cumulative incidence rate of hepatocarcinoma was 0.043%—similar to that reported in the USA [7]. In

Europe, in countries with a high incidence of HCV-associated HCC, the contribution of NAFLD-associated HCC has been less noticeable, and in countries where the prevalence of viral hepatitis is low, a dramatic increase in incidence has been noted for NAFLD-associated HCC [7].

4.2   Mortality in NAFLD/NASH

Long-term outcomes in NAFLD have been evaluated in different studies, and it has been concluded that type 2 diabetes mellitus has increased the risk of liver-related mortality.

A study conducted in Minnesota showed that patients with nonalcoholic liver disease had a 30% increase in mortality compared to the general population. The main cause of death was due to cardiovascular disease, and the second one was due to liver morbidity—cirrhosis and HCC. Liver-related morbidity and mortality were associated with histologically advanced fibrosis [1].

In a recent meta-analysis, Younossi et al. reported that in NASH patients the annual HCC incident rate was 5.29/1000 individuals, and in NAFLD patients, it was 0.44/1000 individuals and the mortality incidence rates were 15.44/1000 person-years versus 0.77/100 person-years [2].

However, cardiovascular events remain the main cause of death in patients with NAFLD/NASH [2].

4.3   Association Between NAFLD and HCC

4.3.1   Genetic Factor

The presence of NAFLD and also the risk of disease progression to advanced fibrosis are related to the single nucleotide polymorphisms (SNPs). The genes encoding patting-like phospholipase domain-containing 3 (PNPLA3) and transmembrane 6 superfamily member 2 (TM6SF2) have been associated with the severity of steatosis, NASH, and fibrosis. Patients who present the PNPLA3 have an important risk of steatohepatitis and fibrosis and also have a more than threefold increased risk of liver cancer [7].

Uncertain data remain about the patients carrying the TM6SF2 polymorphism as an independent risk factor for HCC.

In 2017, a variant in the gene MBOAT1 has also been associated with HCC from a non-cirrhotic UK-Italian study [7].

4.3.2   Environmental Factors

The most important environmental factors associated with NAFLD include alcohol, dietary habits, physical activity, and socio-economic factors.

Several studies suggest that patients with NAFLD adopt unhealthy eating habits such as a high intake of carbohydrates (fructose), high amounts of processed food, sugary sweetened beverages, and high-salt diets and also have a sedentary lifestyle [7].

4.4 Pathogenesis of HCC

Cirrhosis is the precursor lesion and the most important risk factor for HCC, but 20–30% of cases occur in the absence of cirrhosis. The progression from NAFLD to HCC is a continuous process, involving various factors: insulin resistance, lipid accumulation, liver immune microenvironment, and oxidative stress. These determine continuous proliferation and expansion of preneoplastic cells. There are several experimental models for identifying the transition from NAFLD to HCC; in 2022, an isogenic B6/129 hybrid strain of genetically modified mice was described as a new animal NASH-associated HCC preclinical model in this transition of disease [3].

The most important trigger factors for chronic inflammation are represented by insulin resistance, infiltration of proinflammatory cells, and lipotoxicity.

4.4.1 Metabolic Dysregulation

4.4.1.1 Lipid Metabolism and Insulin Resistance

The most important factor toward NASH-derived cancer is represented by a dysregulation of the hepatic lipid metabolism, with triglycerides being the predominant lipid accumulation in NASH. In normal metabolism, the liver is involved in oxidation or exporting of the lipids as very-low-density lipoproteins (VLDLs) and also storage fat by shunting excess lipids for the synthesis of triglycerides. The adipose tissue could produce cytokines, which prevent the absorption of fatty acids and promote the adipose depots to release them. In response, the delivery of fatty acids and triglyceride formation is increased [3].

Insulin resistance suppresses the inhibitory effect of insulin on adipose tissue lipolysis, increases the flux of free fatty acids (FFAs) to the liver, and causes overproduction of VLDLs. It also determines the liver to be overloaded by glucose and insulin. The high values of these promote hepatic de novo lipogenesis by inducing the sterol regulatory element-binding protein 1c (SREBP-1c) and the carbohydrate response element-binding protein (Ch REBP).

The lipid-overloaded liver initiates adaptative changes in free fatty acid metabolism, which increase the secretion of monocyte chemoattractant protein-1 (MCP-1) into circulation and determine the activation of macrophages and release of proinflammatory cytokines (TNF-α, IL-6). TNF-α could promote lipolysis and downregulates triglyceride biosynthesis and triglyceride storage in adipose tissue, which causes more damage to hepatocytes [3].

4.4.1.2 Reactive Oxygen Species (ROS) and Free Fatty Acids (FFAs)

Increase of FFAs (lysophosphatidylcholine, cholesterol, ceramides, palmitic acid) and also lipid accumulation in hepatocytes determine mitochondrial damage and increase the production of mitochondrial reactive oxygen species. The overproduction of these is followed by lipid peroxidation and oxidative damage to mitochondrial DNA, leading to a reduced capacity for mitochondria to oxidize fatty acids. Increasing FFAs and lipid accumulation establish a vicious cycle, which exacerbates oxidative stress and mitochondrial dysfunction [3].

4.4.1.3 Unfolded Protein Response (UPR) and Endoplasmic Reticulum (ER) Stress

Lipid accumulation in hepatocytes and oxidative stress could trigger endoplasmic reticulum stress and activate the unfolded protein response, which fails to restore ER homeostasis and promotes apoptosis [3].

4.4.2 Alteration of the Liver Immune Microenvironment

The immune microenvironment is represented by various immune cells, including dendritic cells (DCs), natural killer (NK) cells, Kupffer cells (KCs), and T and B lymphocytes. The NASH pathogenesis (insulin resistance, reactive oxygen species, endoplasmic reticulum stress, lipid accumulation) induces alteration of the immune microenvironment that causes chronic inflammation and fibrosis [3].

4.4.2.1 Kupffer Cells (KCs)

These cells are resident macrophages in the liver, representing the first line of host defense against invading microorganisms and particles. When a liver injury appears, KCs precede other immune cells by producing cytokines and chemokines, which recruit and instruct other immune cells.

In NASH, metabolic dysregulation leads to liver injury and determines damage to the intestinal barrier. In the early stage of liver injury, Kupffer cells are pushed toward an M1-like proinflammatory phenotype, followed by the change in polarization and wound healing. Once the disease is advanced, dysregulated inflammation and tissue repair response appear, followed by fibrillar connective tissue formation (causing fibrosis and tumorigenic properties) [3].

4.4.2.2 Natural Killer (NK) Cells and Hepatic Stellate Cells (HSCs)

The activation of hepatic stellate cells leads to the formation of a fibrogenic extracellular matrix and fibrosis. Activated NK cells are able to kill hepatic stellate cells (newly activated and senescent), protecting the liver from an excessive fibrogenic response [3].

A cycle of hepatocyte death and hepatic stellate cell proliferation represented the trigger for aberrant proliferation and hepatocytic transformation [3].

4.4.2.3 CD4+ T Cells and Regulatory T (T Reg) Cells

T cells play an important role in the development and progression of NASH (CD4+ helper T and CD8+ cytotoxic). In studies, high levels of fructose diet failed to induce hepatic inflammation and steatosis in T cell-deficient mice. Ma et al. reported that NASH induced a selective loss of intrahepatic CD4+ T cells and accelerated tumor development [7].

Hepatic Treg cells inhibit the immune response and maintain immune homeostasis. In NASH, the number of Treg cells is decreased due to reactive oxygen species-induced apoptosis.

Dysregulation of lipid metabolism produces a selective loss of intrahepatic CD4+ T cells and also an activation of cellular oncogene c-Fos signaling [3].

4.4.2.4 Dendritic Cells (DCs)

Dendritic cells are key antigen-presenting cells that play a role in bridging innate and adaptive immunity. These cells have a dual effect in NASH (produce cytokines that determine adaptive immune response and activation of hepatic stellate cells and increase the secretion of the anti-inflammatory cytokines) that needs to be further studied [3].

4.4.2.5 Natural Killer (NK) Cells and CD8+ T Cells

In NASH, type I NK cells secrete proinflammatory cytokines (INF γ, IL-4, and osteopontin that play an important role in hepatic stellate cell activation and fibrosis) and chemokines (IFN-γ and IL-4 that induce the infiltration of CD8+ T and facilitate NASH to HCC transition) [7]. Also, type I NK cells could cause hepatic cell death [3].

4.4.2.6 B Cells

In NASH, adipocytes secrete B cell-activating factor (BAFF) that promotes B cell maturation, development, and production of proinflammatory cytokines and mediates the activation of T cells, hepatic stellate cells, and Kupffer cells [3].

The increase in the level of immunoglobulin A produced by B cells determines the progression of NASH, favoring the inflammation-to-cancer transition [3].

4.4.2.7 Neutrophils

Infiltration of neutrophils is the most important characteristic of NASH. A lot of studies demonstrated that mice deficient in neutrophils or neutrophil effector molecules were protected from diet-induced nonalcoholic steatohepatitis [3].

HCC in Non-cirrhotic NAFLD/NASH

A significant proportion of patients with NAFLD-associated HCC do not have cirrhosis. The estimated data shows that half of the cases of NASH-induced HCC occur in non-cirrhotic patients [8].

In a study of Kawada et al., they suggested that the presence of cirrhosis in NASH-associated HCC was lower than in HCV-associated HCC. Paradis et al. reported a significant number of patients with NASH who developed liver cancer in the absence of fibrosis compared with other underlying chronic liver diseases [2].

A small number of published reports have suggested that the hepatocellular adenoma, in the presence of metabolic syndrome, may suffer a malignant transformation [2].

HCC can appear associated with metabolic syndrome and NAFLD in the absence of NASH and fibrosis [5].

HCC in Cirrhotic NAFLD/NASH

Cirrhosis is an important risk factor for HCC. An important number of studies published in the last 5 years showed that 60% of HCC-associated NAFLD/NASH had cirrhosis before or at the time of diagnosis [2].

The true prevalence of NASH-related HCC is likely underestimated. The prevalence of NAFLD/NASH-associated HCC is not well defined; the increasing incidence of diabetes and obesity determines the increase of NAFLD/NASH-associated HCC [2].

Some factors are associated with a higher risk of severe/fibrosis cirrhosis and HCC occurrence: the presence of diabetes mellitus, older age, and concurrent alcohol intake all increase the risk of liver cancer [8].

4.5   Diagnosis

The tests used for diagnosis include radiologic studies and pathologic diagnosis through biopsy.

Given the specificity of contrast enhancement for typical lesion (in the presence of cirrhosis), current guidelines (AASLD and EASL) advocate for the use of imaging rather than pathologic diagnosis [7].

When cirrhosis has not been previously diagnosed and NAFLD-associated HCC has been suspected, it is more likely to confirm the diagnosis using biopsy [7].

The EASL criteria establish the following:

1. The diagnosis of HCC in cirrhotic patients should be based on noninvasive criteria and/or pathology (evidence high, recommendation strong).
2. The diagnosis of HCC in non-cirrhotic patients should be confirmed by pathology (evidence moderate, recommendation strong).
3. The pathological diagnosis of HCC should be established on the International Consensus recommendations (evidence high, recommendation strong).
4. Noninvasive criteria (applied to cirrhotic patients for nodule(s) ≥ 1 cm) are based on imaging techniques using multiphasic CT, dynamic contrast-enhanced MRI (evidence high, recommendation strong), or contrast-enhanced ultrasonography (CEUS) (evidence moderate, recommendation weak).
5. Diagnosis is based on the identification of the typical hallmarks of HCC, which differ according to imaging techniques or contrast agents (arterial phase hyperenhancement with washout in the portal venous or delayed phases on computed

tomography (CT) and magnetic resonance imaging (MRI) using extracellular contrast agents or gadobenate dimeglumine, arterial phase hyperenhancement with washout in the portal venous phase on MRI using gadoxetic acid, arterial phase hyperenhancement with late-onset (>60 s) washout of mild intensity on CEUS).

6. Because of their higher sensitivity, CT or MRI should be used first (evidence high, recommendation strong).
7. Positron-emission tomography (PET) scan is not used for early diagnosis because of the high rate of false-negative results (evidence low, recommendation strong) [8].

Due to delay in diagnosis, obese patients may be at an advanced stage, with a poor prognosis of the disease [9].

4.6　Surveillance

The decision to enter into a surveillance program is determined by the level of risk for HCC, age of the patient, functional status, health, and also ability to comply with surveillance program [10].

The ideal interval of surveillance for HCC should be dictated by two main features: rate of tumor growth and tumor incidence in the population.

Based on the available knowledge regarding HCC volume doubling time, guidelines established a 6-month interval for surveillance; a shorter interval of 3 months does not have any clinical benefit, and a longer interval of 12 months is not cost-effective and is associated with fewer early-stage HCC diagnosed [8].

The EASL and AASLD recommended screening for HCC in all patients with NASH-related cirrhosis every 6–12 months using abdominal ultrasonography [2]. According to AASLD guidelines, surveillance benefit is uncertain in the cases of NAFLD without cirrhosis [10]. Also, EASL sustained that the incidence of HCC in these non-advanced patients is expected to be insufficiently high to deserve universal surveillance (Table 4.1) [8].

The sensitivity of ultrasonography is operator dependent and more challenging in overweight patients when cross-sectional imaging with MRI might be appropriate. In this case, the benefit of long-term MRI surveillance is debatable [2].

In a cohort study of 941 patients, three- to eightfold is the higher risk for obese patients to have an inadequate surveillance examination. The delaying in detection determined an advanced stage at diagnosis [9].

Table 4.1 Categories of patients in whom surveillance is recommended [8]

Cirrhotic Child-Pugh A and B	Evidence low, recommendation strong
Cirrhotic Child-Pugh C awaiting liver transplantation	Evidence low, recommendation strong
Non-cirrhotic F3 based on an individual risk assessment	Evidence low, recommendation weak

The patients with metabolic syndrome or NASH who have severe fibrosis or cirrhosis either by histology or by elastography diagnosed should undergo surveillance, whereas the risk of HCC development is insufficiently established in individuals without severe fibrosis/cirrhosis [8].

In patients with high risk of developing HCC, nodule(s) less than 1 cm in diameter detected by ultrasonography should be followed at ≤4-month intervals in the first year. If there is no increase in the size or number, surveillance could be returned to the 6-month interval.

In cirrhotic patients, diagnosis of HCC for nodules of ≥1 cm in diameter can be confirmed with noninvasive criteria and/or biopsy.

In cases of inconclusive histological or discordant findings and in cases of growth or changes in enhancement pattern, repeated biopsy sampling is recommended [8].

4.7 Staging and Treatment

According to EASL guidelines, staging systems in HCC should include tumor burden, performance status, and liver function [8].

The algorithm used by the AASLD and EASL is Barcelona Clinic for Liver Cancer (BCLC) staging system that is recommended for prognostic prediction and treatment selection (Fig. 4.2) [8].

The performance status test (PST) represents a score that estimates the patient's capacity to perform certain activities without the help of others and is an important factor in cancer care:

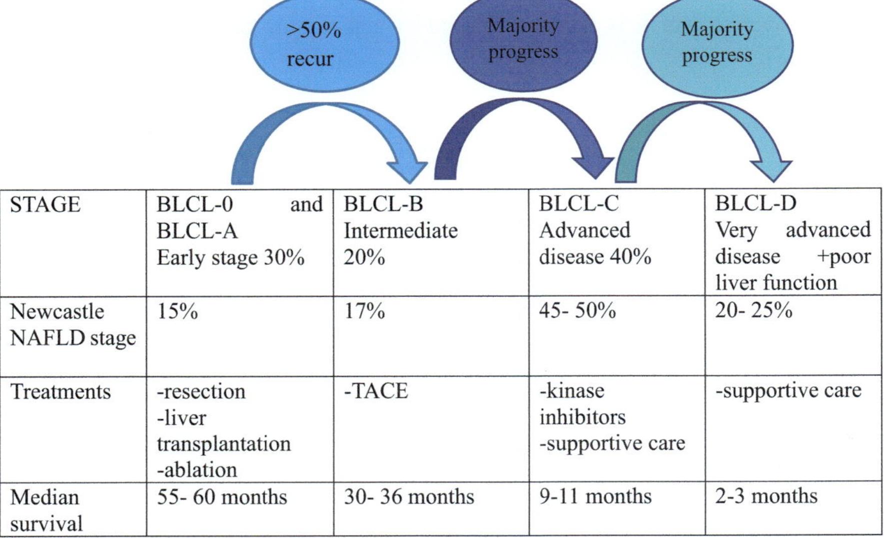

STAGE	BLCL-0 and BLCL-A Early stage 30%	BLCL-B Intermediate 20%	BLCL-C Advanced disease 40%	BLCL-D Very advanced disease +poor liver function
Newcastle NAFLD stage	15%	17%	45- 50%	20- 25%
Treatments	-resection -liver transplantation -ablation	-TACE	-kinase inhibitors -supportive care	-supportive care
Median survival	55- 60 months	30- 36 months	9-11 months	2-3 months

Fig. 4.2 Staging and treatment options for patients with HCC

PST 0: Normal functional activity, without symptoms
PST 1: Minor impairment of normal activity
PST 2: Ambulatory >50% of time, occasional assistance
PST 3: Ambulatory ≤50% of time, nursing care needed
PST 4: Bedridden

However, the BCLC algorithm is less useful for patients with NAFLD-associated cancer because a high number of patients are classified in stage BCLC-C or BCLC-D [7]. Treatment options are illustrated in Table 4.2.

Patients included in early-stage BCLC-0 or BCLC-A had a preserved liver function, a single tumor smaller than 5 cm or three tumors each smaller than 3 cm, and a normal functional activity (performance status test 0). For NAFLD-associated HCC, the detection of an early-stage cancer is rare, and even if tumors are small, advanced age and comorbidities are associated with limited curative procedures [7].

Patients in intermediate stage have multifocal tumors without large-vessel invasion, with PST-0 and preserved liver function. The treatment of these patients is transarterial chemoembolization (TACE)—first-line palliative arterial therapy [7].

An important part of the patients with NAFLD-associated HCC are classified into BCLC-C based on performance status with a major impact of survival. These patients have chronic comorbidities and are often old, with a PST more than 1, so that the effect on survival is less certain, not because of cancer, but because of comorbidities. For a single small growing tumor, when we do not use medical treatment, using TACE is an alternative to supportive care [7].

For patients classified as BCLC-D, the treatment is represented only by supportive care. For this reason, detecting patients at earlier stage represents a major challenge for NAFLD-associated HCC [7].

For all patients with HCC, the treatment should be discussed in multidisciplinary teams to decide which is the first line and when to stop one treatment and start another [8].

Table 4.2 Treatment options for HCC [5]

Surgery	– Partial hepatectomy
	– Liver transplantation
Local ablative therapies	– Cryosurgery
	– Microwave ablation
	– Ethanol, acetic acid injection
	– Radiofrequency ablation
	– Stereotactic body radiation therapy (SBRT)
Regional therapies	– Transarterial radioembolization (TARE)
	– Transarterial chemotherapy
	– Transarterial embolization
	– Transarterial chemoembolization (TACE)
	– Transarterial yttrium-90 microspheres
	– Transarterial I-131-lipiodol
Systemic therapies	– Chemotherapy
	– Immunotherapy
	– Hormonal therapy
Supportive care	

The most important risk factors for NAFLD are represented by obesity, metabolic syndrome, chronic inflammation, and insulin resistance, which are also risk factors for liver cancer. Prevention and control strategies must be developed against these factors [3].

4.7.1 Lifestyle Change

The lifestyle change is the first step in the management of NAFLD for reducing the cardiovascular risk and also for the prevention of progression to fibrosis, cirrhosis, and liver cancer. Weight loss through diet and exercise remains the only evidence-based means of delaying the transition from NAFLD to HCC [3].

In patients with NAFLD and HCC, diet represents a part of standard supportive care, maintaining a well-balanced diet to combat malnutrition and weight loss [7].

There are a lot of treatment options for HCC, which can be divided into curative and noncurative treatment. Curative treatment is represented by surgical resection and orthotopic liver transplant. For small tumors, ablation and radiotherapy may also be curative, improving survival [10].

4.7.2 Surgical Treatment

Liver resection is an important option for the non-cirrhotic patient because they generally have normal liver function with acceptable morbidity and low mortality.

In cases of NAFLD-associated HCC in cirrhotic patients, the degree of hepatic dysfunction and portal hypertension is important for the prognosis and the indication for surgical treatment.

For cirrhotic and non-cirrhotic patients, for surgical treatment, the comorbidities are very important [5].

4.7.3 Allogenic Liver Transplantation

Mazzaferro et al. have defined Milan criteria as a single tumor <5 cm or ≤3 tumors all individually <3 cm with a very favorable outcome, including a 4-year survival rate of 85% [5]. It is the ideal therapy in cirrhotic NAFLD patients because it treats both the underlying parenchymal disease and the liver cancer [5].

4.7.4 Adjuvant and Neoadjuvant Therapy

4.7.4.1 Adjuvant Therapy

Sorafenib used like adjuvant therapy was studied in STORM trial versus placebo after surgery, percutaneous alcohol injection, and radiofrequency ablation. Unfortunately, there was no difference in recurrence-free survival [5].

4.7.4.2 Neoadjuvant Therapy

Two randomized controlled trials which studied preoperative transarterial chemotherapy showed, unfortunately, no survival advantage. Both therapies do not have an important role in NAFL-associated HCC [5].

4.7.5 Ablative Therapy for Localized Tumor

(a) **Chemical ablation**

This technique consists of destroying tumor tissue, frequently used in developing countries, but requires a great number of applications. It has been replaced by thermal ablation.

(b) **Radiofrequency ablation**

This technique is currently the most used ablative technique for the treatment of small tumor, introducing an electrode into the tumor.

(c) **Microwave ablation**

The microwave ablation uses electromagnetic waves to obtain heating; for large tumors, two applicators are needed [5].

4.7.6 Embolic Therapies for Regional Disease

The most commonly used treatments for multifocal liver-predominant disease are represented by transcatheter ablative methods: transarterial chemoembolization (TACE), radioembolization (RAE), and bland hepatic artery embolization.

The chemotherapeutic agents used are doxorubicin, mitomycin C, and aclarubicin [5].

4.7.7 Radiation Therapy (RT) as Local Ablation

Radiation therapy is used when tumors are larger than 3 cm or are located near the diaphragm, gallbladder, or large vessel (not to be treated by radiofrequency ablation) [5].

4.7.8 External Beam Radiotherapy

(a) Fractionated treatment

This technique is used to treat residual disease (after TACE and RT) and to treat tumor thrombus in the portal vein. A study from Taiwan reports a 25% response rate [5].

(b) Stereotactic body radiotherapy (SBRT)

It is a new method of delivering high-precision, high-dose therapy, and the biologic effect is better than other radiation methods [5].

4.7.9 Systemic Therapy

Several drugs are involved in carcinogenic pathways in NASH-associated HCC, suggesting the possibility to be used in prevention strategies: metformin, aspirin, statins, and pioglitazone. But several serious side effects limit their use for long-term prevention, and also international guidelines do not recommend them for NASH-derived HCC (large, randomized, controlled trials are necessary) [3].

4.7.9.1 First-Line Single-Agent Therapies

Systemic chemotherapies did not prove to offer an important increase in survival.

Sorafenib represents a multityrosine kinase inhibitor, which is used in a great number of studies. The survival benefit of sorafenib was independent of the stage of the disease or the performance status.

A lot of receptor tyrosine kinase inhibitors were studied (sunitinib, lenvatinib, brivanib, linifanib), but overall survival was not superior to sorafenib therapy [5].

4.7.9.2 First-Line Combination Therapies

Bevacizumab and erlotinib offer a favorable patient outcome with a median survival of 13.7 months. Oxaliplatin and gemcitabine have proven efficacy in liver cancer and are used with sorafenib in different studies promising encouraging results [5].

4.7.9.3 Second-Line Therapies

Regorafenib, a multityrosine kinase inhibitor, is approved for patients failing sorafenib. There are a lot of drugs used in different studies (tivantinib, cabozantinib, ramucirumab) for second-line treatment [5].

4.7.9.4 Immunotherapy

An important number of drugs have been studied in the treatment of HCC with encouraging results: nivolumab, pembrolizumab, tremelimumab, and durvalumab [5].

For patients with advanced disease (the most part of NAFLD-associated HCC), the treatment with sorafenib had a shorter duration, because studies reported higher rates of hepatic decompensation [5].

4.8 Conclusions

Actually, NAFLD represents the leading cause of chronic liver disease in Europe and also in the USA. Understanding the mechanism of NAFLD-associated HCC is an important step in the management of the disease. Alternative screening modalities may be established for NAFLD patients to increase an accurate diagnosis and early detection of HCC for a better prognosis.

References

1. Libman H, Jiang ZG, Tapper EB, Reynolds E. How would you manage this patient with non-alcoholic fatty liver disease? Ann Intern Med. 2019;171:199–207.
2. Cholankeril G, Patel R, Khurana S, Sarapathy SK. Hepatocellular carcinoma in non-alcoholic steatohepatitis: current knowledge and implications for management. World J Hepatol. 2017;9(11):533–43.
3. Yu S, Wang J, Zheng H, Wang R, Johnson N, Li T, Li P, Lin J, Yan J, Zhang Y, Ding X. Pathogenesis from inflammation to cancer in NASH-derived HCC. J Hepatocellul Carcinoma. 2022;9:855–67.
4. Kanwal F, Kramer JR, Mapakshi S, Natarajan Y, Chayanupatkul M, Richardson PA, Li L, Desiderio R, Thrift AP, Asch SM, Chu J, El-Serag HB. Risk of hepatocellular cancer in patients with non-alcoholic fatty liver disease. Gastroenterology. 2018;155(6):1828–37.
5. DeVita VT, Lawrence TS, Rosenberg SA. Cancer principles and practice of oncology. 11th ed. pp. 837–861; 2019.
6. Younossi Z, Anstee QM, Marietti M, Hardy T, Henry L, Eslam M, George J, Bugianesi E. Global burden of NAFLD and NASH: trends, predictions, risk factors and prevention. Gastroenterol Hepatol. 2018;15:11–20.
7. Anstee QM, Reeves HL, Kotsiliti E, Govaere O, Heikenwalder M. From NASH to HCC: current concepts and future challenges. Gastroenterol Hepatol. 2019;16:411–27.
8. EASL Clinical Practice Guidelines. Management of hepatocellular carcinoma. J Hepatol. 2018;69:182–235.
9. Gupta A, Das A, Majumder K, Arora N, Mayo HG, Singh PP, Beg MS, Singh S. Obesity is independently associated with increased risk of hepatocellular cancer-related mortality: a systematic review and meta-analysis. Am J Clin Oncol. 2018;41:874–81.
10. Marrero JA, Kulik LM, Sirlin CB, Zhu AX, Finn RS, Abecassis MM, Roberts LR, Heimbach JK. Diagnosis, staging and management of hepatocellular carcinoma: 2018 practice guidance by the American Association for the Study of Liver Disease. Hepatology. 68:724–50.

Genetics and Epigenetics in Nonalcoholic Fatty Liver Disease

5

Andra-Iulia Suceveanu, Sergiu-Ioan Micu,
Anca Pantea Stoian, Laura Mazilu, Viorel Gherghina,
Irinel Raluca Parepa, and Adrian-Paul Suceveanu

5.1 Introduction

Although it is a known pathology, described and studied for more than 200 years, nonalcoholic fatty liver disease (NAFLD) remains a complex entity to treat and establish a prognosis.

The marked increase in the prevalence of risk factors among the general population, associated with the asymptomatic nature of this disease, makes NAFLD, for some people, a "silent killer."

NAFLD is an umbrella term for a range of liver conditions. As the name implies, the common feature is excess fat stored in the liver cells. From here, the spectrum can evolve. In some patients, inflammation, necrosis, and fibrosis can be present, or they can be limited only to the fatty loading of the hepatocytes.

The interesting element in the pathogenesis of this disease, which has intrigued clinicians over the years, is its selective character: Why do only some of the patients end up with liver cirrhosis or liver cancer?

A.-I. Suceveanu (✉) · S.-I. Micu · A.-P. Suceveanu
Internal Medicine—Gastroenterology Department, "Ovidius" University, Faculty of
Medicine, Constanta, Romania

A. P. Stoian
Diabetes, Nutrition and Metabolic Diseases Department, "Carol Davila" University of
Medicine and Pharmacy, Bucharest, Romania

L. Mazilu
Oncology Department, Faculty of Medicine, "Ovidius" University, Constanta, Romania

V. Gherghina
Intensive Care Department, Faculty of Medicine, "Ovidius" University, Constanta, Romania

I. R. Parepa
Internal Medicine—Cardiology Department, Faculty of Medicine, "Ovidius" University,
Constanta, Romania

© The Author(s), under exclusive license to Springer Nature
Switzerland AG 2023
A. Trifan et al. (eds.), *Essentials of Non-Alcoholic Fatty Liver Disease*,
https://doi.org/10.1007/978-3-031-33548-8_5

The transition from simple steatosis to fibrosis and cirrhosis is gradual and potentially reversible. This pathogenesis is based on the complex interaction of metabolic, hormonal, nutritional, and genetic factors, with the latter playing a critical role (Fig. 5.1).

A more intensive study of genetic and epigenetic factors can lead to the improvement in the identification of patients at risk as well as the development of new therapeutic tools in the management of this disease.

5.2 Genetic Implications in NAFLD

Even if environmental factors represent an essential link in the etiopathogenesis of NAFLD, the prevalence of the disease varies markedly in various populations, with the highest being in Western countries and Europe, where it reaches 20–30% [1]. The disease spectrum varies from simple fatty loading of hepatocytes to cirrhosis and liver cancer (Fig. 5.1). These inter-individual and inter-ethnic differences and difference in the severity and progression of liver disease among patients with

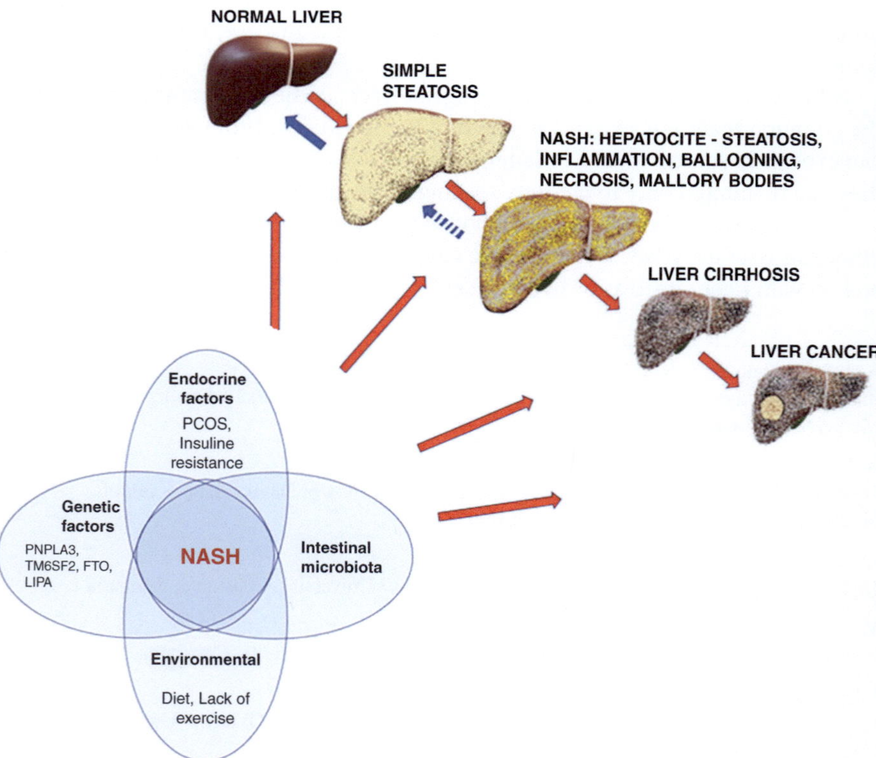

Fig. 5.1 NAFLD spectrum and influencing factors (*created with Paint and Paint 3D softs*)

NAFLD suggest the involvement of factors other than environmental ones in its etiopathogenesis.

The "inherited" side of NAFLD was considered when several studies observed that members of the same family, especially first-degree relatives, presented features suggestive of NAFLD, even liver cirrhosis [2, 3]. Studies conducted on monozygotic and dizygotic twins related to the correlation between serum alanine aminotransferase (ALT) level and liver fat content showed that in approximately 60% of patients, ALT levels were heritable. Also, higher serum ALT levels were found to be more frequent in monozygotic twins versus dizygotic twins. Other studies showed a much higher prevalence of liver fibrosis among monozygotic twins diagnosed with NAFLD. In contrast, researchers revealed a high rate of progression to fibrosis and cirrhosis among first-degree relatives of patients diagnosed with NAFLD-associated cirrhosis, emphasizing the importance of genetic factors, not only in the etiology but also in the progression of this disease [4–6]. Finally, genome-wide association studies have discovered many genes involved in the occurrence and progression of NAFLD. These gene disturbances affect several lipid and carbohydrate metabolism pathways, which ultimately lead, through different mechanisms, to the excess accumulation of triglycerides at the level of the hepatocyte, inflammation, necrosis, and fibrosis (Table 5.1).

5.2.1 Patatin-Like Phospholipase Domain-Containing 3 (PNPLA3) Gene

The polymorphism of the PNPLA3 gene has been the most studied and is considered one of NAFLD's most critical genetic traits. The association between NAFLD and PNPLA3 was described for the first time in 2008 following a genome-wide association study (GWAS) made on individuals with Hispanic, African, American, and European origin. Alterations in PNPLA3 gene are involved in the process of steatosis, inflammation, liver fibrosis, and development of hepatocarcinoma [7].

Table 5.1 Summary of genes and their mutations/variants involved in NAFLD

Gene	Mutation/variant
PNPLA3 gene	Cytosine-to-guanine nucleotide transversion mutation at codon 148, giving rise to the I148M variant
TM6SF2 gene	TM6SF2 E167K variant
HSD17B13 gene	rs72613567 TA, rs6834314 G, rs143404524 variants
LIPA gene	G-to-A transition at position 1 of the exon 8 splice donor (E8SJM, exon 8 splice junction mutation)
MTTP gene	MTTP-493G>T (rs1800591) variant
TNF-α gene	Polymorphisms at position −238
IL-6 gene	174C variant
IRS-1 gene	Substitution glycine-arginine at codon 972

Being located on chromosome 22 (22q13.31), PNPLA3 is known in the literature under several names, including *adiponutrin (ADPN), calcium-independent phospholipase A2-epsilon (IPLA2epsilon),* and *chromosome 22 open reading frame 20 (C22orf20)* and is mainly expressed in the liver and moderately in the adipose tissue, brain, kidney, and skin [8].

Normally, PNPLA3 is mostly bound to lipid droplets and exhibits lipase activity on triglycerides, phospholipids, and retinyl esters, mediating the hydrolytic production of oleate and other unsaturated fatty acids, including arachidonic acid [9]. What ensures susceptibility to the disease is a mutation of this gene, namely a cytosine-to-guanine nucleotide transversion mutation at codon 148, giving rise to the I148M variant [10].

The mutant PNPLA3 I148M impairs, through complex mechanisms, lipid droplet hydrolysis, which will lead to their excessive accumulation at the hepatocyte level. Also, the turnover of this variant is much lower than the normal one, causing excess protein accumulation on lipid droplets' surface [11, 12].

The role of the mutant variant is not limited to the accumulation of lipids on hepatocytes (simple steatosis) but also to the appearance of inflammation and fibrosis. PNPLA3 is also found in Ito stellate liver cells, having an essential role in the metabolism of retinol—a component of these cells. The mutant variant alters the metabolism of retinol. It causes the proliferation and activation of stellate cells, their transformation into myofibroblasts, the synthesis of collagen fibers, and the release of proinflammatory cytokines, leading to inflammation and fibrosis [13, 14].

The presence of the I148M variant is also associated with an increased risk of hepatocarcinoma, this being highlighted by several studies, among which we mention the one carried out by Burza et al., which compared two groups of patients who underwent treatment for obesity (conventional vs. bariatric surgery) [15].

Multiple studies support the hypothesis that the mutant PNPLA3 gene (variant I148M) represents one of NAFLD's most critical genetic traits. It looks to determine susceptibility to the disease through complex mechanisms, being involved in the process of steatosis, inflammation, and fibrosis and even in hepatocarcinoma occurrence (Fig. 5.2).

5.2.2 Transmembrane 6 Superfamily 2 (TM6SF2) Gene

It is a gene found on chromosome 19, more precisely 19p12, consisting of 377 amino acids. Main sites of expression are the liver and intestine, and in smaller amounts, the brain, lungs, kidneys, and adipose tissue. At the intracellular level, it is found within the endoplasmic reticulum and at the level of the Golgi apparatus [16]. The role of this gene is not fully elucidated, being involved in lipid metabolism.

Its role in the pathogenesis of NAFLD is reflected in the metabolism of triglyceride-rich lipoproteins, being considered a gene that regulates their hepatic excretion. The inhibition of this gene, through different mutations, is associated with a decrease in the excretion of triglycerides from the hepatocyte level, with the secondary excess accumulation of them causing the appearance of steatosis. Patients

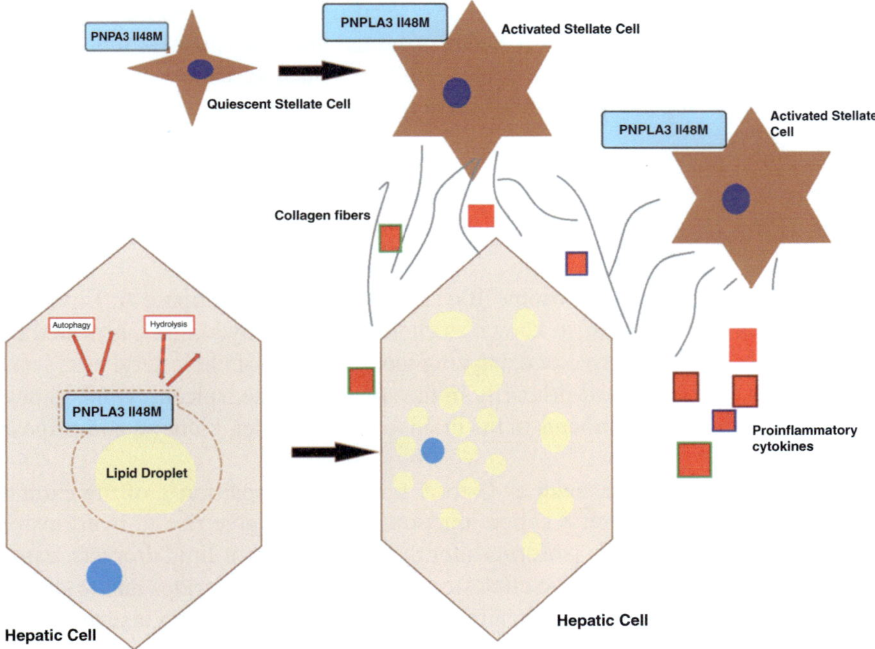

Fig. 5.2 PNPLA3 I148M role in steatosis, inflammation and fibrosis (*created with Paint soft*)

with this gene mutation are characterized by hepatic steatosis and low serum concentrations of triglycerides [16]. Several mutations of this gene were discovered, among which we mention the TM6SF2 E167K variant, which strongly correlates with NAFLD [17].

5.2.3 HSD17B13 Gene

HSD17B13 is a gene found on chromosome 4q22.1, is made up of eight exons and seven introns, and encodes nine different protein isoforms. In humans, HSD17B13 is most abundantly expressed in the liver, with low levels in the ovary, bone marrow, kidney, brain, lung, skeletal muscle, bladder, and testis. Within the liver, genetic sequence analysis showed that HSD17B13 is mainly localized in hepatocytes, with shallow expression in other liver cells such as macrophages, hepatic stellate cells, and liver sinusoidal endothelial cells. This gene is found exclusively on the surface of lipid droplets within the hepatocyte. From a functional point of view, the gene participates in lipid metabolism. It possesses short-chain dehydrogenase/reductase and retinol dehydrogenase activity, being involved in the homeostasis of hepatic lipid droplets [18].

Several studies have shown that the overexpression of HSD17B13 was associated with excessive hepatocyte lipogenesis and accumulation of lipid droplets leading to NAFLD. In contrast, the presence of variants (e.g., rs72613567 TA, rs6834314

G, rs143404524) of this gene shows an inverse correlation with NAFLD. Mutations of this gene reduce the risk of liver steatosis through the mechanism of reducing the synthesis of lipid droplets at the hepatocyte level. Such variants were discovered following different genome-wide association studies in humans and studies on animals [18].

5.2.4 LIPA Gene

It is a gene located on chromosome 10q23.31, which encodes lipase A. Lipase A, the lysosomal acid lipase (also known as cholesterol ester hydrolase), is hosted by the lysosome and has the role of catalyzing the hydrolysis of cholesteryl esters and triglycerides. It is expressed primarily in the small intestine, spleen, lymph nodes, and liver and in smaller amounts in the brain, urinary bladder, kidneys, and adipose tissue [19].

Mutations in this gene, such as G-to-A transition at position 1 of the exon 8 splice donor (E8SJM, exon 8 splice junction mutation), give rise to isoforms of the lipase A enzyme. These isoforms alter the homeostasis of lipid droplets, causing the accumulation of hepatic cholesteryl esters and triglycerides due to defective lysosomal hydrolysis and impaired LD autophagy, generating a severe form of NAFLD called Wolman disease. Wolman disease is caused by the homozygous lysosomal acid lipase D [20]. It is a rare disease, with less than 5000 cases in the USA, which is characterized by excessive accumulation of lipids in the spleen, lymph nodes, and adrenal glands, which leads to hepatosplenomegaly and liver failure [21].

5.2.5 Microsomal Triglyceride Transfer Protein (MTTP) Gene

MTTP is a gene located on chromosome 4q24. It encodes the large subunit of the heterodimeric microsomal triglyceride transfer protein, which has been shown to play a central role in lipoprotein (apolipoprotein B) assembly. In humans, MTTP is most abundantly expressed in the small intestine and the liver. Within the hepatocyte, it is found mainly at the level of the Golgi apparatus and the endoplasmic reticulum [22].

MTTP has an essential role in triglyceride homeostasis; generally, hepatic triglycerides are exported from the liver as VLDL particles mediated through plasma apoB-lipoprotein and MTP.

Studies showed that polymorphism of MTTP gene might contribute to an increased risk of NAFLD. MTTP-493G>T (rs1800591) variant is one of the most common and widely investigated polymorphisms whose presence was strongly associated with NAFLD. MTTP-493G>T polymorphism may decrease its protein and aberrant alterations of MTTP synthesis and secretion and influence the capacity for lipid export and excess accumulation of triglycerides at the hepatocyte level, thus contributing to the occurrence of NAFLD [23].

5.2.6 Polymorphisms of Inflammatory Cytokine Genes

As we have already mentioned, NAFLD encompasses a histopathological spectrum of clinical conditions ranging from the simple fatty loading of hepatocytes to inflammation, necrosis, and fibrosis. Genes influencing inflammation and immune responses modify the susceptibility to NAFLD. Cytokines play an active role in disease development but also in the progression by regulating the inflammatory process [24].

Tumor necrosis factor-α (TNF-α) is part of the TNF superfamily, a cytokine involved in cellular signaling within the immune response. The gene encoding TNF-α is found on chromosome 6 and comprises four exons. TNF-α is a proinflammatory cytokine that mediates hepatic inflammation, oxidative stress, and apoptosis or necrosis of liver cells. Several clinical studies have investigated the role of TNF-α as a marker for NAFLD. They have established a directly proportional positive correlation between the serum levels of this marker and the degree of inflammation and liver fibrosis [25]. A study analyzed TNF-α gene mutations and concluded that TNF-α gene polymorphisms at position −238 are significantly higher in patients with NAFLD than those in the control subject, determining susceptibility for this disease [26].

Interleukin-10 (IL-10) is an anti-inflammatory cytokine encoded by the IL-10 gene on chromosome I, consisting of five exons. The primary routine function of IL-10 appears to limit and ultimately terminate inflammatory responses. Different liver cells, including stellate cells, hepatocytes, and cells, have shown the presence of IL-10. Few studies identified the protective role of IL-10 against hepatic steatosis [27]. In an animal model of diet-induced fatty liver disease, inhibition of IL-10 promoted increased expression of inflammatory cytokines, worsened insulin signaling, and activated gluconeogenic and lipogenic pathways [28].

Interleukin-6 (IL-6) is a cytokine with multiple and varied roles in the immune response, tissue regeneration, and metabolism. Mainly, its role has been studied in the immune response, considered a pleiotropic proinflammatory cytokine specially secreted by monocytes. It is encoded by the IL-6 gene, located on chromosome 7p21. Studies made in animal models and humans showed that IL-6 expression was markedly increased in the NASH livers. In addition, a positive correlation was observed between hepatocyte IL-6 expression, degree of inflammation, and stage of fibrosis [29].

Furthermore, a study conducted on patients with NAFLD showed that the IL-6 polymorphism, specifically the 174C variant, was present in over 80% of the biopsied patients, with the authors concluding that IL-6-174C genetic polymorphisms, involved in inflammation and insulin resistance, are associated with NASH [30].

5.2.7 Insulin Receptor Substrate-1 (IRS-1) Gene

IRS-1 gene is the first discovered member of the family of the insulin receptor substrate (IRS) proteins, cytoplasmic adapter proteins that play a critical role in insulin signaling. The genetic polymorphisms of these receptors lead to alterations in insulin signaling and, consequently, a decrease in cellular sensitivity to this hormone. IRS-1 is encoded by the IRS-1 gene, which is located on chromosome 19. Liver insulin resistance is associated with NAFLD, and it seems that substitution (glycine-arginine) at codon 972 of the IRS-1 gene is associated with reduced insulin sensitivity. This variant was shown to affect insulin receptor activity, predisposing to liver damage and decreased hepatic insulin signaling in patients with NAFLD playing a causal role in the progression of liver damage in these patients [31].

5.2.8　Other Genetic Modifiers in NAFLD

The spectrum of genetic changes involved in the etiopathogenesis of NAFLD is dynamic. Research is constantly coming up with results regarding the genetic alterations associated with this condition. Apart from the established gene polymorphisms, which were debated in the previous sub-chapters, several candidate genes are involved in the occurrence and progression of NAFLD but are waiting to be validated by more extensive studies. *MnSOD* gene mutations look to be associated with excessive oxidation of free fatty acids, leading to oxidative stress, casing apoptosis, and liver injury [32]. *ENPP1 121 Gln* gene mutation is associated with insulin resistance and liver fibrosis [33]. *Glucokinase regulatory protein* (GCKR) polymorphism rs780094 is associated with increased serum triglycerides and liver fibrosis, *SLC2A1* variants promote lipid accumulation and oxidative stress, *MBOAT7* gene variant rs641738 leads to a reduced MBOAT7 expression favoring increase in free arachidonic acid and hepatocyte inflammation, and *SOD2* polymorphism, rs4880 *CD 14 C(−159) T polymorphism, CDKN1A rs762623 variant,* and *KLF6 rs 3,750,861 variant are associated with liver fibrosis* [34–38]. *Uncoupling protein 2 (UCP2)*-866 A/A genotype is associated with increased hepatic UCP2 expression and reduced risk of NASH [39].

5.3　Epigenetic Implications in NAFLD

The term epigenetics occurred in the mid-1900s and was introduced by the biologist Conrad Waddington. The researcher defined the term as *"the branch of biology which studies the causal interactions between genes and their products which bring the phenotype into being"* [40].

Over time, the definition has undergone changes, today being accepted as *"the study of changes in gene function that are mitotically and/or meiotically heritable and that do not entail a change in DNA sequence"* [41].

Epigenetic changes in NAFLD are of great importance because, unlike genetic alterations that cannot be changed, epigenetic factors can be influenced, leading to a broadening of the horizon regarding the treatment of this disease, even its reversibility.

The processes altering the gene activity without changing the DNA sequence target all the molecular pathways that modulate the expression of a genotype in a phenotype and can be represented by alterations in DNA methylation, posttranslational modifications of amino acids, changes in histone proteins, and microRNAs (miR) [38, 42].

5.3.1 DNA Methylation

DNA methylation is a process through which a methyl group is added to cytosine in position C5, giving rise to 5-methylcytosine (5mC). This addition is usually realized in cytosine–guanine dinucleotide-rich regions known as CpG islands. Hypermethylation of CpG islands determines the gene repression because the methyl group blocks the binding of transcription factors to the DNA. It can also act as a binding site for transcriptional repressors [43]. DNA methylation is catalyzed by a family of enzymes called DNA methyltransferases (DNMTs). These enzymes have the role to transfer the methyl group from an S-adenyl methionine (SAM) to DNA [44]. Several studies have analyzed methylation changes in NAFLD patients showing alterations in the methylation signature of many genes involved in lipid and carbohydrate metabolism.

For example, a study using liver biopsies taken before and after bariatric surgery from 45 obese patients with all stages of NAFLD showed methylation and expression differences in nine key enzymes implicated in intermediate metabolism and insulin signaling:

- Pyruvate carboxylase (PC)
- ATP citrate lyase (ACLY)
- Phospholipase C-gamma-1 (PLCG1)
- Insulin-like growth factor 1 (IGF1)
- Insulin-like growth factor-binding protein 2 (IGFBP2)
- Protein kinase C epsilon (PRKCE)
- Putative polypeptide N-acetylgalactosaminyl-transferase-like protein 4 (GALNTL4)
- Glutamate receptor delta-1 (GRID1)
- Inositol hexaphosphate kinase 3 (IP6K3)

The comparison of serial liver biopsies before and after bariatric surgery showed NAFLD-associated methylation changes to be partially reversible, providing an example of treatment-induced epigenetic organ remodeling in humans [45].

Diet habits play an essential role in the occurrence and progression of NAFLD but also determine DNA methylation alterations. A diet rich in processed fats and sugars induces hypermethylation in promoter regions of peroxisome proliferator-activated receptor alpha (PPARA), a transcriptional regulator of genes involved in mitochondrial beta-oxidation, fatty acid transport, and hepatic production of glucose. PPARA hypermethylation showed a decrease in gene expression and induced fatty accumulation in the liver in a rat model [46]. In human models, a study conducted on 120 participants who followed a low-fat and low-carbohydrate diet for 18 months analyzed the intrahepatic fat accumulation and the CpG-specific DNA methylation levels of 41 selected genes known to be associated with NAFLD. After an 18-month lifestyle intervention, different DNA methylation patterns were observed [47].

5.3.2 Modifications in Histone Proteins

Histones are a family of structural proteins that condense DNA into chromatin, which can undergo acetylation, methylation, and phosphorylation under the action of different enzymes.

Acetylation is a process that causes the activation of gene transcription and deacetylation repression. The imbalance between enzymes causing acetylation and deacetylation may influence phenotypic gene expression [38].

This is the case of cyclic AMP-responsive element-binding protein 3-like 3 (CREBH), a hepatocyte-specific transcription factor localized in the endoplasmic reticulum membrane activated by endoplasmic reticulum, stress, or inflammation. CREBH enters the cell nucleus and activates the expression of genes involved in the acute-phase response, gluconeogenesis, lipogenesis, fatty acid oxidation, and lipolysis. Modulation of CREBH acetylation can lead to altered lipid homeostasis associated with NAFLD [38, 48].

5.3.3 MicroRNAs

MicroRNAs (miRNAs) are single-stranded noncoding RNAs made up of 18–25 nucleotides long that can regulate gene expression at the posttranscriptional level by inhibiting translation or inducing degradation of target messenger RNAs. More than 2000 human miRNAs have been discovered, accounting for 1–5% of the human genome. These are predicted to regulate up to 60% of human genes [43, 49].

miRNAs play a role in many cellular processes. miRNA dysregulation looks to be associated with several liver diseases, including NAFLD, viral hepatitis, fibrosis, and liver cancer. Data in NAFLD patients suggests that miR-21, miR-34a, and miR-182 are upregulated in NAFLD while miR-122 is downregulated [38].

5.4 Conclusions

In an era where metabolic disorders are alarmingly high, NAFLD represents the worldwide most common liver disease and is considered the leading cause of liver-related morbidity and mortality. Hence, the new terminology "metabolic associated fatty liver disease" starts to be more and more accepted.

Although initially considered a disease primarily determined by environmental factors (diet, physical exercise), in the last decades, research has shown impressive results regarding the genetic and epigenetic alterations found in this broad spectrum of conditions that represent NAFLD. Knowing them is the first step in drawing new directives regarding managing patients at risk of developing NAFLD, its treatment, and achieving a degree of reversibility of the characteristic liver lesions.

References

1. Bellentani S, Scaglioni F, Marino M, Bedogni G. Epidemiology of non-alcoholic fatty liver disease. Dig Dis. 2010;28:155–61.
2. Willner IR, Waters B, Patil SR, Reuben A, Morelli J, Riely CA. Ninety patients with nonalcoholic steatohepatitis: insulin resistance, familial tendency, and severity of disease. Am J Gastroenterol. 2001;96:2957–61.
3. Truben VM, Hespenheide EE, Caldwell SH. Nonalcoholic steatohepatitis and cryptogenic cirrhosis within kindreds. Am J Med. 2000;108:9–13.
4. Makkonen J, Pietilainen KH, Rissanen A, Kaprio J, Yki-Jarvinen H. Genetic factors contribute to variation in serum alanine aminotransferase activity independent of obesity and alcohol: a study in monozygotic and dizygotic twins. J Hepatol. 2009;50:1035–42.
5. Loomba R, Schork N, Chen CH, Bettencourt R, Bhatt A, Ang B, Nguyen P, et al. Heritability of hepatic fibrosis and steatosis based on a prospective twin study. Gastroenterology. 2015;149:1784–93.
6. Caussy C, Soni M, Cui J, Bettencourt R, Schork N, Chen CH, Ikhwan MA, et al. Nonalcoholic fatty liver disease with cirrhosis increases familial risk for advanced fibrosis. J Clin Invest. 2017;127:2697–704.
7. Romeo S, Kozlitina J, Xing C, Pertsemlidis A, Cox D, Pennacchio LA, Boerwinkle E, Cohen JC, Hobbs HH. Genetic variation in PNPLA3 confers susceptibility to nonalcoholic fatty liver disease. Nat Genet. 2008;40(12):1461–5. https://doi.org/10.1038/ng.257.
8. Dong XC. PNPLA3-a potential therapeutic target for personalized treatment of chronic liver disease. Front Med (Lausanne). 2019;17(6):304. https://doi.org/10.3389/fmed.2019.00304.
9. Sookoian S, Pirola CJ, Valenti L, Davidson NO. Genetic pathways in nonalcoholic fatty liver disease: insights from systems biology. Hepatology. 2020;72(1):330–46. https://doi.org/10.1002/hep.31229.
10. Anstee QM, Seth D, Day CP, et al. Genetic factors that affect risk of alcoholic and nonalcoholic fatty liver disease. Gastroenterology. 2016;150:1728–44.
11. BasuRay S, Wang Y, Smagris E, Cohen JC, Hobbs HH. Accumulation of PNPLA3 on lipid droplets is the basis of associated hepatic steatosis. Proc Natl Acad Sci U S A. 2019;116:9521–6.
12. BasuRay S, Smagris E, Cohen JC, Hobbs HH. The PNPLA3 variant associated with fatty liver disease (I148M) accumulates on lipid droplets by evading ubiquitylation. Hepatology. 2017;66:1111–24.
13. Pingitore P, Dongiovanni P, Motta BM, et al. PNPLA3 overexpression results in reduction of proteins predisposing to fibrosis. Hum Mol Genet. 2016;25:5212–22.
14. Pirazzi C, Valenti L, Motta BM, et al. PNPLA3 has retinyl-palmitate lipase activity in human hepatic stellate cells. Hum Mol Genet. 2014;23:4077–85.
15. Burza MA, Pirazzi C, Maglio C, et al. PNPLA3 I148M (rs738409) genetic variant is associated with hepatocellular carcinoma in obese individuals. Dig Liver Dis. 2012;44:1037–41.
16. Mahdessian H, Taxiarchis A, Popov S, Silveira A, Franco-Cereceda A, Hamsten A, Eriksson P, van't Hooft F. TM6SF2 is a regulator of liver fat metabolism influencing triglyceride secretion and hepatic lipid droplet content. Proc Natl Acad Sci U S A. 2014;111(24):8913–8.
17. Prill S, Caddeo A, Baselli G, et al. The TM6SF2 E167K genetic variant induces lipid biosynthesis and reduces apolipoprotein B secretion in human hepatic 3D spheroids. Sci Rep. 2019;9:11,585.

18. Zhang HB, Su W, Xu H, Zhang XY, Guan YF. HSD17B13: a potential therapeutic target for NAFLD. Front Mol Biosci. 2022;7(8):824776. https://doi.org/10.3389/fmolb.2021.824776.

19. https://www.ncbi.nlm.nih.gov/gene/

20. Pericleous M, Kelly C, Wang T, Livingstone C, Ala A. Wolman's disease and cholesteryl ester storage disorder: the phenotypic spectrum of lysosomal acid lipase deficiency. Lancet Gastroenterol Hepatol. 2017;2:670–9.

21. https://rarediseases.info.nih.gov/diseases/7899/wolman-disease

22. https://www.genecards.org/cgi-bin/carddisp.pl?gene=MTTP#localization

23. Gouda W, Ashour E, Shaker Y, Ezzat W. MTP genetic variants associated with non-alcoholic fatty liver in metabolic syndrome patients. Genes Dis. 16, 4(4):222–8. https://doi.org/10.1016/j.gendis.2017.09.002.

24. Braunersreuther V, Viviani GL, Mach F, Montecucco F. Role of cytokines and chemokines in non-alcoholic fatty liver disease. World J Gastroenterol. 2012;18:727–35.

25. Seo YY, Cho YK, Bae JC, Seo MH, Park SE, Rhee EJ, Park CY, Oh KW, Park SW, Lee WY. Tumor necrosis factor-α as a predictor for the development of nonalcoholic fatty liver disease: a 4-year follow-up study. Endocrinol Metab (Seoul). 2013;28(1):41–5. https://doi.org/10.3803/EnM.2013.28.1.41.

26. Hu ZW, Luo HB, Xu YM, Guo JW, Deng XL, Tong YW, Tang X. Tumor necrosis factor-alpha gene promoter polymorphisms in Chinese patients with nonalcoholic fatty liver diseases. Acta Gastroenterol Belg. 2009;72(2):215–21.

27. en Boer MA, Voshol PJ, Schröder-van der Elst JP, Korsheninnikova E, Ouwens DM, Kuipers F, Havekes LM, Romijn JA. Endogenous interleukin-10 protects against hepatic steatosis but does not improve insulin sensitivity during high-fat feeding in mice. Endocrinology. 2006;147:4553–8.

28. Cintra DE, Pauli JR, Araújo EP, Moraes JC, de Souza CT, Milanski M, Morari J, Gambero A, Saad MJ, Velloso LA. Interleukin-10 is a protective factor against diet-induced insulin resistance in liver. J Hepatol. 2008;48:628–37.

29. Wieckowska A, Papouchado BG, Li Z, Lopez R, Zein NN, Feldstein AE. Increased hepatic and circulating interleukin-6 levels in human nonalcoholic steatohepatitis. Am J Gastroenterol. 2008;103(6):1372–9. https://doi.org/10.1111/j.1572-0241.2007.01774.x.

30. Carulli L, Canedi I, Rondinella S, Lombardini S, Ganazzi D, Fargion S, De Palma M, Lonardo A, Ricchi M, Bertolotti M, Carulli N, Loria P. Genetic polymorphisms in non-alcoholic fatty liver disease: interleukin-6-174G/C polymorphism is associated with non-alcoholic steatohepatitis. Dig Liver Dis. 2009;41(11):823–8. https://doi.org/10.1016/j.dld.2009.03.005.

31. Dongiovanni P, Valenti L, Rametta R, Daly AK, Nobili V, Mozzi E, Leathart JB, Pietrobattista A, Burt AD, Maggioni M, et al. Genetic variants regulating insulin receptor signalling are associated with the severity of liver damage in patients with non-alcoholic fatty liver disease. Gut. 2010;59:267–73.

32. Wang K. Molecular mechanisms of hepatic apoptosis. Cell Death Dis. 2014;5:e996.

33. Dongiovanni P, Valenti L, Rametta R, et al. Genetic variants regulating insulin receptor signalling are associated with the severity of liver damage in patients with non-alcoholic fatty liver disease. Gut. 2010;59:267–73.

34. Petta S, Miele L, Bugianesi E, et al. Glucokinase regulatory protein gene polymorphism affects liver fibrosis in non-alcoholic fatty liver disease. PLoS One. 2014;9:e87523.

35. Vazquez-Chantada M, Gonzalez-Lahera A, Martinez-Arranz I, et al. Solute carrier family 2 member 1 is involved in the development of nonalcoholic fatty liver disease. Hepatology. 2013;57:505–14.

36. Meroni M, Longo M, Rametta R, et al. Genetic and epigenetic modifiers of alcoholic liver disease. Int J Mol Sci. 2018;19:3857.

37. Al-Serri A, Anstee QM, Valenti L, et al. The SOD2 C47T polymorphism influences NAFLD fibrosis severity: evidence from case-control and intra-familial allele association studies. J Hepatol. 2012;56:448–54.

38. Choudhary NS, Duseja A. Genetic and epigenetic disease modifiers: non-alcoholic fatty liver disease (NAFLD) and alcoholic liver disease (ALD). Transl Gastroenterol Hepatol. 2021;6:2. https://doi.org/10.21037/tgh.2019.09.06.
39. Fares R, Petta S, Lombardi R, et al. The UCP2 -866 G>A promoter region polymorphism is associated with nonalcoholic steatohepatitis. Liver Int. 35:1574–80.
40. Waddington CH. The epigenotype. Endeavour. 1942;2015(1):18–20.
41. Ct W, Morris JR. Genes, genetics, and epigenetics: a correspondence. Science. 2001;293(5532):1103–5.
42. Dupont C, Armant DR, Brenner CA. Epigenetics: definition, mechanisms and clinical perspective. Semin Reprod Med. 2009;27(5):351–7. https://doi.org/10.1055/s-0029-1237423.
43. Rodríguez-Sanabria JS, Escutia-Gutiérrez R, Rosas-Campos R, Armendáriz-Borunda JS, Sandoval-Rodríguez A. An update in epigenetics in metabolic-associated fatty liver disease. Front Med (Lausanne). 2022;8:770504. https://doi.org/10.3389/fmed.2021.770504.
44. Angeloni A, Bogdanovic O. Enhancer DNA methylation: implications for gene regulation. Essays Biochem. 2019;63:707–15. https://doi.org/10.1042/EBC20190030.
45. Ahrens M, Ammerpohl O, von Schönfels W, Kolarova J, Bens S, Itzel T, Teufel A, Herrmann A, Brosch M, Hinrichsen H, Erhart W, Egberts J, Sipos B, Schreiber S, Häsler R, Stickel F, Becker T, Krawczak M, Röcken C, Siebert R, Schafmayer C, Hampe J. DNA methylation analysis in nonalcoholic fatty liver disease suggests distinct disease-specific and remodeling signatures after bariatric surgery. Cell Metab. 2013;18(2):296–302. https://doi.org/10.1016/j.cmet.2013.07.004.
46. Li YY, Tang D, Du YL, Cao CY, Nie YQ, Cao J, et al. Fatty liver mediated by peroxisome proliferator-activated receptor-α DNA methylation can be reversed by a methylation inhibitor and curcumin. J Dig Dis. 2018;19:421–30. https://doi.org/10.1111/1751-2980.12610.
47. Yaskolka Meir A, Keller M, Müller L, Bernhart SH, Tsaban G, Zelicha H, et al. Effects of lifestyle interventions on epigenetic signatures of liver fat: central randomized controlled trial. Liver Int. 2021;41:2101–11. https://doi.org/10.1111/liv.14916.
48. Kim H, Mendez R, Chen X, Fang D, Zhang K. Lysine acetylation of CREBH regulates fasting-induced hepatic lipid metabolism. Mol Cell Biol. 2015;35(24):4121–34. https://doi.org/10.1128/MCB.00665-15.
49. Bartel DP. MicroRNAs: genomics, biogenesis, mechanism, and function. Cell. 2004;116:281–97. https://doi.org/10.1016/s0092-8674(04)00045-5.

The Place of Transabdominal Liver Biopsy in Nonalcoholic Fatty Liver Disease

6

Cristina Muzica, Anca Trifan, Irina Girleanu,
Camelia Cojocariu, and Carol Stanciu

6.1 Introduction

The medical field of hepatology encompasses a wide range of diseases which are characterized by a large variability regarding etiologies and risk factors; thus, liver diseases have different ways of development and disease course, which consequently need different therapeutical approach. During the recent years, liver diseases have been intensely studied with great results in terms of not only diagnosis but also treatment and prognostic factors, prolonging both the life expectancy and quality of life in patients. The discovery of direct-acting antivirals for the therapy of hepatitis C virus, the development of new targeted agents for hepatocellular carcinoma, and the implementation of noninvasive scoring systems for liver fibrosis in clinical practice are a few cornerstone discoveries that changed the course of these diseases. Furthermore, recent years brought new definitions and classifications that made it easier for clinicians to diagnose and treat liver diseases. Such an example is represented by nonalcoholic fatty liver disease (NAFLD), which has gained major attention since it was first described in 1980 [1]. Accordingly, there is large data coming from many studies regarding the epidemiology, risk factors, diagnosis, therapy, and prognosis of NAFLD. In terms of diagnosis, there are various tests with varying sensitivities and specificities.

According to current guidelines, the initial evaluation of patients with NAFLD should include a comprehensive assessment of all associated metabolic disorders (i.e., type 2 diabetes mellitus, obesity, sleep apnea, insulin resistance, hypothyroidism) and exclude other competing etiologies (viral hepatitis, metabolic hepatitis,

C. Muzica (✉) · A. Trifan · I. Girleanu · C. Cojocariu · C. Stanciu
Gastroenterology Department, Grigore T. Popa University of Medicine and Pharmacy, Iasi, Romania

St. Spiridon Emergency Hospital, Institute of Gastroenterology and Hepatology, Iasi, Romania

© The Author(s), under exclusive license to Springer Nature Switzerland AG 2023
A. Trifan et al. (eds.), *Essentials of Non-Alcoholic Fatty Liver Disease*,
https://doi.org/10.1007/978-3-031-33548-8_6

alcoholic liver disease, etc.) [2]. Next steps in the diagnosis workup of NAFLD should include blood tests for liver function, liver enzymes, complete blood count, lipid and glycemic profile, uric acid, testing for viral hepatitis, and ultrasound.

A very important part in the evaluation of NAFLD is establishing the presence/grade of liver fibrosis. Currently, there are numerous noninvasive tests based on several scores for the prediction of liver fibrosis in patients with NAFLD, such as AST to platelet ratio index (APRI), the NAFLD fibrosis score, BARD score, fibrosis-4 score (FIB-4), enhanced liver fibrosis (ELF) score, HAIR score, Palekar's score, and BAAT score [3–7]. Furthermore, the high accuracy in predicting the liver fibrosis in NAFLD patients by advanced imaging techniques such as vibration-controlled transient elastography, 2D shear wave elastography, and acoustic radiation force impulse has led to their immediate acceptance in daily practice by hepatologists [8]. However, the liver biopsy (LB) has been used as a standard for diagnosing and grading NAFLD among these tests and techniques, being currently the gold standard. The diagnosis of NAFLD is based on the presence of macrovesicular steatosis in at least 5% of hepatocytes, and, moreover, LB is the only method to document NASH.

There are three different techniques for liver tissue sampling: transabdominal LB, transjugular LB, and surgical LB.

6.2 Principles of Transabdominal LB

6.2.1 Indications of Transabdominal LB

The indications for LB in general include those of transabdominal LB. A liver biopsy serves three main purposes: (1) making a diagnosis, (2) determining the prognosis or disease stage, and (3) assisting with clinical management and therapeutic options.

Numerous liver diseases can be diagnosed via a liver biopsy, which also provides extra information that blood tests may not be able to provide. If another workup is unremarkable, a biopsy, for instance, can help with analyzing abnormal liver function tests [9].

Transabdominal LB aids in the confirmation of the diagnosis and directs treatment in patients in whom autoimmune hepatitis (AIH) is highly suspected despite negative autoantibodies and/or normal IgG levels. Those who have an "overlap" syndrome combining primary biliary cirrhosis (PBC) and AIH can also be identified through a biopsy [10]. The degree of fibrosis can help guide treatment decisions for people with PBC [11].

Other liver diseases whose diagnosis could benefit from LB are drug-induced liver injury (DILI), acute or chronic rejection in patients after liver transplantation, and infiltrative and/or storage disease.

Furthermore, it is important to assess the degree of inflammation and fibrosis in people with chronic viral hepatitis. Additionally, among individuals with hemochromatosis, those whose biopsy revealed advanced fibrosis had a higher risk of developing hepatocellular carcinoma (HCC) than those whose biopsy revealed no fibrosis [12].

6.2.2 Contraindications of Transabdominal LB

There are a few contraindications that limit the use of transabdominal LB in certain patients. The contraindications are relative and absolute (Table 6.1). Relative contraindications in patients with urgent need of LB need careful considerations of the benefits and risks and a judicious decision regarding whether to perform the procedure or search for another noninvasive surrogate for LB.

6.2.3 Technique of Transabdominal LB

In a percutaneous liver biopsy, a needle is inserted through the skin and eventually into the liver tissue to collect a sample for use in staging, diagnosing, and/or developing therapy options for a range of liver illnesses. Since the very first report of transabdominal LB use in the year of 1923 [13], advances in the field allowed for a more precise target of liver lesion by using imaging techniques such as ultrasound, computed tomography (CT), and magnetic resonance imaging (MRI). Furthermore, with the use of imaging technique-guided transabdominal LB, there is a lower risk of complications and a higher rate of success in attaining the targeted liver tissue [14]. Transabdominal LB is the most common type of LB chosen in clinical practice.

6.2.3.1 Description of the Technique
Three alternative methods can be used to do a percutaneous liver biopsy: real-time image guidance, image guidance, and palpation/percussion guidance.

The most popular technique is the palpation/percussion method, which is based on physical examination. Before inserting the needle for the image-guided procedure, the biopsy site is marked using ultrasound. The real-time image-guided method uses tissue samples and the US concurrently. The patient is lying on his or

Table 6.1 Contraindications for transabdominal LB

Absolute contraindications	Relative contraindications
• The inability of a patient to fully cooperate with the procedure • Significant coagulopathy or thrombocytopenia (unless corrected before the liver biopsy) • Large ascites • NSAID use (including aspirin) within the last 5–7 days • Patient refusal to accept blood transfusion or inability to provide blood transfusion support • Hemangioma, vascular tumor, or echinococcal cyst • Extrahepatic biliary obstruction	• Morbid obesity • Mild ascites • Hemophilia • Infection within the right pleural cavity • Infection below the right hemidiaphragm • Amyloidosis

her right side, close to the edge of the bed, in a supine position. The lower extremities should be shifted away from the torso to best allow for intercostal space expansion before the patient's right arm is raised over the head. The skin is uncovered, and percussion is applied to the upper right quadrant. The midaxillary line, which is the location of maximum dullness, is normally between the seventh and eighth intercostal spaces and serves as the typical biopsy site. After designating the location, a bedside ultrasonography can verify its suitability and rule out the possibility of intestinal tissue covering the biopsy tract. The skin is then prepared and sterilely draped. To avoid the neurovasculature that runs along the lower border of each rib, lidocaine solution (1% or 2% solution is an alternative) is injected along the top border of the rib. At the location of the biopsy, a small surgical incision is performed. The chosen biopsy needle is then inserted through the skin incision parallel to the floor and toward the xiphoid process (Fig. 6.1). In the phase of expiration, a tissue sample is obtained. Following the removal of the needle, the biopsy site is subjected to pressure for a short period of time before being bandaged. After that, the patient is positioned in the right lateral decubitus position, likely to stop bleeding by applying pressure on the liver against the abdominal wall.

Following the procedure, the patient's vital signs—including their blood pressure, heart rate, and level of pain—are checked every 15 min for the first hour, every 30 min for the following, and then every hour until they are ready to be released. The American Association for the Study of Liver Diseases states that patients should be monitored between 2 and 4 h after the procedure [15]. Patients are advised not to carry more than 4.5–7 kg for 1 week following the procedure.

6.2.3.2 The Choice of the Needle

There are three primary groups of needles, each with different sizes and varieties: suction needles, cutting needles, and spring-loaded cutting needles with triggering

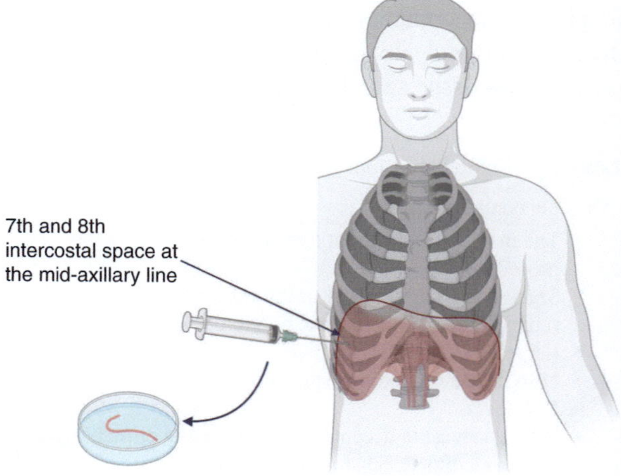

Fig. 6.1 The technique of transabdominal liver biopsy

mechanisms The operator's desire, the availability of the device, and the clinical picture essentially determine the needle to use [16]. For instance, if there is a strong suspicion of cirrhosis, a cutting needle may be preferable over a suction needle since suction needles have a tendency to fracture fibrotic tissue [17].

6.2.4   Complications of Transabdominal LB

Complications can rarely occur after transabdominal LB, but the risk exists and can result in death. Approximately 60% of the complications happen during the first 2 h, and 96% happen within the first 24 h after transabdominal LB [13]. A cohort study which included about 60,000 individuals which were evaluated for various liver diseases by LB demonstrated that the overall mortality risk was approximately 0.2% [16]. Pain at the biopsy site or pain that refers to the right shoulder is the most typical consequence [17]. Other complications are illustrated in Table 6.2.

6.2.5   The Place of Transabdominal LB in the Diagnostic Workup for NAFLD

The gold standard for distinguishing steatohepatitis from simple steatosis and determining the stage of fibrosis is still liver histology. Thus, LB remains an important diagnostic tool, particularly in patients with NASH in which the diagnosis as well as the staging of the disease is difficult to be done with only the use of noninvasive tests. All recommendations concur that LB should only be taken into consideration in a small number of people due to its invasive nature and related costs. But furthermore, the limitations of LB are not related only to the invasive nature of the

Table 6.2 Complications of transabdominal LB

Complication	Commentary
Transient hypotension	As a result of vasovagal response or hemorrhage
Hemorrhage	Subscapular, intrahepatic, intraperitoneal, hemobilia*, hemothorax
Pneumothorax	After the injury of pleura or lung or right diaphragm
Biliary peritonitis	Standard care of biliary peritonitis requires a multidisciplinary approach with endoscopic and surgical management
Portal vein thrombosis	Probably as a result of the damage to a branch of portal vein during biopsy
Transient bacteremia	Can occur in patients with biliary obstruction and cholangitis or when the colon is incidentally punctured
Subphrenic abscess	
Carcinoid crisis	The main manifestations are hypotension or hypertension, diarrhea, bronchoconstriction, flushing, and an acidosis
Death	The main cause of death is intraperitoneal bleeding

*Quincke's triad: Gastrointestinal bleeding, biliary pain, and jaundice

procedure; it has also been associated with a high inter- and intraobserver variability, sampling errors, and poor patient acceptance [8].

The American and European recommendations concur that patients with NAFLD suspected of advanced fibrosis should undergo a liver biopsy to confirm findings because this would have prognostic implications and result in therapy adjustments [2, 18]. The Asian recommendations are different in that they only advocate for LB when it is impossible to rule out the existence or severity of concomitant chronic liver disease or when the assessment of fibrosis by noninvasive tests is unclear [19].

All guidelines acknowledge that noninvasive methods should be performed to categorize individuals as low or high risk for advanced fibrosis; however, the American and Asian guidelines do not provide a preferred order of testing. The European recommendation offers a suggested diagnostic algorithm with recommendations to help with hepatology referral. Additionally, it offers a suggested follow-up plan to keep track of illness development with the caution that the best follow-up method has not yet been established.

The detection of NASH is crucial from a therapeutic standpoint since it signals a higher risk of fibrosis progression and the requirement for prompt treatment and vigilant monitoring. Currently, there are no reliable noninvasive methods to distinguish between simple steatosis and steatohepatitis. The US guidelines advise doing an LB in patients with the metabolic syndrome since it raises the risk for steatohepatitis. However, this strategy is clinically unworkable because the majority of NAFLD patients have at least one metabolic syndrome component. Furthermore, many clinicians are still hesitant to perform a biopsy because there is currently no pharmaceutical therapy for NASH approved by regulatory authorities.

6.3 Conclusions

Despite all limitations of LB, it remains the gold standard for the differentiation of steatohepatitis from simple steatosis, which is a mandatory step in the evaluation of patients suspected of NASH. Transabdominal LB should be performed only in a small proportion of patients, particularly in those included in a high-risk group, after a close evaluation of all indications and contraindications stated above.

References

1. Ludwig J, Viggiano TR, McGill DB, Oh BJ. Nonalcoholic steatohepatitis: Mayo Clinic experiences with a hitherto unnamed disease. Mayo Clin Proc. 1980;55(7):434–8.
2. Chalasani N, Younossi Z, Lavine JE, Charlton M, Cusi K, Rinella M, Harrison SA, Brunt EM, Sanyal AJ. The diagnosis and management of nonalcoholic fatty liver disease: practice guidance from the American Association for the Study of Liver Diseases. Hepatology. 2018;67(1):328–57. https://doi.org/10.1002/hep.29367. Epub 2017 Sep 29.
3. Harrison SA, Oliver D, Arnold HL, et al. Development and validation of a simple NAFLD clinical scoring system for identifying patients without advanced disease. Gut. 2008;57:1441–7.

4. Angulo P, Hui JM, Marchesini G, et al. The NAFLD fibrosis score: a noninvasive system that identifies liver fibrosis in patients with NAFLD. Hepatology. 2007;45:846–54.
5. Guha IN, Parkes J, Roderick P, et al. Noninvasive markers of fibrosis in nonalcoholic fatty liver disease: validating the European Liver Fibrosis Panel and exploring simple markers. Hepatology. 2008;47:455–60.
6. Dixon JB, Bhathal PS, O'Brien PE. Nonalcoholic fatty liver disease: predictors of nonalcoholic steatohepatitis and liver fibrosis in the severely obese. Gastroenterology. 2001;121:91–100.
7. Palekar NA, Naus R, Larson SP, et al. Clinical model for distinguishing nonalcoholic steatohepatitis from simple steatosis in patients with nonalcoholic fatty liver disease. Liver Int. 2006;26:151–6.
8. Zenovia S, Stanciu C, Sfarti C, et al. Vibration-controlled transient Elastography and controlled attenuation parameter for the diagnosis of liver steatosis and fibrosis in patients with nonalcoholic fatty liver disease. Diagnostics (Basel). 2021;11(5):787.
9. Skelly MM, James PD, Ryder SD. Findings on liver biopsy to investigate abnormal liver function tests in the absence of diagnostic serology. J Hepatol. 2001;35(2):195–9.
10. Zein CO, Angulo P, Lindor KD. When is liver biopsy needed in the diagnosis of primary biliary cirrhosis? Clin Gastroenterol Hepatol. 2003;1(2):89–95.
11. Rockey DC, Caldwell SH, Goodman ZD, Nelson RC, Smith AD, American Association for the Study of Liver Diseases. Liver biopsy. Hepatology. 2009;49(3):1017–44.
12. Niederau C, Fischer R, Pürschel A, Stremmel W, Häussinger D, Strohmeyer G. Long-term survival in patients with hereditary hemochromatosis. Gastroenterology. 1996;110(4):1107–19.
13. Grant A, Neuberger J. Guidelines on the use of liver biopsy in clinical practice. British Society of Gastroenterology. Gut. 1999;45(Suppl 4):IV1–IV11.
14. Midia M, Odedra D, Shuster A, Midia R, Muir J. Predictors of bleeding complications following percutaneous image-guided liver biopsy: a scoping review. Diagn Interv Radiol. 2019;25(1):71–80.
15. Rockey DC, Caldwell SH, Goodman ZD, Nelson RC, Smith AD. Liver biopsy. Hepatology. 2009;49:1017–44.
16. Sporea I, Popescu A, Sirli R. Why, who and how should perform liver biopsy in chronic liver diseases. World J Gastroenterol. 2008;14(21):3396–402.
17. Colombo M, Del Ninno E, de Franchis R, De Fazio C, Festorazzi S, Ronchi G, Tommasini MA. Ultrasound-assisted percutaneous liver biopsy: superiority of the Tru-cut over the Menghini needle for diagnosis of cirrhosis. Gastroenterology. 1988;95(2):487–9.
18. European Association for the Study of the Liver, European Association for the Study of Diabetes, European Association for the Study of Obesity. EASL-EASD-EASO clinical practice guidelines for the management of non-alcoholic fatty liver disease. J Hepatol. 2016;64:1388–402.
19. Wong VW, Chan WK, Chitturi S, et al. Asia-Pacific working party on non-alcoholic fatty liver disease guidelines 2017-part 1: definition, risk factors and assessment. J Gastroenterol Hepatol. 2018;33:70–85.

Alternative Methods for Liver Biopsy: Endoscopic Ultrasound-Guided and Transjugular Liver Biopsy

Catalin Victor Sfarti, Stefan Chiriac, and Gheorghe G. Balan

7.1 Introduction

Liver biopsy (LB) has long been considered the gold standard for the diagnosis of liver fibrosis in patients with nonalcoholic fatty liver disease (NAFLD) [1]. The traditional percutaneous method is the most preferred approach. However, alternative LB methods can be used in certain settings. Transjugular liver biopsy (TJLB) can reduce the risks of complications in patients with coagulopathy and ascites and can provide simultaneous portal pressure measurement if indicated [2].

Another recently introduced technique for LB is endoscopic ultrasound (EUS)-guided LB. Although initially designed to improve the visualization of the pancreaticobiliary system, endoscopic ultrasound (EUS) has been increasingly used for the diagnostic and treatment of various conditions in the field of hepatology [3].

7.2 Endoscopic Ultrasound-Guided Liver Biopsy (EUS-Guided LB)

EUS-guided LB can present several advantages compared to the other methods, such as decreased post-procedure pain, better patient tolerance, as well as possibility of performing several parenchymal passes without puncturing the liver capsule multiple times [4]. It seems that EUS-guided LB gains more and more popularity as patients tend to consider an endoscopic procedure under deep sedation preferable to

C. V. Sfarti (✉) · S. Chiriac · G. G. Balan
Grigore T. Popa University of Medicine and Pharmacy, Gastroenterology Department, Iasi, Romania

St. Spiridon Emergency Hospital, Institute of Gastroenterology and Hepatology, Iasi, Romania

A. Trifan et al. (eds.), *Essentials of Non-Alcoholic Fatty Liver Disease*, https://doi.org/10.1007/978-3-031-33548-8_7

the conventional endovascular approach. Nevertheless, EUS-guided LB combines the advantages of tissue acquisition to those of a high-resolution ultrasonographic examination of the liver parenchyma that can involve additional features like elastometry and contrast enhancement analyses.

7.2.1 Indications and Contraindications for EUS-Guided LB

EUS-guided LB can be offered to all patients that require an LB. However, the most adequate and judicious use of this procedure would be in patients that also require endoscopic or EUS evaluation for associated indications. The main advantages and disadvantages of the procedure are presented in Table 7.1. EUS-guided LB is contraindicated in patients with coagulopathy, defined as platelets <50,000/microliter or an international normalized ratio >1.5. Patients that are not sedation candidates should be offered alternative LB methods [6].

7.2.2 EUS-Guided LB Technique

7.2.2.1 Description of the Technique

The procedure should be carried out with moderate or deep sedation, in accordance with the American Society of Anesthesiologists (ASA) score as well as with local and national endoscopy sedation protocols [5, 8, 9]. There are various techniques used for EUS-guided LB. As in all EUS-guided tissue acquisition procedures, the search for the optimal needle and method has led to an ample debate that has not yet produced a definite conclusion [10]. Ultimately, the choice of needle as well as method is in the hands of the endoscopists, in accordance with personal preference and expertise.

The patients rest in general in prone position. The echoendoscope is advanced at the level of the cardia, and endosonographic examination is used in order to identify the left lobe of the liver. The echoendoscope can be slowly advanced distally and

Table 7.1 Advantages and disadvantages of EUS-guided LB [5–7]

Advantages	Disadvantages

• Less post-procedure pain
• Faster recovery time
• Adequate specimen
• Real-time assessment and possibility to target and to avoid specific areas of the liver
• Access of both the liver lobes
• Can be performed in obese patients
• Can be performed in patients with ascites
• Can be performed in the same setting in patients that require:
  – Portal pressure gradient measurement
  – Screening and/or treatment of esophageal and/or gastric varices
  – EUS-guided biliary drainage
	• High cost
	• Need for experienced operator
	• Requires sedation
	• Low availability

gently torqued as needed to visualize the hepatic parenchyma. If access to the right lobe of the liver is desired, the echoendoscope should be positioned at the level of the duodenal bulb. Counterclockwise torque should then be applied until the liver parenchyma is visualized. In cases of altered anatomy, such as Roux-en-Y gastric bypass, EUS-guided LB can be performed from the transgastric route [5–7].

When the position of the echoendoscope is deemed stable and the liver parenchyma intended to be punctured is visualized, the needle is advanced through the working channel of the echoendoscope and fixed with the Luer-lock system. Color Doppler can be used to ensure that no visible vessels are interposed in the needle trajectory. The sheath is consequently advanced until it is seen on the endosonographic image and locked. The needle is then advanced into the liver parenchyma with a rapid motion. Several passes can be performed. After each pass, the needle should be removed and the tissue obtained should be placed in formalin [6, 7].

7.2.2.2 The Choice of the Technique

Various techniques have been proposed in order to maximize the quantity as well as the quality of the tissue obtained [5]. Traditionally, dry suction has been used for EUS-guided tissue acquisition [10]. This implies the attachment of an empty negative pressure syringe at the proximal end of the needle after it has been passed into the parenchyma. However, recent prospective data concerning EUS-guided LB showed that the wet suction technique allows better results in terms of the length of the biopsy obtained as well as the number of complete portal tracts (CPTs) when compared to dry suction [11]. In this setting, the needle is primed either with saline solution or with heparin prior to its use [10]. Several authors have used either the no-suction or the slow-pull techniques, which consist of completely removing the stylet before the procedure or slowly removing the stylet during the procedure, with different but overall good outcomes [12].

7.2.2.3 The Choice of the Needle

There are many needles commercially available, both for fine needle aspiration (FNA) or fine needle biopsy (FNB), with different calibers, ranging from 19 to 25 gauge. There is much published data regarding the quality of the sample obtained by FNA or by FNB with different types of needles. A recent meta-analysis including 23 studies and a total of 1488 liver biopsies performed in 1326 patients concluded that FNB needles, especially third-generation ones, were superior in terms of CPTs than FNA. However, in terms of caliber, the authors did not find any significant difference when comparing 19–22 gauge FNB needles [13].

7.2.3 Adverse Events of EUS-Guided LB

Adverse effect (AE) rate after EUS-guided LB is under 10%; significant AEs are found in about 1% of the cases [13]. The most common adverse effect is post-procedural abdominal pain. Rare AEs include bleeding, subcapsular hematoma, bile leak, and death [13].

7.3 Transjugular Liver Biopsy

Transjugular liver biopsy (TJLB) has long been one of the main tools used in liver tissue acquisition in patients with acute or chronic liver diseases, especially in cases which are associated with severe coagulopathy or ascites [14]. Such method is an alternative to classic liver biopsy and includes obtaining liver tissue through a rigid cannula introduced into one of the hepatic veins, by means of jugular venous access, most frequently through the right internal jugular vein. It was first described by Dotter in 1964 and clinically performed for the first time by Hanafee in 1967. The method is characterized by several advantages, with the most important one being decreasing the risk of hemorrhage after biopsy since bleeding secondary to liver injury will drain into the hepatic veins [15].

Quality standards in TJLB include obtaining a tissue specimen of at least 15 mm long and/or containing at least six complete portal tracts (CPTs) as minimal standards [14, 16]; nevertheless, at least 20 mm specimens and/or 11 CPTs have been associated with best results and optimal reliability in staging and grading [17–19]. Furthermore, the number of CPTs has been regarded as the most reliable tool for assessing the adequacy of a tissue specimen mainly because specimens obtained by a transjugular technique used to be viewed as suboptimal compared with the samples obtained with percutaneous approach as they were smaller and relatively more fragmented [14, 20]. The quality core tissue obtained by TJLB has significantly improved once automatic cutting-type Tru-cut needles entered the market, and now samples obtained by transjugular approach are considered comparable to those obtained by percutaneous technique [20, 21].

7.3.1 Indications and Contraindications of TJLB

The most determinant aspect regarding indications of TJLB is the fact that it can be used in patients where percutaneous approach is either challenging or contraindicated. Thus, the main indication is tissue acquisition in diffuse liver diseases, which is associated with severe coagulopathy and/or ascites where standard percutaneous, endosonographic, or surgical approach is associated with a higher risk of severe coagulation abnormalities or ascites, where standard percutaneous liver biopsy is associated with a high risk of a potentially life-threatening hemoperitoneum [14, 22, 23]. Thus, as shown in Table 7.2, indications for TJLB may be either absolute or relative.

TJLB may also be used as an adjacent technique for the measurement of hepatic venous pressure gradient (HVPG)—a reliable prognostic marker for survival and response to pharmacologic treatment in patients with clinically significant portal hypertension [24]. Moreover, TJLB plays an important role in the workup of patients who received liver transplantation to histologically assess recipients with HCV reinfection or suspected acute rejection and preservation-reperfusion injury and to measure HVPG [25]. However, the main indication of TJLB has always been represented by the histological assessment of acute alcoholic hepatitis, to guide early corticosteroid therapy [26].

Table 7.2 Absolute and relative indications for transjugular liver biopsy (after Dohan et al., 2014)

Absolute
1. Abnormalities of coagulation
(a) Platelets <50,000 per mm³
(b) Prothrombin time >4 s over control
2. Massive ascites
3. Anticoagulant or antiplatelet aggregation treatment that cannot be interrupted
4. Vascular tumors, hereditary hemorrhagic telangiectasia, or liver peliosis

Relative
1. Need to perform other vascular procedures (hemodynamic study and portography)
2. Inability to perform percutaneous liver biopsy or previously failed percutaneous biopsy
3. Evaluation prior to cardiac and kidney transplant
4. Severe obesity
5. Budd-Chiari syndrome
6. Atrophic liver
7. Suspected amyloidosis
8. Cardiac liver
9. Hemodialysis and chronic kidney disease

While no specific contraindication of TJLB has so far been cited, common recommendations state that the risk-benefit ratio should always be assessed in a case-by-case scenario. However, it is commonly acknowledged that TJLB should not be performed when there is no central venous access available (inferior vena cava obstruction). Moreover, TJLB is contraindicated due to the lack of feasibility in case of thromboses of the right jugular vein [19, 21, 22]. In such cases, expert opinions suggest several alternative access routes like the right external jugular vein, the left internal jugular vein, or the femoral vein. Nevertheless, such techniques are associated with a higher risk for adverse events and should be referred to expert and high-volume centers.

There are some other clinical conditions considered as relative contraindications where TJLB should be avoided due to the increased likelihood for adverse events and complications. Among such conditions are the following [19, 21]: polycystic liver disease, hepatic hydatid disease, acute cholangitis, uncontrolled sepsis and septic shock, focal hepatic lesions and liver trauma, and not the least allergy to contrast agent. Proper patient cooperation and full disclosure and informed consent are also prerequisites for proper TJLB procedure quality.

7.3.2 Technique and Puncture Procedure

Proper preparation requires abdominal ultrasound prior to the procedure to assess liver size, identify any focal lesions, and assess the hepatic veins. Procedure details should be presented to patients, and a written informed consent form should be provided and signed. Using a pre-procedural checklist is encouraged, and it should include (i) ruling out contrast allergy, (ii) 6-h fasting to reduce the chances of aspiration, (iii) ruling out coagulopathy and proper management of antithrombotic agents, and (iv) assessing kidney function. The patient may receive by mouth light sedation using a premedication consisting of anxiolytics and/or antalgics administered 2 h before the procedure. An anesthetic patch may be applied to the puncture site on the neck 1 h before the procedure.

The biopsy should be performed in an interventional radiology room, under strictly aseptic conditions, and the patient's vital signs need to be checked repeatedly by recording arterial pressure and continuous heart monitoring to detect transient arrhythmias which might occur during the transit through the right atrium [23]. In order to increase patient safety, ultrasonographic localization of the right internal jugular vein and real-time guidance of puncture are mandatory as they avoid accidental puncture of the carotid artery and pneumothorax [27]. After the puncture, a guide wire (0.035 in. for 18G) is passed through the needle and a 9Fr sheath is placed. The wire is advanced along the superior vena cava-right atrium-inferior vena cava and into the right hepatic vein. Suitable specimens should be at least 15 mm long and contain at least 6 CPTs, and reliable grading and staging of liver disease require a biopsy of at least 20 mm in length and at least 11 portal tracts [19, 20].

7.3.3 Adverse Events of TJLB

The overall adverse event rate of TJLB is relatively low, with most studies reporting cumulative incidences of under 10%, with minor complications occurring in up to 6.5% of patients, major complications in no more than 1%, and extremely rare cases of death in up to 0.1% of patients [19, 28]. Nevertheless, when pain, abdominal discomfort, and patient intolerance are added on, adverse event rates may reach 30% [23]. Moreover, high-intensity new-onset right upper quadrant pain and worsening of previous dyspnea are highly suggestive for complicated TJLB, and appropriate workup should be indicated to early detect such events. The most frequent adverse events are related to the venous access and puncture and include neck pain, local hematoma, and accidental puncture of carotid artery. Hence, the use of US guidance for venous access has substantially decreased the incidence of such events.

7.4 The Specific Role of EUS-Guided LB and TJLB in NAFLD

Histologic evaluation with liver biopsy is still considered by most authors as the gold standard to diagnose NAFLD as tissue acquisition adds on the diagnosis through its findings that can range from triglyceride deposition as droplets in the hepatocyte to more extensive forms of nonalcoholic steatohepatitis [29]. However, a preemptive diagnosis that would include the medical history, physical examination, and laboratory and imagistic workup seems mandatory. Thus, main indications for tissue acquisition in patients with NAFLD are to confirm or exclude the diagnosis in patients that still have an unclear diagnosis after noninvasive assessments and, in specific cases, to assess the extent of histologic liver damage [30–32].

7.5   Conclusions

Given the constantly growing obesity pandemics and the higher and higher prevalence of metabolic comorbidities, achieving proper workup and management of patients with NAFLD and its complications will clearly require all the complex tools. Among these, EUS-guided LB and TJLB will not only hold their position and gold standard for NAFLD diagnosis but also gain an extension to their applications towards achieving proper differential diagnosis and risk stratification of liver histologic damage.

References

1. Ando Y, Jou JH. Nonalcoholic fatty liver disease and recent guideline updates. Clin Liver Dis (Hoboken). 2021;17(1):23–8.
2. Sue MJ, Lee EW, Saab S, McWilliams JP, Durazo F, El-Kabany M, et al. Transjugular liver biopsy: safe even in patients with severe coagulopathies and multiple biopsies. Clin Transl Gastroenterol [Internet]. 2019;10(7):63. Available from: /pmc/articles/PMC6708667/. [cited 2022 Oct 29].
3. Dhar J, Samanta J. Role of endoscopic ultrasound in the field of hepatology: recent advances and future trends. World J Hepatol [Internet]. 2021;13(11):1459. Available from: /pmc/articles/PMC8637671/. [cited 2022 Oct 29].
4. Jearth V, Sundaram S, Rana S. Diagnostic and interventional EUS in hepatology: an updated review. Endosc Ultrasound [Internet]. 2022;11(5):355. Available from: http://www.eusjournal.com/text.asp?2022/11/5/355/357886
5. Madhok IK, Parsa N, Nieto JM. Endoscopic ultrasound-guided liver biopsy. Clin Liver Dis [Internet]. 2022;26(1):127–38. Available from: https://pubmed.ncbi.nlm.nih.gov/34802658/. [cited 2022 Oct 30].
6. Mohan BP, Shakhatreh M, Garg R, Ponnada S, Adler DG. Efficacy and safety of EUS-guided liver biopsy: a systematic review and meta-analysis. Gastrointest Endosc [Internet]. 2019;89(2):238–246.e3. Available from: https://pubmed.ncbi.nlm.nih.gov/30389469/. [cited 2022 Oct 30].
7. Rangwani S, Ardeshna DR, Mumtaz K, Kelly SG, Han SY, Krishna SG. Update on endoscopic ultrasound-guided liver biopsy. World J Gastroenterol [Internet]. 2022;28(28):3586. Available from: /pmc/articles/PMC9372801/. [cited 2022 Oct 30].
8. Dumonceau JM, Riphaus A, Schreiber F, Vilmann P, Beilenhoff U, Aparicio JR, et al. Non-anesthesiologist administration of propofol for gastrointestinal endoscopy: European Society of Gastrointestinal Endoscopy, European Society of Gastroenterology and Endoscopy Nurses and Associates Guideline—updated June 2015. Endoscopy [Internet]. 2015;47:1175–89. Available from: http://www.esge.com/. [cited 2022 Nov 6].
9. Early DS, Lightdale JR, Vargo JJ, Acosta RD, Chandrasekhara V, Chathadi KV, et al. Guidelines for sedation and anesthesia in GI endoscopy ASGE standards of practice committee. Gastrointest Endosc [Internet]. 2018;87:327–37. https://doi.org/10.1016/j.gie.2017.07.018. [cited 2022 Nov 6].
10. Kovacevic B, Vilmann P. EUS tissue acquisition: from A to B. Endosc Ultrasound [Internet]. 2020;9(4):–225. Available from: http://www.eusjournal.com/article.asp?issn=2303-9027;year=2020;volume=9;issue=4;spage=225;epage=231;aulast=Kovacevic. [cited 2022 Nov 6].
11. Mok SRS, Diehl DL, Johal AS, Khara HS, Confer BD, Mudireddy PR, et al. A prospective pilot comparison of wet and dry heparinized suction for EUS-guided liver biopsy (with videos). Gastrointest Endosc [Internet]. 2018, 88;(6):919–25. Available from: https://pubmed.ncbi.nlm.nih.gov/30120956/. [cited 2022 Nov 6].

12. Madhok IK, Parsa N, Nieto JM. Endoscopic ultrasound-guided liver biopsy. Vol. 26, Clinics in liver disease. W.B. Saunders; 2022. p. 127–38.

13. Baran B, Kale S, Patil P, Kannadath B, Ramireddy S, Badillo R, et al. Endoscopic ultrasound-guided parenchymal liver biopsy: a systematic review and meta-analysis. Surg Endosc [Internet]. 2021;35:–10, 5546, 57. Available from: https://pubmed-ncbi-nlm-nih-gov.dbproxy.umfiasi.ro/33052529/. [cited 2022 Nov 6].

14. Bravo AA, Sheth SG, Chopra S. Liver biopsy. N Engl J Med. 2001;344(7):495–500.

15. Nousbaum JB, Cadranel JF, Bonnemaison G, Bourlière M, Chiche L, Chor H, Denninger MH, Degos F, Jacquemin E, Le Bail B, Loustaud-Ratti V. Clinical practice guidelines on the use of liver biopsy. Gastroenterologie clinique et biologique. 2002;26(10):848–78.

16. Cadranel JF, Nousbaum JB, Gouillou M, Hanslik B. Major changes in the number and indications of liver biopsy for chronic liver diseases over one decade in France. Eur J Gastroenterol Hepatol. 2016;28(9):e26–32.

17. Colloredo G, Guido M, Sonzogni A, Leandro G. Impact of liver biopsy size on histological evaluation of chronic viral hepatitis: the smaller the sample, the milder the disease. J Hepatol. 2003;39(2):239–44.

18. Guido M, Rugge M. Liver biopsy sampling in chronic viral hepatitis. Semin Liver Dis. 2004;24(01):89–97. Copyright© 2004 by Thieme Medical Publishers, Inc.

19. Kalambokis G, Manousou P, Vibhakorn S, Marelli L, Cholongitas E, Senzolo M, Patch D, Burroughs AK. Transjugular liver biopsy–indications, adequacy, quality of specimens, and complications–a systematic review. J Hepatol. 2007;47(2):284–94.

20. Cholongitas E, Quaglia A, Samonakis D, Senzolo M, Triantos C, Patch D, Leandro G, Dhillon AP, Burroughs AK. Transjugular liver biopsy: how good is it for accurate histological interpretation? Gut. 2006;55(12):1789–94.

21. Ble M, Procopet B, Miquel R, Hernandez-Gea V, García-Pagán JC. Transjugular liver biopsy. Clin Liver Dis. 2014;18(4):767–78.

22. Keshava SN, Mammen T, Surendrababu NR, Moses V. Transjugular liver biopsy: what to do and what not to do. Indian J Radiol Imaging. 2008;18(03):245–8.

23. Dohan A, Guerrache Y, Boudiaf M, Gavini JP, Kaci R, Soyer P. Transjugular liver biopsy: indications, technique and results. Diagn Interv Imaging. 2014;95(1):11–5.

24. Reiberger T, Schwabl P, Trauner M, Peck-Radosavljevic M, Mandorfer M. Measurement of the hepatic venous pressure gradient and transjugular liver biopsy. JoVE. 2020;18(160):e58819.

25. Geramizadeh B, Malek-Hosseini SA. Role of histopathologist in liver transplantation. Int J Organ Transpl Med. 2017;8(1):1.

26. Dhanda AD, Collins PL, McCune CA. Is liver biopsy necessary in the management of alcoholic hepatitis? World J Gastroenterol: WJG. 2013;19(44):7825.

27. Soyer P, Fargeaudou Y, Boudiaf M, Rymer R. Transjugular liver biopsy using ultrasonographic guidance for jugular vein puncture and an automated device for hepatic tissue sampling: a retrospective analysis of 200 consecutive cases. Abdom Imaging. 2008;33(6):627–32.

28. Kis B, Pamarthi V, Fan CM, Rabkin D, Baum RA. Safety and utility of transjugular liver biopsy in hematopoietic stem cell transplant recipients. J Vasc Interv Radiol. 2013;24(1):85–9.

29. Pouwels S, Sakran N, Graham Y, Leal A, Pintar T, Yang W, Kassir R, Singhal R, Mahawar K, Ramnarain D. Non-alcoholic fatty liver disease (NAFLD): a review of pathophysiology, clinical management and effects of weight loss. BMC Endocr Disord. 2022;22(1):1–9.

30. Ratziu V, Charlotte F, Heurtier A, Gombert S, Giral P, Bruckert E, Grimaldi A, Capron F, Poynard T, LIDO Study Group. Sampling variability of liver biopsy in nonalcoholic fatty liver disease. Gastroenterology. 2005;128(7):1898–906.

31. Merriman RB, Ferrell LD, Patti MG, Weston SR, Pabst MS, Aouizerat BE, Bass NM. Correlation of paired liver biopsies in morbidly obese patients with suspected nonalcoholic fatty liver disease. Hepatology. 2006;44(4):874–80.

32. Arun J, Jhala N, Lazenby AJ, Clements R, Abrams GA. Influence of liver biopsy heterogeneity and diagnosis of nonalcoholic steatohepatitis in subjects undergoing gastric bypass. Obes Surg. 2007;17(2):155–61.

Morphopathology of Nonalcoholic Fatty Liver Disease

8

Mirela Marinela Florescu and Dan Ionuț Gheonea

8.1 Introduction

Nonalcoholic fatty liver disease (NAFLD) is a disorder outlined by redundant conglomeration of triglycerides within the hepatocytes that outstrip 5% of liver weight, in a liver with no history of alcohol abuse. NAFLD includes a large spectrum of disease such as simple steatosis or even nonalcoholic steatohepatitis (NASH).

Past studies considered that these entities can rarely lead to cirrhosis and hepatocellular carcinoma, but as chronic viral hepatitis C is targeted for worldwide elimination, NAFLD and NASH are expected to lead to more and more cases of cirrhosis and even hepatocellular carcinoma [1, 2].

Histopathologically, lobular inflammation, macrovesicular steatosis, and hepatocyte ballooning determinate the presence of NASH. In most of the cases, the pathology of NASH is not much different from alcoholic fatty liver disease. Therefore, the diagnosis can only be made in the total or significant absence of alcohol consumption or in the case of ingestion of less than 30 g/day of alcohol for men and 20 g/day of alcohol for women [3].

NAFLD is becoming one of the most common liver diseases today, being identified by imaging studies in approximately 20–33% of the adults [3–5]. NAFLD is frequently diagnosed from the fourth to the sixth decades of life, although the increase in childhood obesity has also influenced the increased rate of NAFLD in children.

The prevalence of this disease also varies according to the ethnicity of the patients, affecting ~45% of the Hispanic population, 33% of the white population, and 24% of the African American population. Among the white population, NAFLD

M. M. Florescu · D. I. Gheonea (✉)
University of Medicine and Pharmacy of Craiova, Craiova, Romania
e-mail: mirela.florescu@umfcv.ro; dan.gheonea@umfcv.com

A. Trifan et al. (eds.), *Essentials of Non-Alcoholic Fatty Liver Disease*,
https://doi.org/10.1007/978-3-031-33548-8_8

Table 8.1 Secondary causes of NAFLD

Disorders of lipid metabolism	Medications	Nutritional causes	Other causes
Abetalipoproteinemia	Highly active antiretroviral therapy	Total parenteral nutrition	Celiac disease
Familial hypobetalipoproteinemia	Tamoxifen	Severe surgical weight loss	Hepatitis C infection
Familial combined hyperlipidemia	Amiodarone	Starvation	Wilson's disease
Glycogen storage disease	Methotrexate		Environmental toxicity
Weber–Christian syndrome	Corticosteroids		
Lipodystrophy			

is more common in men than in women, in contrast to the Hispanic and African American population where the ratio between men and women is 1:1 [6].

NAFLD is included in the metabolic syndrome, being considered a hepatic manifestation of it. From an etiological point of view, NAFLD is associated with hepatic and systemic insulin resistance, obesity, type 2 diabetes, and dyslipidemia [1, 2].

However, quite a few cases of NAFLD result from various specific secondary causes (Table 8.1) [7–13].

8.2 Histopathological Diagnosis of NAFLD/NASH

In order to be able to diagnose NAFLD/NASH, we usually have to clinically exclude other liver diseases such as alcoholic hepatic steatosis, Wilson's disease, acute and chronic viral hepatitis, or liver lesions caused by medication (antiretroviral therapies, amiodarone, tamoxifen, corticosteroids, methotrexate). From a histopathological point of view, the diagnosis of NAFLD/NASH is highlighted by the presence of macronodular steatosis accentuated in zone 3 (Figs. 8.1 and 8.2) and the presence of a slight polymorphic inflammation and hepatocellular ballooning, also most frequently found in zone 3. The presence of fibrosis can also be observed quite frequently but does not represent a diagnostic criterion for this type of disease [14–16].

Histopathological aspects of NAFLD/NASH include:

- Steatosis
- Portal and lobular inflammation
- Mallory-Denk bodies
- Hepatocellular ballooning
- Apoptotic hepatocytes
- Glycogenated nuclei
- Megamitochondria
- Iron deposits
- Fibrosis

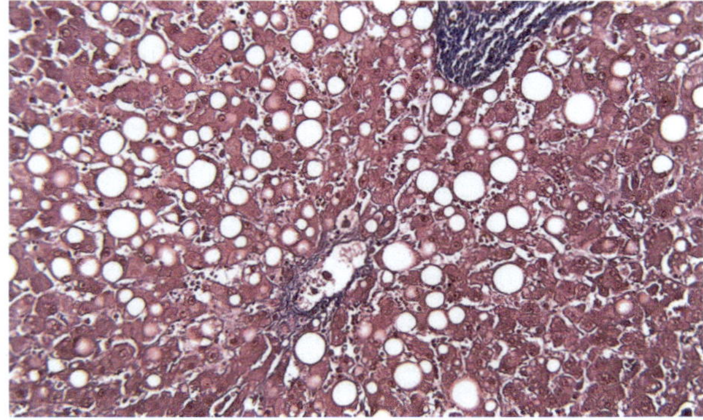

Fig. 8.1 Macrovesicular steatosis in nonalcoholic fatty liver disease. Masson's trichrome staining. Macrovesicular steatosis predominant in zone 3

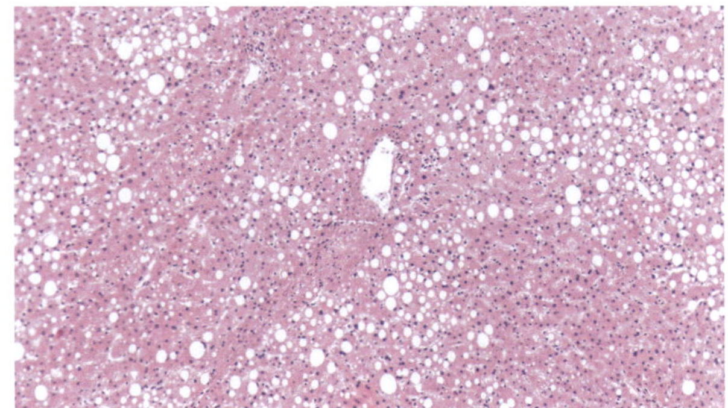

Fig. 8.2 Macrovesicular steatosis in nonalcoholic fatty liver disease. Hematoxylin and eosin staining. Macrovesicular steatosis predominant in zone 3

8.2.1 Steatosis

Steatosis represents the most important aspect of NAFLD. Hepatocellular steatosis can be of two types: microvesicular steatosis (hepatocytes contain small fat vacuoles in the cytoplasm, with the nucleus located centrally) and macrovesicular steatosis (hepatocytes contain large or small well-defined fat vacuoles that can converge and push the nucleus to the periphery). In most cases of NAFLD, the steatosis is macrovesicular. In order to make a diagnosis of NAFLD, it is necessary that steatosis is present in more than 5% of hepatocytes [17–20].

8.2.2 Portal and Lobular Inflammation

Also, both intralobular inflammation and portal inflammation are present in NAFLD/NASH. The intralobular inflammation is frequently mild and is expressed by a polymorphic inflammatory infiltrate that contains both neutrophils and lymphocytes, plasma cells, Kupffer cells, and eosinophils. This type of inflammation is more common in NASH [20]. Moreover, also in NASH, agglomerations of sinusoidal Kupffer cells and lipogranulomas consisting of fat vacuoles, collagen fibers, and a polymorphic inflammatory infiltrate are observed. Portal inflammation is usually mild or even absent in NAFLD/NASH, composed mainly of chronic inflammatory cells (lymphocytes). In cases where the portal inflammation is severe, several studies have shown that the possibility of autoimmune hepatitis or even a viral hepatitis with virus C should be considered. Medium or severe chronic portal inflammation has always been associated with the localization of steatosis, hepatocyte ballooning, and appearance of advanced fibrosis [21, 22]. Thus, in an untreated NAFLD, moderate or even severe chronic portal inflammation can be perceived as a marker of advanced liver diseases [22, 23].

8.2.3   Mallory-Denk Bodies

Mallory-Denk bodies (MDBs) are frequently observed in ballooned hepatocytes, especially in zone 3 (centrolobular). These structures are represented by cytokeratin 8 and 18, p16, and ubiquitin. They stand out as eosinophilic aggregates with an irregular shape that are found in the cytoplasm of hepatocyte cells, with their role being still unclear [24]. The immunohistochemical examination helps to identify these aggregates of cytokeratins 8 and 18 if they are present in the ballooned cells. The presence of MDBs is very useful in the diagnosis of NASH, but these structures are also found in other liver pathologies such as chronic cholestasis or alcoholic hepatitis [25]. For a differential diagnosis, we can take into account the presence of MBDs in non-ballooned cells in the case of alcoholic hepatitis [8, 21].

8.2.4   Hepatocellular Ballooning

The process by which ballooned hepatocytes appear was highlighted following the alteration of the intermediate filament of the cytoskeleton. Thus, cytokeratins 8 and 18 (hepatocyte keratins) are dispersed and are found only in the periphery of the cytoplasm [26]. Hepatocyte ballooning is highlighted in hematoxylin-eosin staining by large, swollen hepatocytes with rarefied cytoplasm. Fat vacuoles and/or MDBs can be highlighted inside them. Because in hematoxylin-eosin staining ballooned hepatocyte cells can be recognized with difficulty, it is important to use the immunohistochemical marker cytokeratin 8/18 to highlight the lack of immunostaining. This is considered an objective marker of ballooned hepatocytes [27].

8.2.5   Apoptotic Hepatocytes

In NASH, apoptotic hepatocytes can also be present, which are frequently found in the sinusoids. These acidophilic bodies are represented by intensely eosinophilic and round bodies, with/or without the presence of hyperchromatic nuclear fragments [28].

8.2.6 Glycogenated Nuclei

The presence of glycogenated nuclei is frequently found in NAFLD. These are visible vacuolated nuclei in the periportal hepatocytes. The identification of these nuclei is important in differentiating NASH from alcoholic steatohepatitis (ASH), because in ASH they are rarely found [29].

8.2.7 Megamitochondria

Megamitochondria are frequently found in hepatocytes with microvesicular steatosis. They are represented by the round structure or in the form of crystals, as eosinophils located in the cytoplasm of liver cells. Although the mechanism of production of these lesions is poorly understood in NASH, they could represent an adapted change of mitochondria or may be caused by lipid peroxidation [30].

8.2.8 Iron Deposits

Iron deposits can be present in NAFLD/NASH both in liver cells and in sinusoidal lining cells of the reticuloendothelial system [21, 31, 32]. Some specialized studies highlight the fact that the accumulation of iron predominantly in hepatocytes leads to the appearance of advanced fibrosis in NASH. There are also studies that demonstrated that iron accumulations at the level of the reticuloendothelial system were associated with advanced fibrosis, compared to patients in which iron accumulations were at the level of hepatocytes [33, 34].

8.2.9 Fibrosis

Perisinusoidal or pericellular fibrosis (chicken wire) is characteristic in NASH and is frequently found in zone 3. To highlight the fibrosis, special stains can be used such as Masson's trichrome stain or stains for reticulin fibers. In NAFLD, fibrosis is often accompanied by an active necroinflammatory reaction. In the evolution of NASH, portal/periportal fibrosis may appear, afterwards bridging fibrosis, and finally liver cirrhosis may also develop [35, 36]. In a meta-analysis of ten histological studies carried out by Argo CK et al. in 2009, the following were highlighted as independent markers of progression to advanced fibrosis in NASH: parenchymal inflammation or portal inflammation, but also the older age of patients in the case of the first biopsies performed [37]. There is also the notion of burnout NASH, which is used in the event that during the onset of advanced fibrosis or cirrhosis, necroinflammatory reactions and steatosis disappear [26, 38]. NAFLD/NASH is one of the main causes of cryptogenic cirrhosis [39], and the macroscopic appearance of cirrhosis associated with NASH can be both macronodular and mixed [40, 41].

Table 8.2 Grading and staging system of NASH

Grading

	Steatosis	Ballooning	Intralobular inflammation	Portal inflammation
Grade 1 (mild)	+++	± In zone 3	+ Polymorphs ± Lymphocytes	±
Grade 2 (moderate)	+++	++ In zone 3	+ Polymorphs + Lymphocytes	+/++
Grade 3 (severe)	++++	+++ In zone 3	+ Polymorphs ± Lymphocytes	+/++

Staging

Stage 1	Perisinusoidal fibrosis, focal/extensive
Stage 2	Perisinusoidal and periportal fibrosis, focal/extensive
Stage 3	Perisinusoidal and periportal fibrosis + bridging fibrosis
Stage 4	Cirrhosis

8.3 Grading and Staging System of NASH

In 1999, Brunt et al. classified NASH into three grades, in which hepatocellular steatosis, presence of portal or intralobular inflammation, and ballooning of hepatocytes are analyzed. Grade 1 was described as the mild form, grade 2 as the moderate form, and grade 3 as the severe form (Table 8.2). At the same time, the same authors proposed a score based on the location and extent of the fibrosis. Thus, three stages resulted: stage 1 in which the fibrosis is located in perisinusoidal zone 3, stage 2 in which the fibrosis is located both perisinusoidally and at the periportal level, stage 3 in which bridges of porto-portal and porto-centrolobular fibrosis are formed, and stage 4 cirrhosis (Table 8.2) [14]. Several years later from the classification made by Brunt et al., the NASH Clinical Research Network (NASH CRN) subclassified stage 1 into stage 1A in which mild fibrosis is observed in zone 3, perisinusoidal; stage 1B in which a moderate fibrosis appears in zone 3; and stage 1C in which only portal and periportal fibrosis can be noted (Table 8.2) [14, 17].

8.4 Differential Diagnosis

NAFLD requires histological differentiation from alcoholic liver disease, which can be a demanding task even when considering anamnesis and clinical aspects of the patients. There are a few histological dissimilarities that have been outlined.

More regular aspects in ASH embrace canalicular cholestasis, frequent and well-proportioned MDBs, prominent ductular reaction, as well as acute inflammation and fibrosis in the portal extent. In a few occasions, other aspects can be noticed in alcoholic liver disease such as sclerosing hyaline, necrosis, and veno-occlusive lesions, whereas in NAFLD, such lesions have not been reported [21].

Regarding the necroinflammatory activity, data reports suggest that it is more severe in ASH than in NASH [27]. On the other hand, there are histological aspects like glycogenated nuclei or lipogranulomas that are more common in NASH. In a similar manner, severe steatosis is a common feature as well; hence, steatosis is a prime pathological aspect of NASH, which can be absent in some cases of ASH.

There are differences regarding fibrosis in both ASH and NASH that show distinct patterns. Fibrosis pattern in ASH is a firm pattern on reticulin-strained slides, whereas in NASH, the fibrosis reveals in a lattice pattern [41].

8.5   Evolution

NASH is considered to be involved in the development of liver cirrhosis and hepatocellular carcinoma. In the course of developing antiviral treatment of chronic hepatitis B and elimination of chronic hepatitis C through interferon-free treatment, 5-year incidence estimates of HCC suggest increasing cases for cirrhotic NASH compared to viral hepatitis in the past [42, 43].

There is undergoing research to fully clarify specific pathological aspects regarding HCC development in patients with NASH. Past research indicated a characteristic HCC histological type developed in cases of extensive steatosis.

These variants were described as steatohepatitis hepatocellular carcinoma (SH-HCC), and several histological aspects were enhanced such as large droplet steatosis, ballooning of malignant hepatocytes, MDBs, as well as chronic inflammation or pericellular fibrosis [42]. Other reports also indicate that the prevalence of SH-HCC is increasing in patients with NASH or ASH, and most cases develop on severe steatohepatitis, hence the hefty interconnection of SH-HCC and NASH. Also, new data shows that SH-HCC tends to develop more often in cirrhotic NAFLD patients in contrast with ASH [43].

There are literature reports that suggest the possibility of NAFLD regression, but at the same, it is estimated that over 20% of patients with NASH and bridging fibrosis progress to liver cirrhosis and first liver decompensation within the first 2 years of the diagnosis [44].

References

1. Marchesini G, Bugianesi E, Forlani G, Cerrelli F, Lenzi M, Manini R, Natale S, Vanni E, Villanova N, Melchionda N, et al. Nonalcoholic fatty liver, steatohepatitis, and the metabolic syndrome. Hepatology. 2003;37:917–23.
2. Abdelmalek MF, Diehl AM. Nonalcoholic fatty liver disease as a complication of insulin resistance. Med Clin North Am. 2007;91:1125–49, ix.
3. Sanyal AJ, Brunt EM, Kleiner DE, Kowdley KV, Chalasani N, Lavine JE, Ratziu V, McCullough A. Endpoints and clinical trial design for nonalcoholic steatohepatitis. Hepatology. 2011;54(1):344–53. https://doi.org/10.1002/hep.24376.
4. Younossi ZM, Koenig AB, Abdelatif D, Fazel Y, Henry L, Wymer M. Global epidemiology of nonalcoholic fatty liver disease-meta-analytic assessment of prevalence, incidence, and outcomes. Hepatology. 2016;64(1):73–84.
5. Ratziu V, Bellentani S, Cortez-Pinto H, Day C, Marchesini G. A position statement on NAFLD/NASH based on the EASL 2009 special conference. J Hepatol. 2010;53(2):372–84. https://doi.org/10.1016/j.jhep.2010.04.008.

 6. Angulo P. GI epidemiology: nonalcoholic fatty liver disease. Aliment Pharmacol Ther. 2007;25(8):883–9. https://doi.org/10.1111/j.1365-2036.2007.03246.x.
 7. Zeissig S, Dougan SK, Barral DC, Junker Y, Chen Z, Kaser A, Ho M, Mandel H, McIntyre A, Kennedy SM, Painter GF, Veerapen N, Besra GS, Cerundolo V, Yue S, Beladi S, Behar SM, Chen X, Gumperz JE, Breckpot K, Raper A, Baer A, Exley MA, Hegele RA, Cuchel M, Rader DJ, Davidson NO, Blumberg RS. Primary deficiency of microsomal triglyceride transfer protein in human abetalipoproteinemia is associated with loss of CD1 function. J Clin Invest. 2010;120(8):2889–99. https://doi.org/10.1172/JCI42703.
 8. de Bruin TW, Georgieva AM, Brouwers MC, Heitink MV, van der Kallen CJ, van Greevenbroek MM. Radiological evidence of nonalcoholic fatty liver disease in familial combined hyperlipidemia. Am J Med. 2004;116(12):847–9. https://doi.org/10.1016/j.amjmed.2003.12.031.
 9. Kishnani PS, Austin SL, Arn P, Bali DS, Boney A, Case LE, Chung WK, Desai DM, El-Gharbawy A, Haller R, Smit GP, Smith AD, Hobson-Webb LD, Wechsler SB, Weinstein DA, Watson MS, ACMG. Glycogen storage disease type III diagnosis and management guidelines. Genet Med. 2010;12(7):446–63. https://doi.org/10.1097/GIM.0b013e3181e655b6. Erratum in: Genet Med.
10. Herranz P, de Lucas R, Pérez-España L, Mayor M. Lipodystrophy syndromes. Dermatol Clin. 2008;26(4):569–78, ix. https://doi.org/10.1016/j.det.2008.05.004.
11. Gan SK, Watts GF. Is adipose tissue lipolysis always an adaptive response to starvation?: Implications for non-alcoholic fatty liver disease. Clin Sci (Lond). 2008;114(8):543–5. https://doi.org/10.1042/CS20070461.
12. Allard JP. Other disease associations with non-alcoholic fatty liver disease (NAFLD). Best Pract Res Clin Gastroenterol. 2002;16(5):783–95. https://doi.org/10.1053/bega.2002.0330.
13. Kneeman JM, Misdraji J, Corey KE. Secondary causes of nonalcoholic fatty liver disease. Ther Adv Gastroenterol. 2012;5(3):199–207.
14. Brunt EM, Tiniakos DG. Alcoholic and non-alcoholic fatty liver disease. In: Odze RD, Goldblum JR, Crawford JM, editors. Pathology of the GI tract, liver, biliary tract and pancreas. Philadelphia: Saunders; 2009. p. 1087–114.
15. Brunt EM, Janney CG, Di Bisceglie AM, NeuschwanderTetri BA, Bacon BR. Nonalcoholic steatohepatitis: a proposal for grading and staging the histological lesions. Am J Gastroenterol. 1999;94:2467–74.
16. Brunt EM, Kleiner DE, Wilson LA, Belt P, NeuschwanderTetri BA. Nonalcoholic fatty liver disease (NAFLD) activity score and the histopathologic diagnosis in NAFLD: distinct clinico-pathologic meanings. Hepatology. 2011;53:810–20.
17. Kleiner DE, Brunt EM, Van Natta M, Behling C, Contos MJ, Cummings OW, Ferrell LD, Liu YC, Torbenson MS, UnalpArida A, Yeh M, McCullough AJ, Sanyal AJ. Design and validation of a histological scoring system for nonalcoholic fatty liver disease. Hepatology. 2005;41:1313–21. https://doi.org/10.1002/hep.20701.
18. Yeh MM, Brunt EM. Pathology of nonalcoholic fatty liver disease. Am J Clin Pathol. 2007;128:837–47. https://doi.org/10.1309/RTPM1PY6YGBL2G2R.
19. Patton HM, Lavine JE, Van Natta ML, Schwimmer JB, Kleiner D, Molleston J. Clinical correlates of histopathology in pediatric nonalcoholic steatohepatitis. Gastroenterology. 2008;135:1961–1971.e2. https://doi.org/10.1053/j.gastro.2008.08.050.
20. Tandra S, Yeh MM, Brunt EM, Vuppalanchi R, Cummings OW, Unalp-Arida A, Wilson LA, Chalasani N. Presence and significance of microvesicular steatosis in nonalcoholic fatty liver disease. J Hepatol. 2011;55:654–9. https://doi.org/10.1016/j.jhep.2010.11.021.
21. Takahashi Y, Fukusato T. Histopathology of nonalcoholic fatty liver disease/nonalcoholic steatohepatitis. World J Gastroenterol. 2014;20(42):15539–48. https://doi.org/10.3748/wjg.v20.i42.15539.
22. Brunt EM, Kleiner DE, Wilson LA, Unalp A, Behling CE, Lavine JE, Neuschwander-Tetri BA. Portal chronic inflammation in nonalcoholic fatty liver disease (NAFLD): a histologic marker of advanced NAFLD-Clinicopathologic correlations from the nonalcoholic steatohepatitis clinical research network. Hepatology. 2009;49:809–20. https://doi.org/10.1002/hep.22724.

23. Rakha EA, Adamson L, Bell E, Neal K, Ryder SD, Kaye PV, Aithal GP. Portal inflammation is associated with advanced histological changes in alcoholic and non-alcoholic fatty liver disease. J Clin Pathol. 2010;63:790–5. https://doi.org/10.1136/jcp.2010.079145.
24. Zatloukal K, French SW, Stumptner C, Strnad P, Harada M, Toivola DM, Cadrin M, Omary MB. From Mallory to Mallory-Denk bodies: what, how and why? Exp Cell Res. 2007;313:2033–49. https://doi.org/10.1016/j.yexcr.2007.04.024.
25. Denk H, Stumptner C, Zatloukal K. Mallory bodies revisited. J Hepatol. 2000;32:689–702. https://doi.org/10.1016/S0168-8278(00)80233-0.
26. Brunt EM. Pathology of nonalcoholic fatty liver disease. Nat Rev Gastroenterol Hepatol. 2010;7:195–203. https://doi.org/10.1038/nrgastro.2010.21.
27. Lackner C, Gogg-Kamerer M, Zatloukal K, Stumptner C, Brunt EM, Denk H. Ballooned hepatocytes in steatohepatitis: the value of keratin immunohistochemistry for diagnosis. J Hepatol. 2008;48:82. https://doi.org/10.1016/j.jhep.2008.01.026.
28. Feldstein AE, Gores GJ. Apoptosis in alcoholic and nonalcoholic steatohepatitis. Front Biosci. 2005;10:3093–9.
29. Pinto HC, Baptista A, Camilo ME, Valente A, Saragoça A, de Moura MC, Nonalcoholic steatohepatitis. Clinicopathological comparison with alcoholic hepatitis in ambulatory and hospitalized patients. Dig Dis Sci. 1996;41:172–9.
30. Le TH, Caldwell SH, Redick JA, Sheppard BL, Davis CA, Arseneau KO, Iezzoni JC, Hespenheide EE, Al-Osaimi A, Peterson TC. The zonal distribution of megamitochondria with crystalline inclusions in nonalcoholic steatohepatitis. Hepatology. 2004;39:1423–9. https://doi.org/10.1002/hep.20202.
31. Struben VM, Hespenheide EE, Caldwell SH. Nonalcoholic steatohepatitis and cryptogenic cirrhosis within kindreds. Am J Med. 2000;108:9–13. https://doi.org/10.1016/S0002-9343(99)00315-0.
32. Brunt EM. Non-alcoholic fatty liver disease: what's new under the microscope? Gut. 2011;60:1152–8. https://doi.org/10.1136/gut.2010.218214.
33. Valenti L, Fracanzani AL, Bugianesi E, Dongiovanni P, Galmozzi E, Vanni E, Canavesi E, Lattuada E, Roviaro G, Marchesini G, Fargion S. HFE genotype, parenchymal iron accumulation, and liver fibrosis in patients with nonalcoholic fatty liver disease. Gastroenterology. 2010;138:905–12. https://doi.org/10.1053/j.gastro.2009.11.013.
34. Nelson JE, Wilson L, Brunt EM, Yeh MM, Kleiner DE, Unalp-Arida A, Kowdley KV. Relationship between the pattern of hepatic iron deposition and histological severity in nonalcoholic fatty liver disease. Hepatology. 2011;53:448–57. https://doi.org/10.1002/hep.24038.
35. Skoien R, Richardson MM, Jonsson JR, Powell EE, Brunt EM, Neuschwander-Tetri BA, Bhathal PS, Dixon JB, O'Brien PE, Tilg H, Moschen AR, Baumann U, Brown RM, Couper RT, Manton ND, Ee LC, Weltman M, Clouston AD. Heterogeneity of fibrosis patterns in nonalcoholic fatty liver disease supports the presence of multiple fibrogenic pathways. Liver Int. 2013;33:624–32. https://doi.org/10.1111/liv.12100.
36. Tiniakos DG. Nonalcoholic fatty liver disease/nonalcoholic steatohepatitis: histological diagnostic criteria and scoring systems. Eur J Gastroenterol Hepatol. 2010;22:643–50. https://doi.org/10.1097/MEG.0b013e32832ca0cb.
37. Argo CK, Northup PG, Al-Osaimi AM, Caldwell SH. Systematic review of risk factors for fibrosis progression in nonalcoholic steatohepatitis. J Hepatol. 2009;51:371–9. https://doi.org/10.1016/j.jhep.2009.03.019.
38. Caldwell SH, Lee VD, Kleiner DE, Al-Osaimi AM, Argo CK, Northup PG, Berg CL. NASH and cryptogenic cirrhosis: a histological analysis. Ann Hepatol. 2009;8:346–52.
39. Caldwell SH, Oelsner DH, Iezzoni JC, Hespenheide EE, Battle EH, Driscoll CJ. Cryptogenic cirrhosis: clinical characterization and risk factors for underlying disease. Hepatology. 1999;29:664–9.
40. Poonawala A, Nair SP, Thuluvath PJ. Prevalence of obesity and diabetes in patients with cryptogenic cirrhosis: a case-control study. Hepatology. 2000:689–92.

41. Nakano M, Fukusato T. Histological study on comparison between NASH and ALD. Hepatol Res. 2005;33:110–5.
42. Yatsuji S, Hashimoto E, Tobari M, Taniai M, Tokushige K, Shiratori K. Clinical features and outcomes of cirrhosis due to non-alcoholic steatohepatitis compared with cirrhosis caused by chronic hepatitis C. J Gastroenterol Hepatol. 2009;24:248–54. https://doi.org/10.1111/j.1440-1746.2008.05640.x.
43. Salomao M, Remotti H, Vaughan R, Siegel AB, Lefkowitch JH, Moreira RK. The steatohepatitic variant of hepatocellular carcinoma and its association with underlying steatohepatitis. Hum Pathol. 2012;43:737–46. https://doi.org/10.1016/j.humpath.2011.07.005.
44. Loomba R, Adams LA. The 20% rule of NASH progression: the natural history of advanced fibrosis and cirrhosis caused by NASH. Hepatology. 2019;70(6):1885–8. https://doi.org/10.1002/hep.30946.

2D Shear Wave Elastography Performance in the Diagnosis of Nonalcoholic Fatty Liver Disease

9

Ioan Sporea and Alina Popescu

9.1 Introduction

Nonalcoholic fatty liver disease (NAFLD) currently represents an important public health problem, due to its high and increasing frequency in the general population [1]. It can be divided from the point of view of prognosis into simple hepatic steatosis, generally without the potential of progression to liver cirrhosis, and nonalcoholic steatohepatitis (NASH), in which the central element is inflammation [2]. The prognosis, however, in this last category, is given by the presence of fibrosis, with potential evolution towards cirrhosis and hepatocellular carcinoma, respectively, hence the importance of evaluating the severity of liver fibrosis in NAFLD, for the stratification of the prognosis and the modulation of therapeutic interventions.

The method currently considered the "gold standard" for evaluating liver fibrosis is liver biopsy, an invasive procedure, burdened by the possibility of complications [3] and generally being more difficult to be accepted by patients. However, there are currently noninvasive evaluation methods, which have the advantage of much easier acceptance by patients, being free of complications, and having elements that recommend them also in the case of the need for repetitive evaluations.

The role of noninvasive assessment would be to identify people at risk of NAFLD among people at increased metabolic risk, among those with NAFLD, to

I. Sporea (✉) · A. Popescu
Department of Internal Medicine II, Division of Gastroenterology and Hepatology, Center for Advanced Research in Gastroenterology and Hepatology, "Victor Babeş" University of Medicine and Pharmacy, Timişoara, Romania

Department of Gastroenterology and Hepatology, "Pius Brânzeu" Clinical Emergency County Hospital, Timişoara, Romania

Regional Center of Research in Advanced Hepatology, Academy of Medical Sciences, Timişoara, Romania
e-mail: isporea@umft.ro

A. Trifan et al. (eds.), *Essentials of Non-Alcoholic Fatty Liver Disease*,
https://doi.org/10.1007/978-3-031-33548-8_9

identify those with a more severe prognosis requiring specific interventions, to monitor the evolution of the disease, and to assess the response to therapeutic interventions [2].

Ultrasound-based elastography is a method that has developed rapidly recently, due to its applications in multiple liver pathologies, due to the fact that it is a fast method, and due to it being easily accepted by patients, which can be repeated and is not very expensive [4]. It is also the most frequently used method at present, for the noninvasive evaluation of liver fibrosis.

International guidelines classify these US elastography techniques into strain elastography (developed mainly for breast, thyroid, and prostate nodule assessment) and shear wave elastography (SWE—in which the speed of shear waves generated inside the liver is measured by ultrasound) [4, 5].

Based on the type of external impulse and the technology used to measure the shear wave speed, SWE elastography is subdivided into transient elastography (TE), point SWE (pSWE), and real-time elastography which includes 2D-SWE and 3D-SWE [4, 5].

9.2   2D-SWE Technique

For 2D-SWE, acoustic radiation force impulse (ARFI) is used to interrogate the tissue and create tissue displacement at multiple points [4, 5]. A large quantitative color-coded elasticity map (elastogram) is displayed, usually overlaid on the conventional B-mode ultrasound image, and, in addition, a quantitative measurement can be obtained by placing smaller regions of interest (ROIs) inside the color-coded elasticity map (Figs. 9.1 and 9.2). The result of one measurement is displayed usually as the mean and standard deviation, either in m/s or in kPa. This technique is available on multiple ultrasound systems including Aixplorer SuperSonic Imagine (Hologic), General Electric Healthcare, Canon, Philips, Siemens, Samsung, Mindray, and others.

The technique is simple; for the measurements, patients will be held in a supine position with their right arm in maximal abduction for a better approach of the right liver lobe through the intercostal spaces. Patients should be fasting (for at least 3 h) and rest for a minimum of 10 min before the assessment, and large vessels, artifacts, and respiratory movements should be avoided [4, 5]. Compared to other elastography techniques, for 2D-SWE, ultrasound experience is useful for better performance of the examiner [6]. The technique has the advantage that can be performed also in patients with ascites, but an adequate B-mode conventional ultrasound image is necessary for reliable results.

The technique is the most recent one available implemented in ultrasound systems, and already several studies have showed its good accuracy for predicting significant fibrosis and liver cirrhosis, in chronic liver diseases of different etiologies.

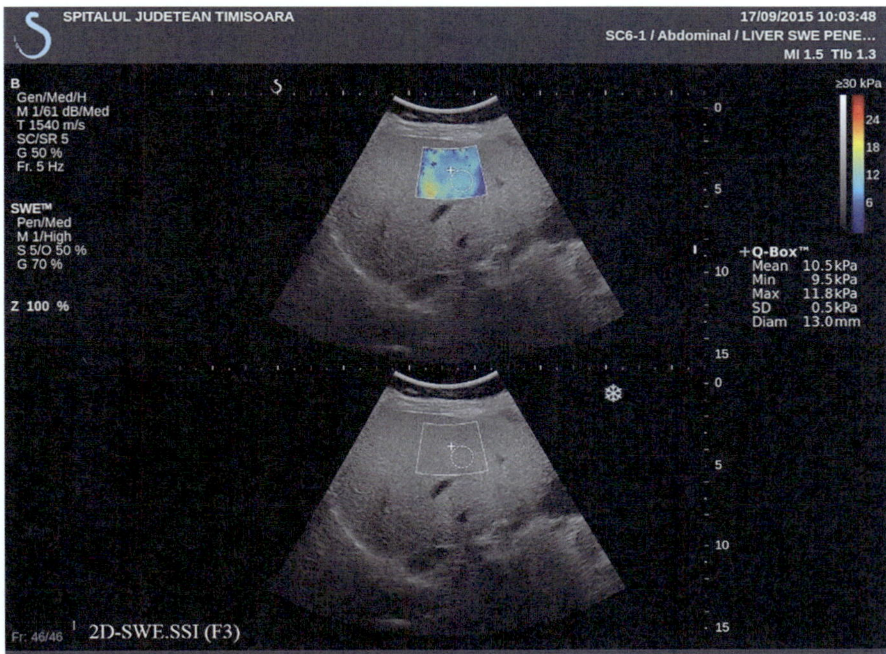

Fig. 9.1 Liver stiffness measurement by 2D-SWE using Aixplorer system (SuperSonic Imagine) (Hologic)

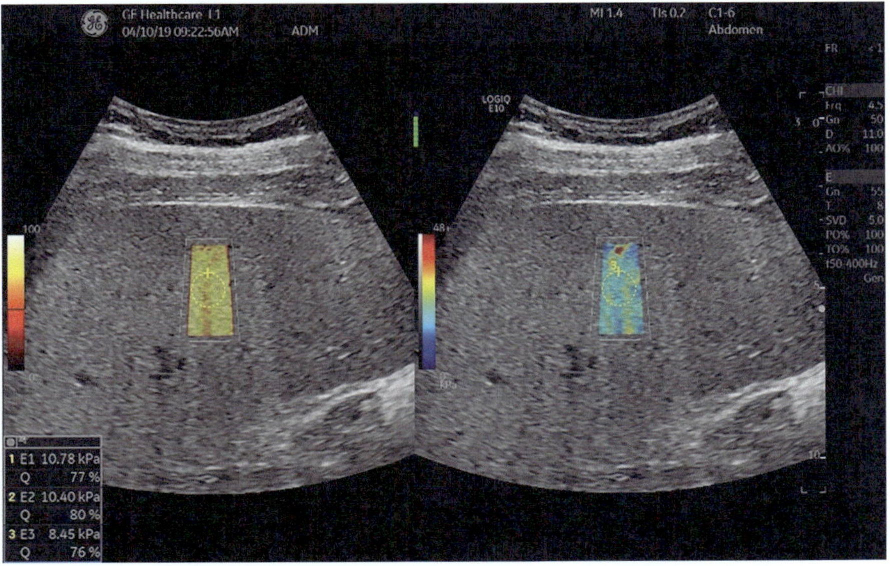

Fig. 9.2 Liver stiffness measurement by 2D-SWE using E10 system (General Electric Healthcare)

9.3 Accuracy of 2D-SWE for Liver Fibrosis Assessment in NAFLD Patients

Several studies evaluated the accuracy of 2D-SWE techniques for liver fibrosis assessment in NAFLD patients. Table 9.1 summarizes these studies and the proposed cutoff values for the different stages of fibrosis.

One of the first studies that compared 2D-SWE, TE, and pSWE with liver biopsy in 291 NAFLD patients [7] showed similar good accuracies for all three techniques, slightly better for 2D-SWE: the AUROCs for 2D-SWE, TE, and pSWE (VTQ) were 0.86, 0.82, and 0.77 for diagnosing $\geq$F2; 0.89, 0.86, and 0.84 for $\geq$F3; and 0.88, 0.87, and 0.84 for F4, respectively. The cutoff values for 2D-SWE and TE for predicting different stages of fibrosis with a sensitivity $\geq$90% were very close: 6.3/6.2 kPa for $\geq$F2, 8.3/8.2 kPa for $\geq$F3, and 10.5/9.5 kPa for F4.

Several other studies had similar results for different 2D-SWE techniques. Table 9.2 summarizes the accuracy of 2D-SWE for diagnosing different stages of fibrosis reported by different studies.

In a study performed by our group [18], that included 204 consecutive adult patients with NAFLD, liver fibrosis was evaluated by the 2D-SWE technique embedded on the Aixplorer MACH 30 system-shear wave elastography (2D-SWE PLUS), using TE as reference method. A strong correlation between LSMs by 2D-SWE PLUS and TE ($r = 0.89$) was found, with a best 2D-SWE PLUS cutoff value for the presence of significant fibrosis ($F \geq 2$) of 7 kPa, and the assessment of steatosis and inflammation was also possible by the same system.

Table 9.1 Cutoff values of 2D-SWE for liver fibrosis assessment in NAFLD patients

Study	No. of patients	Elastography	Cutoff values for each fibrosis stage			
			F1	F2	F3	F4
Cassinotto (2016) [7]	291	2D-SWE	–	>6.3 kPa	>8.3 kPa	>10.5 kPa
Herrmann (2017) [8]	156	2D-SWE	–	>7.1 kPa	>9.2 kPa	>13 kPa
Lee (2017) [9]	94	2D-SWE	–	>8.3 kPa	>10.7 kPa	>15.1 kPa
Takeuchi (2018) [10]	71	2D-SWE	>6.6 kPa	>11.6 kPa	>13.1 kPa	>15.7 kPa
Jamialahmadi (2019) [11]	90	2D-SWE	>5.6 kPa	>6.6 kPa	>6.8 kPa	>6.8 kPa
Imajo (2020) [12]	221	2D-SWE	>6.65 kPa	>8.04 kPa	>10.6 kPa	>12.37 kPa
Furlan (2020) [13]	57	2D-SWE	–	>5.7 kPa	>8.1 kPa	–
Sharpton (2021) [14]	114	2D-SWE	>7.5 kPa	>7.7 kPa	>7.7 kPa	>9.3 kPa
Podrug (2021) [15]	164	2D-SWE		>7.9 kPa	>10 kPa	>11.4 kPa

METAVIR fibrosis stage: F1: mild fibrosis; F2: significant fibrosis; F3: severe fibrosis; F4: cirrhosis

Table 9.2 Accuracy of 2D-SWE for liver fibrosis assessment in NAFLD patients

Study	No. of patients	Fibrosis stage	AUROC
Cassinotto (2016) [7]	291	≥F2	0.86
		≥F3	0.89
		F4	0.88
Herrmann (2017) [8]	156	≥F2	0.86
		≥F3	0.93
		F4	0.92
Takeuchi (2018) [10]	71	≥F1	0.82
		≥F2	0.75
		≥F3	0.82
		F4	0.90
Jamialahmadi (2019) [11]	90	≥F1	0.77
		≥F2	0.72
		≥F3	0.77
		F4	0.70
Furlan (2020) [13]	57	≥F2	0.80
		≥F3	0.89
Sugimoto (2020) [16]	111	≥F1	0.79
		≥F2	0.88
		≥F3	0.90
		F4	0.95
Podrug (2021) [15]	164	≥F2	0.91
		≥F3	0.92
		F4	0.95
Zhou (2022) [17]	116	≥F2	0.86
		≥F3	0.89
		F4	0.90

METAVIR fibrosis stage: F1: mild fibrosis; F2: significant fibrosis; F3: severe fibrosis; F4: cirrhosis. n: sample size. AUROC: area under receiver operating characteristics curve

In a more recent study [19] that included 104 patients with NAFLD evaluated by TE and 2D-SWE, with liver biopsy as reference method, the correlation between fibrosis based on histology and liver stiffness measurements (LSMs) was significantly stronger for 2D-SWE as compared to TE (Spearman's correlation coefficient of 0.71; $P < 0.001$ vs. 0.51, $P < 0.001$; $Z = 2.21$, $P = 0.027$). Inflammatory activity was an independent predictor of LSM by TE, but not of LSM by 2D-SWE.

Similar to all elastography techniques, 2D-SWE has better accuracy for diagnosing severe stages of fibrosis. In a study that included 552 patients with NAFLD that underwent LSM by 2D-SWE and TE at the same visit [20], the median LSMs were 5.5 (2.8–75) kPa for TE and 6.2 (3.7–46.2) kPa for 2D-SWE. LSMs by TE and 2D-SWE were correlated regardless of the obesity status ($r = 0.774$; $P < 0.001$; $r = 0.774$; $P < 0.001$; $r = 0.75$; $P < 0.001$ in BMI <25, 25–30, and ≥30 kg/m^2, respectively) or the degree of liver steatosis ($r = 0.63$; $P < 0.001$ and $r = 0.743$; $P < 0.001$ in mild and moderate/severe steatosis, respectively). The correlation between the two methods was strong in patients with at least severe fibrosis ($r = 0.84$; $P < 0.001$) or cirrhosis ($r = 0.658$; $P < 0.001$), with an excellent accuracy of 98.8 and 99.8% in diagnosing severe fibrosis and cirrhosis for 2D-SWE using TE as reference.

9.4   Conclusions

Thus, 2D-SWE techniques are proved to be reliable also for the evaluation of liver fibrosis in NAFLD patients, and the guidelines recommend to use them especially for ruling out liver cirrhosis [4, 5, 21]. To avoid the confusion created by the different cutoff values available in the literature, the experts suggested the use of "rule of four" for the interpretation of liver stiffness values obtained also by 2D-SWE in NAFLD patients: ≤ 5 kPa—normal, <9 kPa—excludes advanced fibrosis, 9–13 kPa—suggests advanced fibrosis, >13 kPa—diagnostic for cACLD (advanced fibrosis), and >17 kPa—suggests CSPH [22].

References

1. Sporea I, Popescu A, Dumitraşcu D, Brisc C, Nedelcu L, Trifan A, Gheorghe L, Fierbinţeanu BC. Nonalcoholic fatty liver disease: status quo. J Gastrointestin Liver Dis. 2018;27(4):439–48. https://doi.org/10.15403/jgld.2014.1121.274.quo.
2. European Association for the Study of the Liver (EASL), European Association for the Study of Diabetes (EASD), European Association for the Study of Obesity (EASO). EASL-EASD-EASO clinical practice guidelines for the management of non-alcoholic fatty liver disease. J Hepatol. 2016;64(6):1388–402. https://doi.org/10.1016/j.jhep.2015.11.004.
3. Seeff LB, Everson GT, Morgan TR, Curto TM, Lee WM, Ghany MG, Shiffman ML, Fontana RJ, Di Bisceglie AM, Bonkovsky HL, Dienstag JL, HALT–C Trial Group. Complication rate of percutaneous liver biopsies among persons with advanced chronic liver disease in the HALT-C trial. Clin Gastroenterol Hepatol. 2010;8(10):877–83. https://doi.org/10.1016/j.cgh.2010.03.025. Epub 2010 Apr 1.
4. Dietrich CF, Bamber J, Berzigotti A, Bota S, Cantisani V, Castera L, Cosgrove D, Ferraioli G, Friedrich-Rust M, Gilja OH, Goertz RS, Karlas T, de Knegt R, de Ledinghen V, Piscaglia F, Procopet B, Saftoiu A, Sidhu PS, Sporea I, Thiele M. EFSUMB Guidelines and Recommendations on the Clinical Use of Liver Ultrasound Elastography, Update 2017 (Long Version). Ultraschall Med. 2017;38(4):e16–47. https://doi.org/10.1055/s-0043-103952. English. Epub 2017 Apr 13. Erratum in: Ultraschall Med. 2017 Aug;38(4):e48.
5. Ferraioli G, Wong VW, Castera L, Berzigotti A, Sporea I, Dietrich CF, Choi BI, Wilson SR, Kudo M, Barr RG. Liver ultrasound elastography: an update to the world federation for ultrasound in medicine and biology guidelines and recommendations. Ultrasound Med Biol. 2018;44(12):2419–40. https://doi.org/10.1016/j.ultrasmedbio.2018.07.008. Epub 2018 Sep 9.
6. Grădinaru-Taşcău O, Sporea I, Bota S, Jurchiş A, Popescu A, Popescu M, Şirli R, Szilaski M. Does experience play a role in the ability to perform liver stiffness measurements by means of supersonic shear imaging (SSI)? Med Ultrason. 2013;15(3):180–3. https://doi.org/10.11152/mu.2013.2066.153.ogt1is2.
7. Cassinotto C, Boursier J, de Lédinghen V, Lebigot J, Lapuyade B, Cales P, Hiriart JB, Michalak S, Bail BL, Cartier V, Mouries A, Oberti F, Fouchard-Hubert I, Vergniol J, Aubé C. Liver stiffness in nonalcoholic fatty liver disease: a comparison of supersonic shear imaging, FibroScan, and ARFI with liver biopsy. Hepatology. 2016;63(6):1817–27. https://doi.org/10.1002/hep.28394. Epub 2016 Jan 22.
8. Herrmann E, de Lédinghen V, Cassinotto C, Chu WC, Leung VY, Ferraioli G, Filice C, Castera L, Vilgrain V, Ronot M, Dumortier J, Guibal A, Pol S, Trebicka J, Jansen C, Strassburg C, Zheng R, Zheng J, Francque S, Vanwolleghem T, Vonghia L, Manesis EK, Zoumpoulis P, Sporea I, Thiele M, Krag A, Cohen-Bacrie C, Criton A, Gay J, Deffieux T, Friedrich-Rust M. Assessment of biopsy-proven liver fibrosis by two-dimensional shear wave elastography:

an individual patient data-based meta-analysis. Hepatology. 2018;67(1):260–72. https://doi.org/10.1002/hep.29179. Epub 2017 Nov 15.

9. Lee MS, Bae JM, Joo SK, Woo H, Lee DH, Jung YJ, Kim BG, Lee KL, Kim W. Prospective comparison among transient elastography, supersonic shear imaging, and ARFI imaging for predicting fibrosis in nonalcoholic fatty liver disease. PLoS One. 2017;12(11):e0188321. https://doi.org/10.1371/journal.pone.0188321. Erratum in: PLoS One 2018;13(6):e0200055.

10. Takeuchi H, Sugimoto K, Oshiro H, Iwatsuka K, Kono S, Yoshimasu Y, Kasai Y, Furuichi Y, Sakamaki K, Itoi T. Liver fibrosis: noninvasive assessment using supersonic shear imaging and FIB4 index in patients with non-alcoholic fatty liver disease. J Med Ultrason (2001). 2018;45(2):243–9. https://doi.org/10.1007/s10396-017-0840-3. Epub 2017 Nov 11.

11. Jamialahmadi T, Nematy M, Jangjoo A, Goshayeshi L, Rezvani R, Ghaffarzadegan K, Nooghabi MJ, Shalchian P, Zangui M, Javid Z, Doaei S, Rajabzadeh F. Measurement of liver stiffness with 2D-shear wave Elastography (2D-SWE) in bariatric surgery candidates reveals acceptable diagnostic yield compared to liver biopsy. Obes Surg. 2019;29(8):2585–92. https://doi.org/10.1007/s11695-019-03889-2.

12. Imajo K, Honda Y, Kobayashi T, Nagai K, Ozaki A, Iwaki M, Kessoku T, Ogawa Y, Takahashi H, Saigusa Y, Yoneda M, Kirikoshi H, Utsunomiya D, Aishima S, Saito S, Nakajima A. Direct comparison of US and MR Elastography for staging liver fibrosis in patients with nonalcoholic fatty liver disease. Clin Gastroenterol Hepatol. 2020;S1542-3565(20):31673–6. https://doi.org/10.1016/j.cgh.2020.12.016. Epub ahead of print.

13. Furlan A, Tublin ME, Yu L, Chopra KB, Lippello A, Behari J. Comparison of 2D shear wave elastography, transient elastography, and MR elastography for the diagnosis of fibrosis in patients with nonalcoholic fatty liver disease. AJR Am J Roentgenol. 2020;214(1):W20–6. https://doi.org/10.2214/AJR.19.21267. Epub 2019 Nov 12.

14. Sharpton SR, Tamaki N, Bettencourt R, Madamba E, Jung J, Liu A, Behling C, Valasek MA, Loomba R. Diagnostic accuracy of two-dimensional shear wave elastography and transient elastography in nonalcoholic fatty liver disease. Ther Adv Gastroenterol. 2021;14:17562848211050436. https://doi.org/10.1177/17562848211050436.

15. Podrug K, Sporea I, Lupusoru R, Pastrovic F, Mustapic S, Bâldea V, Bozin T, Bokun T, Salkic N, Şirli R, Popescu A, Puljiz Z, Grgurevic I. Diagnostic performance of 2-D shear-wave elastography with propagation maps and attenuation imaging in patients with non-alcoholic fatty liver disease. Ultrasound Med Biol. 2021;47(8):2128–37. https://doi.org/10.1016/j.ultrasmedbio.2021.03.025. Epub 2021 May 10.

16. Sugimoto K, Moriyasu F, Oshiro H, Takeuchi H, Abe M, Yoshimasu Y, Kasai Y, Sakamaki K, Hara T, Itoi T. The role of multiparametric US of the liver for the evaluation of nonalcoholic steatohepatitis. Radiology. 2020;296(3):532–40. https://doi.org/10.1148/radiol.2020192665. Epub 2020 Jun 23.

17. Zhou J, Yan F, Xu J, Lu Q, Zhu X, Gao B, Zhang H, Yang R, Luo Y. Diagnosis of steatohepatitis and fibrosis in biopsy-proven nonalcoholic fatty liver diseases: including two-dimension real-time shear wave elastography and noninvasive fibrotic biomarker scores. Quant Imaging Med Surg. 2022;12(3):1800–14. https://doi.org/10.21037/qims-21-700.

18. Popa A, Bende F, Şirli R, Popescu A, Bâldea V, Lupuşoru R, Cotrău R, Fofiu R, Foncea C, Sporea I. Quantification of liver fibrosis, steatosis, and viscosity using multiparametric ultrasound in patients with non-alcoholic liver disease: a "real-life" cohort study. Diagnostics (Basel). 2021;11(5):783. https://doi.org/10.3390/diagnostics11050783.

19. Mendoza YP, Rodrigues SG, Delgado MG, Murgia G, Lange NF, Schropp J, Montani M, Dufour JF, Berzigotti A. Inflammatory activity affects the accuracy of liver stiffness measurement by transient elastography but not by two-dimensional shear wave elastography in nonalcoholic fatty liver disease. Liver Int. 2022;42(1):102–11. https://doi.org/10.1111/liv.15116. Epub 2021 Dec 3.

20. Karagiannakis DS, Markakis G, Lakiotaki D, Cholongitas E, Vlachogiannakos J, Papatheodoridis G. Comparing 2D-shear wave to transient elastography for the evaluation of liver fibrosis in nonalcoholic fatty liver disease. Eur J Gastroenterol Hepatol. 2022;34(9):961–6. https://doi.org/10.1097/MEG.0000000000002412. Epub 2022 Jul 19.

21. European Association for the Study of the Liver. EASL clinical practice guidelines on non-invasive tests for evaluation of liver disease severity and prognosis—2021 update. J Hepatol. 2021;75(3):659–89. https://doi.org/10.1016/j.jhep.2021.05.025. Epub 2021 Jun 21.
22. Barr RG, Wilson SR, Rubens D, Garcia-Tsao G, Ferraioli G. Update to the Society of Radiologists in ultrasound liver elastography consensus statement. Radiology. 2020;296(2):263–74. https://doi.org/10.1148/radiol.2020192437. Epub 2020 Jun 9.

Sebastian Zenovia, Cristina Muzica, and Mihaela Dimache

10.1 Introduction

According to most recent epidemiologic data, the most widespread chronic liver condition is nonalcoholic fatty liver disease (NAFLD). The prevalence of NAFLD is much more common than previously believed and is increasing at an alarming rate, according to a recent study [1]. Men have a much greater incidence and prevalence of NAFLD compared to women. Greater awareness of NAFLD and development of cost-effective risk stratification techniques are required to combat the increasing prevalence of NAFLD. Although, formerly, the prevalence of NAFLD was estimated to be 32.4% globally (95% CI: 29.9–34.0%), prevalence has grown considerably over time, from 25.5% (20.1–31.0) before 2005 to 37.8% (32.4–43.3) after 2016 [1], becoming a significant cause of hepatocellular carcinoma (HCC) in the United States and the second cause of liver transplantation, respectively [2].

Nonalcoholic steatohepatitis (NASH) is the driver of disease progression among the NAFLD severity characteristics, while liver fibrosis is the connection between liver damage and cirrhosis and associated consequences. Multiple meta-analyses have conclusively revealed a substantial dose-response connection between the stage of histologic fibrosis and liver-related morbidity and death [3]. In addition, a recent prospective research revealed that the overall mortality rate of NAFLD patients rose with increasing fibrosis stage [4]. Although liver biopsy (LB) is the sole acknowledged approach for diagnosing NASH and the gold standard for evaluating fibrosis, it is an intrusive operation that cannot be used on a large scale [5]. Additionally, it is unsuitable as a monitoring test. In addition to being a substandard

S. Zenovia (✉) · C. Muzica · M. Dimache
Gastroenterology Department, Grigore T. Popa University of Medicine and Pharmacy,
Iasi, Romania

St. Spiridon Emergency Hospital, Institute of Gastroenterology and Hepatology,
Iasi, Romania

A. Trifan et al. (eds.), *Essentials of Non-Alcoholic Fatty Liver Disease*,
https://doi.org/10.1007/978-3-031-33548-8_10

reference standard, LB exhibits substantial sample bias and intra- and interobserver variability.

Therefore, noninvasive diagnostics for hepatic steatosis, steatohepatitis, and fibrosis have been a subject of intense study. For clinical usage, several noninvasive diagnostics have been developed in recent years. In deciding which tests to utilize in different clinical circumstances, doctors may encounter ambiguity. It is necessary to create and verify a consensus scoring system for clinical use [6]. Noninvasive tests are preferred for early detection due to the enormous number of NAFLD patients and the fact that only a small proportion of people experience liver-related illness and death. Among the several noninvasive procedures, hepatologists in Europe, the United States, and Asia frequently use vibration-controlled transient elastography (VCTE) (FibroScan®, Echosens, Paris, France) [7]. The machine was certified by the Food and Drug Administration of the United States in 2013 and has since been swiftly implemented in several countries. Various probe sizes (S, M, and XL) are available on the most recent versions of TE to accommodate individuals of various sizes.

10.2 Vibration-Controlled Transient Elastography (VCTE) and Controlled Attenuation Parameter (CAP)

10.2.1 CAP: Mechanism

The most recent model of TE concurrently with CAP assesses liver stiffness and severity of hepatic steatosis [8]. Ultrasound energy dissipates more rapidly in a liver with steatosis. On abdominal ultrasonography, fatty liver is characterized by a bright liver echotexture, profound signal attenuation, and vascular blunting [7]. The latter two characteristics are a result of the quicker attenuation of ultrasonic wave amplitude in a liver with steatosis. CAP makes use of this physical attribute to calculate the ultrasonic attenuation at the central frequency of TE, assuming a uniform fat distribution and appropriate penetration in order to determine the severity of hepatic steatosis [9].

10.2.2 CAP: Performance

Although abdominal ultrasound is frequently the initial diagnostic procedure for NAFLD, it is operator dependent and insensitive to mild hepatic steatosis [8]. Typically, more than 30% of hepatocytes must be affected by hepatic steatosis for ultrasonography to accurately detect fatty liver [10]. Table 10.1 provides a summary of studies comparing the performance of CAP and liver histology in detecting various stages of steatosis [9–22]. Overall, the areas under receiver-operating characteristics (AUROCs) curves for S1 (steatosis ≥5–10% of hepatocytes), S2 (33%), and S3 (66%) steatosis are 81–84%, 85–88%, and 86–91%, respectively. The observed sensitivities (Ss) for S1, S2, and S3 are, correspondingly, 60–75%, 69–84%, and

Table 10.1 Performance of controlled attenuation parameter in studies using histology as reference

Study (year)	Number of patients included in studies according to etiologies	Histological percentage of fat hepatocytes	Cutoff (dB/m)	Sn (%)	Sp (%)	PPV (%)	NPV (%)
Sasso et al. [10] (2012)	CHC: 615	S1–S3 (S1 11–33% steatosis) S2–S3 S3	222 233 290	43 26 78	93 99 93	71 77 15	79 90 100
de Lédinghen et al. [11] (2012)	ALD: 6 NAFLD: 28 CHC: 40 Other etiologies: 38	S1–S3 (S1 11–33% steatosis) S2–S3 S3	263 311 318	71 57 87	93 94 91	81 81 65	74 83 97
Myers et al. [9] (2012)	Viral hepatitis: 67 NAFLD: 72 Other etiologies: 14	S1–S3 (S1 5–33% steatosis) S2–S3 S3	289 288 283	68 85 94	88 62 47	94 55 17	49 88 98
Chan et al. [12] (2014)	CHB: 133 NAFLD: 93 Other etiologies: 12	S1–S3 (S1 5–33% steatosis) S2–S3 S3	263 281 283	92 89 93	94 74 54	96 70 16	88 91 99
Shen et al. [13] (2014)	CHB: 100 NAFLD: 52	S1–S3 (S1 5–33% steatosis) S2–S3 S3	253 285 310	89 93 92	83 83 79	88 70 29	84 97 99
Chon et al. [14] (2014)	NAFLD: 56 CHB: 47 CHC: 12 Other etiologies: 20	S1–S3 (S1 5–33% steatosis) S2–S3 S3	250 299 327	73 82 78	95 86 84	97 67 26	62 94 98
Mi et al. [15] (2015)	CHB: 340	S1–S3 (S1 5–33% steatosis) S2–S3 S3	224 236 285	76 92 1	75 70 93	68 21 23	80 99 1
Imajo et al. [16] (2016)	NAFLD: 127	S1–S3 (S1 5–33% steatosis) S2–S3 S3	236 270 302	82 78 64	91 81 74	99 73 76	67 76 94

(continued)

Table 10.1 (continued)

Study (year)	Number of patients included in studies according to etiologies	Histological percentage of fat hepatocytes	Cutoff (dB/m)	Sn (%)	Sp (%)	PPV (%)	NPV (%)
de Lédinghen et al. [17] (2016)	NAFLD: 261	S1–S3 (S1 5–33% steatosis) S2–S3 S3	– 310 311	– 79 87	– 71 47	– 86 43	– 59 88
Park et al. [18] (2017)	NAFLD: 104	S1–S3 (S1 5–33% steatosis) S2–S3 S3	261 305 312	72 63 64	86 69 70	98 56 26	23 75 92
Chan et al. [19] (2018)	NAFLD: 156 CHB: 7 CHC: 3 Other etiologies: 14	S1–S3 (S1 5–33% steatosis) S2–S3 S3	253 294 294	93 85 88	71 59 36	97 77 24	50 70 93
Garg et al. [20] (2018)	NAFLD: 124	S1–S3 (S1 5–33% steatosis) S2–S3 S3	323 336 357	59 74 100	83 76 78	97 57 20	15 87 1
Siddiqui et al. [21] (2019)	NAFLD: 393	S1–S3 (S1 5–33% steatosis) S2–S3 S3	285 311 306	80 77 80	77 57 40	99 70 32	16 66 85
Eddowes et al. [22] (2019)	NAFLD: 415	S1–S3 (S1 5–33% steatosis) S2–S3 S3	302 331 337	80 70 72	83 76 63	97 84 52	37 58 80

Steatosis was graded according to the percentage of hepatocytes containing fat: S0 5% or 10%, S1: 5–33% or 11–33%, S2: 34–66%, S3 67%; *Sn* Sensitivity, *Sp* Specificity, *PPV* Positive predictive value, *NPV* Negative predictive value, *CHC* Chronic hepatitis C, *ALD* Alcoholic liver disease, *NAFLD* Nonalcoholic fatty liver disease

77–96%. The associated specificities (Sp) are between 76 and 90%, 75 and 88%, and 72 and 82%. A meta-analysis with 19 trials including 2735 patients reveals comparable results, with pooled Ss and Sp of 69% and 82% for S1, 77% and 81% for S2, and 88% and 77% for S3. CAP's ideal cutoffs for S1 and S2 are 248 dB/m and 280 dB/m, respectively [23]. It should be emphasized that in certain studies, liver steatosis-free controls consisted of individuals with various liver disorders. Due to the fact that these individuals received LB for various reasons, they do not reflect a healthy population. This may have had an impact on the determination of appropriate cutoffs and the evaluation of test performance. Moreover, patient composition affects the test assessment. In Europe and North America, research based on more obese NAFLD cohorts often suggests higher cutoff values for each steatosis degree [21, 22].

The CAP threshold is also a topic of dispute. In the two meta-analyses, the best cutoffs for detecting fatty liver using the M and XL probes were 248 dB/m and 297 dB/m, respectively [23, 24]. Two recent prospective investigations reported detection thresholds of 244 and 295 dB/m for S1 steatosis, respectively [25, 26]. However, investigations conducted in the United States have consistently shown appropriate cutoffs of roughly 300 dB/m [27]. It is uncertain if the greater BMI in American cohorts caused the disparity. Patients with an interquartile range of CAP of >40 dB/m were more likely to have erroneous results, according to a multicenter international investigation, although these findings require independent validation [28]. The most recent version of VCTE supports the SmartExam and continuous CAP assessment. In the original model, CAP measurements are obtained and the median value is used to reflect the degree of steatosis. The new continuous CAP enables continuous CAP measurements during the whole examination and takes around 200 CAP readings in the same amount of time. According to preliminary statistics, continuous CAP offers less measurement variability than the traditional approach [29].

10.2.3 CAP: Clinical Use

Although MRI-PDFF offers higher performance to CAP, its cost and availability restrict its use. When 30% of hepatocytes are lipidic inclusions, abdominal ultrasound may be mistakenly negative in clinical settings [30]. CAP has a high connection with metabolic syndrome, body mass index (BMI), and chronic hepatitis C (CHC), according to studies [10, 23]. Therefore, CAP is an essential and noninvasive approach for screening for fatty liver in the general population or high-risk population, such as individuals with type 2 diabetes (T2DM), obesity, and other chronic liver disorders (Fig. 10.1).

10.2.4 VCTE: Liver Stiffness Measurement (LSM)—Mechanism

During LSM via TE, the transducer transmits vibrations of moderate amplitude and low frequency (50 Hz), creating an elastic shear wave that propagates through the underlying tissues [31]. Pulse-echo ultrasonic acquisition is utilized to determine the velocity of the shear wave, which is directly proportional to tissue stiffness: the stiffer the tissue is, the quicker the shear wave propagates, and lower LSM levels suggest a more elastic liver [8] (Fig. 10.2). LSM values vary from 1.5 to 75 kPa [32]. TE assesses liver stiffness in a volume of at least 100 times larger than a biopsy sample and is thus considerably more representative and accurate compared to LB [33].

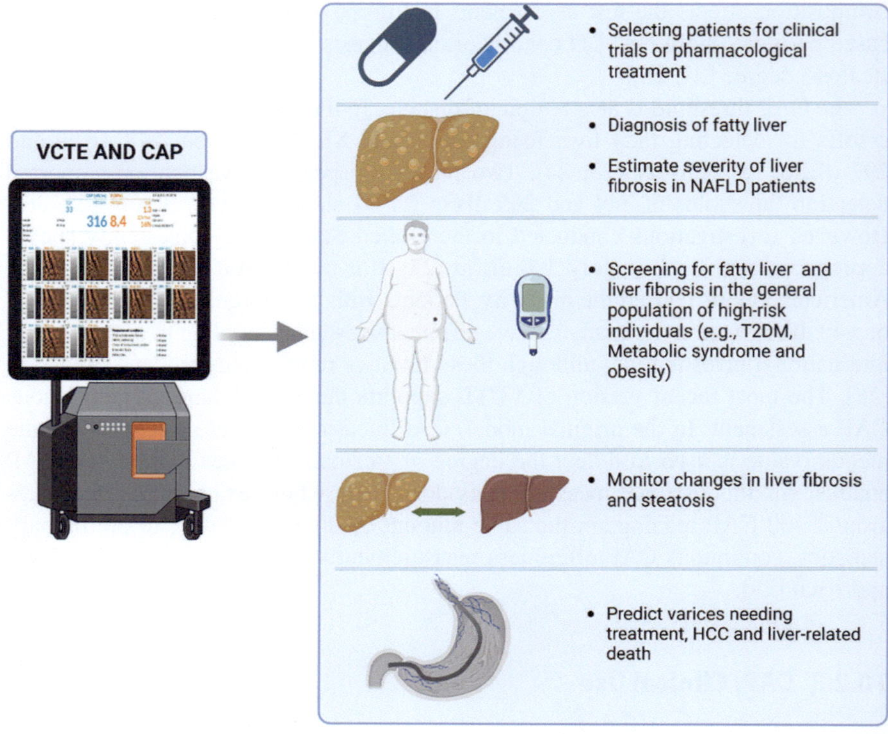

Fig. 10.1 Clinical applications of vibration-controlled transient elastography and controlled attenuation parameter

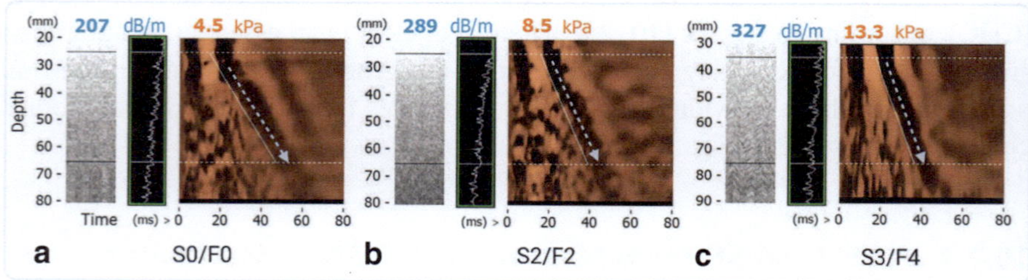

Fig. 10.2 Elastic wave propagation in hepatic parenchyma with different fibrosis degrees and steatosis stages: (**a**) S0/F0, (**b**) S2/F2, (**c**) S3/F4. The blue slope dotted arrow line represents the propagation of velocity of the wave pattern that increases from an oblique to vertical line as a function of fibrosis degree

10.2.5 VCTE: Performance

TE is noninvasive, quick, and simple to conduct in the hospital or clinic. It permits noninvasive and fast assessment of hepatic fibrosis in patients with chronic liver disorders such as CHC, chronic hepatitis B (CHB), and NAFLD [34–36]. Studies comparing the performance of LSM and LB in NAFLD patients are included in Table 10.2 [16, 18, 20–22, 38–42]. Overall, the AUROCs of LSM were 0.82, 0.85, 0.94, and 0.96 for stages F1, F2, F3, and F4, respectively. The LSM cutoff values for F2–4 fibrosis vary between 6.2 and 11 kPa, with 62–90% Ss and 74–100% Sp. For

Table 10.2 Performance of liver stiffness measurement in NAFLD studies using histology as reference

Study (year)	Number of patients	VCTE probe	Liver fibrosis histology	Cutoff (kPa)	Sn (%)	Sp (%)	PPV (%)	NPV (%)
Yoneda et al. [37] (2007)	67	M	F1–F4	5.6	83	81	94	59
			F2–F4	6.7	82	91	90	84
			F3–F4	8.0	88	84	64	96
			F4	17.0	100	98	83	100
Yoneda et al. [36] (2008)	97	M	F1–F4	5.9	86	89	97	59
			F2–F4	6.7	88	74	79	85
			F3–F4	9.8	85	81	64	83
			F4	17.5	100	97	75	100
Wong et al. [38] (2010)	246	M	F2–F4	7.0	79	76	70	84
			F3–F4	8.7	84	83	60	95
			F4	10.3	92	88	46	99
Gaia et al. [39] (2011)	72	M	F1–F4	5.5	84	57	80	62
			F2–F4	7.0	76	80	75	78
			F3–F4	8.0	65	80	48	86
Wong et al. [40] (2012)	193	M	F2–F4	5.8	94	42	54	90
			F3–F4	7.9	88	68	51	94
			F4	103	81	83	35	98
		XL	F2–F4	4.8	92	37	54	84
			F3–F4	5.7	91	54	45	93
			F4	7.2	92	70	31	98
Kumar et al. [41] (2013)	120	M	F1–F4	6.1	78	68	87	53
			F2–F4	7.0	77	78	75	81
			F3–F4	9.0	85	88	68	95
			F4	11.8	90	88	41	98
Imajo et al. [16] (2016)	142	M	F1–F4	7.0	62	100	100	87
			F2–F4	11.0	65	89	88	66
			F3–F4	11.4	86	84	75	92
			F4	14.0	100	76	73	100
Lee et al. [42] (2016)	183	M	F1–F4	6.7	66	85	88	63
			F2–F4	8.0	83	85	64	94
			F3–F4	9.0	96	86	55	99
			F4	11.0	100	90	45	100
Park et al. [18] (2017)	104	M	F1–F4	6.1	67	65	69	62
			F2–F4	6.9	79	85	70	90
			F3–F4	7.3	78	78	45	94
			F4	6.9	63	66	15	95
Garg et al. [20] (2018)	124	XL	F1–F4	6.0	80	56	87	43
			F2–F4	7.3	70	59	53	76
			F3–F4	12.5	64	88	47	93

(continued)

Table 10.2 (continued)

Study (year)	Number of patients	VCTE probe	Liver fibrosis histology	Cutoff (kPa)	Sn (%)	Sp (%)	PPV (%)	NPV (%)
Siddiqui et al. [21] (2019)	393	M	F1–F4	8.6	53	87	93	37
			F2–F4	8.6	66	80	78	70
			F3–F4	8.6	80	74	59	89
			F4	13.1	89	86	39	99
Eddowes et al. [22] (2019)	415	M + XL	F2–F4	8.2	71	70	78	61
			F3–F4	9.7	71	75	63	81
			F4	13.6	85	79	29	98

NAFLD Nonalcoholic fatty liver disease, *Sn* Sensitivity, *Sp* Specificity, *PPV* Positive predictive value, *NPV* Negative predictive value

F3–4 fibrosis, the LSM cutoff values range between 8 and 12 kPa, with an Ss of 84–100% and an Sp of 83–97%. The LSM cutoff values for F4 vary from 9.5 to 20 kPa, with 90–100% Ss and 74.9–98.4% Sp. The appropriate threshold differs between studies because it is a compromise between Ss and Sp, and it may be affected by the underlying liver diseases. Magnetic resonance elastography (MRE) is an MRI-based technique for measuring tissue stiffness quantitatively. Multiple studies have demonstrated that MRE is an effective approach for the early detection of liver fibrosis in NAFLD patients. Imajo et al. compared TE and MRE in 142 Japanese patients with biopsy-proven NAFLD in a cross-sectional investigation [16]. Using MRE and TE, the AUROC curves for diagnosing liver fibrosis stages 1, 2, 3, and 4 were 0.80 vs. 0.78, 0.89 vs. 0.82, 0.89 vs. 0.88, and 0.97 vs. 0.92, respectively. The observed Ss for F1–4, F2–4, F3–4, and F4 fibrosis were 75% compared to 61.7%, 87.3% compared to 65.2%, 74.5% compared to 85.7%, and 90.9% compared to 100%, respectively. The comparable Sp were 85.7% vs. 100%, 85% versus 88.7%, 86.9% versus 83.8%, and 94.5% versus 75.9%. The findings were supported by a second American research that compared the two procedures head-to-head [18]. The results show that MRE is more accurate than TE in assessing liver fibrosis, while the absolute difference is minimal. LSM by use of TE is remarkably repeatable. In the research by Fraquelli and colleagues, 800 TE exams were done on 200 patients with chronic liver disorders, and the overall intraclass correlation coefficient (ICC) for interobserver agreement was 0.98 [43].

10.2.6 VCTE: Predicting Liver-Related Complications

Not only does TE allow for early identification of patients with fibrosis and cirrhosis, but it also plays a crucial role in predicting complications of compensated advanced chronic liver disease (cACLD), such as gastroesophageal varices, HCC, and liver-related deaths. Hemorrhage from varices is a common and serious consequence of cACLD. Current recommendations advocate screening for the existence of esophageal varices (EV) using esophagogastroduodenoscopy (EGD, the gold standard), although EGD is expensive and cumbersome. Numerous investigations have demonstrated that TE may be useful for EV prediction. Patients with LSM 20 kPa with a normal platelet count ($\geq$150 $\times$ 10^9/L) are unlikely to have varices requiring therapy and may be avoided endoscopy, according to the Baveno VII agreement [44]. This concept is based on previous studies, such as Petta and colleagues established the relevance of probe-specific LSM and platelet count in a large multicenter cohort of patients with NASH-related cirrhosis. The study also recommends that the criteria might be loosened (LSM 30 kPa for M probe and 25 kPa for XL probe; platelet count 110 $\times$ 10^9/L) to lower the number of patients undergoing endoscopy without compromising the false-negative rate. In addition to EV, HCC is one of the most significant consequences of liver fibrosis advancement. Based on the considerable link between the risk of HCC development and the degree of liver fibrosis, several studies have shown that TE can be used to evaluate the risk of HCC development. Singh et al. conducted a systematic review and meta-analysis that supports these findings [45]. In addition, recent research have demonstrated a correlation between LSM and survival rate. Pang and colleagues found that in 2052 patients with chronic liver disease, LSM by TE accurately predicted the likelihood of mortality [46]. CAP did not appear to predict liver-related outcomes, however. This is consistent with LB studies indicating that steatosis is not as significant a prognostic indicator as other histological characteristics [47].

10.2.7 VCTE: Clinical Applications

TE can evaluate the degree of liver fibrosis in NAFLD patients in both primary and secondary care settings. A recent meta-analysis of nine studies involving 1047 NAFLD patients indicates that TE is excellent for diagnosing F3–4 (85% Ss, 82% Sp) and F4 fibrosis (92% Ss, 92% Sp) and has moderate accuracy for diagnosing F2–4 fibrosis (79% Ss, 75% Sp) [48]. Second, TE can aid in the selection of individuals for clinical trials or pharmaceutical therapy. Not only does TE have strong accuracy and high repeatability in the detection of liver fibrosis, but it is also noninvasive, easy to learn, and well accepted by patients, which makes it frequently used in scientific study [49]. Thirdly, TE can be utilized to screen the general population of high-risk patients (e.g., T2DM and obesity) for liver fibrosis. Current practice grossly underestimates the influence of obesity, T2DM, and other metabolic risk factors on liver fibrosis. Both BMI >30 kg/m^2 and T2DM were substantially linked with liver stiffness $\geq$8 kPa, as determined by TE in a population-based investigation of adults aged 45 and older [50]. In another research including 1918 individuals with T2DM, 72.8% had fatty liver and 17.7% had significant liver stiffness indicative of advanced fibrosis, underscoring the necessity of case discovery or even screening in this group at high risk [51]. Varices, HCC, and liver-related mortality may be predicted with LSM in patients with cirrhosis caused by NASH. The Baveno VII criteria and their adaptations are excellent beginning points for patient selection for endoscopic screening. Some studies suggest that TE can be used to monitor fibrosis changes following therapy; however, this needs to be validated by additional research utilizing paired LB [52].

10.2.8 VCTE: M and XL Probes, Reliability Criteria, and Confounding Factors

The reduced success rate of TE examinations in obese people is one of its greatest obstacles. This is especially pertinent for NAFLD because of its tight relationship with obesity. To address this issue, the producer of TE has developed several probes to accommodate individuals of varying body types. The M probe is designed for average-sized adults, while the S probe is designed for children and adolescents and the XL probe is designed for obese population. Using a lower frequency than the M probe (2.5 MHz as opposed to 3.5 MHz), the XL probe assesses CAP and liver stiffness at a larger depth (35–75 vs. 25–65 mm) [22, 53]. In the majority of instances, the XL probe enables accurate readings in obese subjects. Because ultrasound-based TE evaluates Young's modulus and is anticipated to be impacted by ultrasound frequency, prospective tests revealed that the XL probe will produce a lower liver stiffness result than the M probe when the evaluation is performed on the same patient [31]. Nonetheless, as a high BMI is also associated with increased liver stiffness, the effects of obesity and XL probing on LSM tend to cancel out [40, 54]. When the M probe was used in patients with a body mass index <30 kg/m^2 and the XL probe was used in patients with a BMI ≥30 kg/m^2, the median liver stiffness values by both probes were nearly identical at each fibrosis stage, indicating that the same interpretation may be adopted when the appropriate probe is used for the appropriate patient [55]. The most recent model of TE has an automatic probe selection tool that suggests the M or XL probes based on the distance between the skin and liver capsule. Following the probe selection tool, it appears that no cutoff modifications are necessary for the two probes [22].

After an overnight or at least 8-h fast, patients are evaluated in a supine position with the arm maximally abducted, focusing on the right hepatic lobe in one of the intercostal spaces (from 9th to 11th on the midaxillary line) (Fig. 10.3). During a typical TE study, ten measures are taken. The median values of CAP and liver stiffness reflect the degree of hepatic steatosis and fibrosis, whereas the interquartile range (IQR) of the ten measures shows the variability of measurements. Highly varied measurements are indicative of a difficult examination, inadequate methodology, or diverse liver parenchymal disease. In accordance with the original manufacturer's specifications, a reliable LSM is characterized by ten valid measurements, a success rate (number of valid acquisitions divided by the number of tries) of at least 60%, and an interquartile range-to-median ratio (IQR/M) of less than 0.30 [38, 40]. However, further research has shown that success rate is not a reliable indicator of examination validity. In a study of 1165 French patients with chronic liver diseases (798—chronic hepatitis C), Boursier et al. established new reliability criteria based on both the IQR/M and median values for liver stiffness. IQR/M >0.30 and liver stiffness ≥7.1 kPa (F2–3 fibrosis) and ≥12.5 kPa (F4 fibrosis essentially) constitute unreliable LSM [56]. Given that LSM has a strong negative predictive value but a minor positive predictive value, it is acceptable to assume that a patient with a liver stiffness of 7.1 kPa or less does not have severe fibrosis, independent of the other quality markers. This method also has the benefit of decreasing the number of

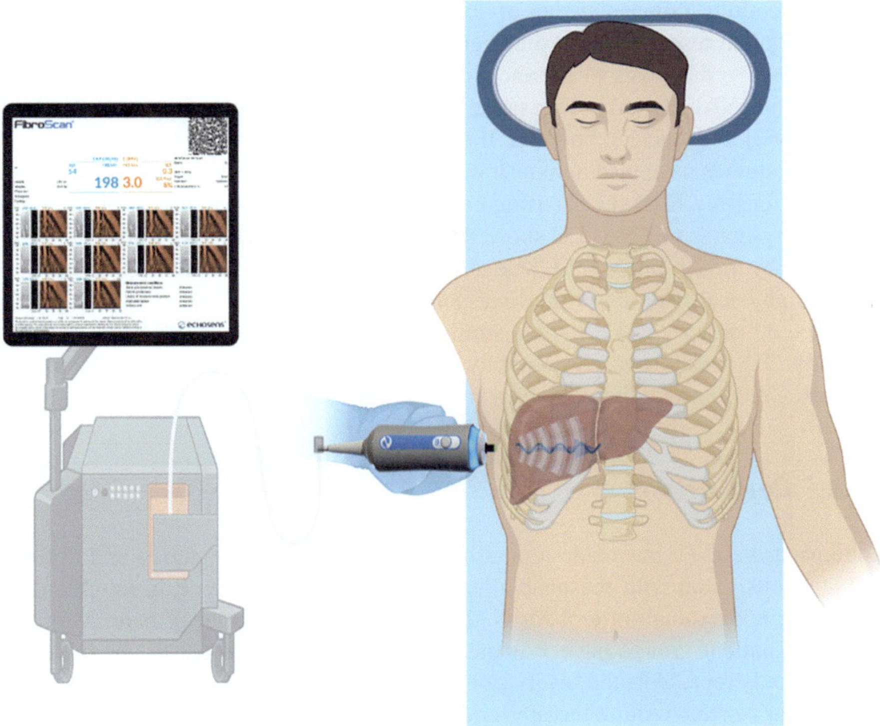

Fig. 10.3 An illustration regarding the positioning of the patient and the probe during the VCTE examination

patients with unreliable exams. In a study of 754 individuals with chronic liver disease and liver histology (349 of whom had NAFLD), our team found that an absolute CAP IQR of >40 dB/m with M probe measurement was linked with a less accurate diagnosis of hepatic steatosis [57].

Hepatic congestion, biliary blockage, amyloidosis, and benign and malignant liver lesions are well-studied confounding variables for LSM that contribute to a false-positive diagnosis of advanced fibrosis. Moreover, after a meal, the liver stiffness rises by 1–5 kPa, likely due to increased portal blood flow [58]. The rigidity of the liver normally reaches its peak between 20 and 40 min, although it may rise by 180 min. Acute viral hepatitis and acute aggravation of chronic viral hepatitis both significantly increase liver stiffness [59]. In fact, people with CHB with blood alanine aminotransferase (ALT) elevations between one and five times the usual upper limit had a stiffer liver than those with normal ALT levels [35]. However, it does not appear that ALT increase affects LSM in NAFLD patients. Two factors may explain this distinction. First, NASH is a condition that is not often characterized by abrupt exacerbations. In general, NASH is associated with a lesser degree of hepatic necro-inflammation than viral or autoimmune hepatitis. Second, the correlation between the ALT level and histological necroinflammation in NAFLD patients is low [60].

A contentious issue is whether or not severe hepatic steatosis impacts liver stiffness. An Italian research found that significant steatosis enhanced the likelihood of a false-positive diagnosis of advanced fibrosis by LSM with the M probe in individuals with NAFLD [61]. The same holds true for patients with elevated CAP readings [62]. It is unclear, however, if the impact is a direct result of hepatic steatosis. Other studies have also demonstrated that an extremely high BMI is connected with a stiffer liver. Recent tests using both the M and XL probes on 496 individuals with biopsy-confirmed NAFLD showed that severe steatosis did not impair LSM as measured by the XL probe [55]. Due to the fact that the aforementioned parameters describe physical features of the liver parenchyma, it is anticipated that they will influence other types of LSMs in a similar manner, such as point-shear wave elastography, 2D-shear wave elastography, and magnetic resonance elastography. In contrast, CAP confounding variables have not been investigated as thoroughly.

10.3 Conclusions

The invention of TE has made it possible to measure hepatic steatosis and fibrosis simultaneously and with reasonable accuracy. Thus, the approach is suitable as a diagnostic and evaluation tool for NAFLD patients at the point of care. Multiple areas and patient groups have validated CAP and LSM with consistent findings. LSM not only represents the severity of liver fibrosis, but also predicts portal hypertension, varices that require therapy, cirrhotic development, and HCC. Obesity used to be a typical cause of measurement failure; however, when the XL probe is used in obese NAFLD patients, it is feasible to acquire correct measurements in the majority of cases. Importantly, the automated probe selection tool enables operators to use the same liver stiffness cutoffs when the M and XL probes are utilized on the appropriate patients. However, whether the same applies to CAP interpretation merits more research. Despite the fact that two research imply that the IQR also represents the dependability of CAP, findings are inconsistent and require additional clarity. As pharmaceutical therapy for NASH is anticipated to become accessible in the near future, it is crucial to evaluate the use of noninvasive diagnostics in various clinical contexts. Several prospective studies have demonstrated the use of basic fibrosis scores, fibrosis biomarkers, and TE for detecting severe liver disorders in primary care settings and certain patient groups. A step-by-step strategy employing basic fibrosis scores followed by fibrosis biomarkers or LSM will likely be the best course of action but must be tailored to the local context.

References

1. Riazi K, Azhari H, Charette JH, Underwood FE, King JA, Afshar EE, Swain MG, Congly SE, Kaplan GG, Shaheen AA. The prevalence and incidence of NAFLD worldwide: a systematic review and meta-analysis. Lancet Gastroenterol Hepatol. 2022;7(9):851–61. https://doi.org/10.1016/S2468-1253(22)00165-0. Epub 2022 Jul 5.

2. Younossi Z, Stepanova M, Ong JP, Jacobson IM, Bugianesi E, Duseja A, et al. Nonalcoholic steatohepatitis is the fastest growing cause of hepatocellular carcinoma in liver transplant candidates. Clin Gastroenterol Hepatol. 2019;17:748–755.e3. https://doi.org/10.1016/j.cgh.2018.05.057.

3. Taylor RS, Taylor RJ, Bayliss S, Hagstrom H, Nasr P, Schattenberg JM, et al. Association between fibrosis stage and outcomes of patients with nonalcoholic fatty liver disease: a systematic review and meta-analysis. Gastroenterology. 2020;158:1611–1625.e12. https://doi.org/10.1053/j.gastro.2020.01.043.

4. Sanyal AJ, Van Natta ML, Clark J, Neuschwander-Tetri BA, Diehl A, Dasarathy S, et al. Prospective study of outcomes in adults with nonalcoholic fatty liver disease. N Engl J Med. 2021;385:1559–69. https://doi.org/10.1056/NEJMoa2029349.

5. Davison BA, Harrison SA, Cotter G, Alkhouri N, Sanyal A, Edwards C, et al. Suboptimal reliability of liver biopsy evaluation has implications for randomized clinical trials. J Hepatol. 2020;73:1322–32. https://doi.org/10.1016/j.jhep.2020.06.025.

6. Zhou YJ, Wong VWS, Zheng MH. Consensus scoring systems for nonalcoholic fatty liver disease: an unmet clinical need. Hepatobiliary Surg Nutr. 2021;10:388–90. https://doi.org/10.21037/hbsn-21-80.

7. Wong VW, Adams LA, de Lédinghen V, Wong GL, Sookoian S. Noninvasive biomarkers in NAFLD and NASH—current progress and future promise. Nat Rev Gastroenterol Hepatol. 2018;15:461–78.

8. Mikolasevic I, Orlic L, Franjic N, Hauser G, Stimac D, Milic S. Transient elastography (FibroScan(®)) with controlled attenuation parameter in the assessment of liver steatosis and fibrosis in patients with nonalcoholic fatty liver disease—where do we stand? World J Gastroenterol. 2016;22:7236–51.

9. Myers RP, Pollett A, Kirsch R, Pomier-Layrargues G, Beaton M, Levstik M, et al. Controlled attenuation parameter (CAP): a noninvasive method for the detection of hepatic steatosis based on transient elastography. Liver Int. 2012;32:902–10.

10. Sasso M, Tengher-Barna I, Ziol M, Miette V, Fournier C, Sandrin L, et al. Novel controlled attenuation parameter for noninvasive assessment of steatosis using Fibroscan(®): validation in chronic hepatitis C. J Viral Hepat. 2012;19:244–53.

11. de Lédinghen V, Vergniol J, Foucher J, Merrouche W, le Bail B. Noninvasive diagnosis of liver steatosis using controlled attenuation parameter (CAP) and transient elastography. Liver Int. 2012;32:911–8.

12. Chan WK, Nik Mustapha NR, Mahadeva S. Controlled attenuation parameter for the detection and quantification of hepatic steatosis in nonalcoholic fatty liver disease. J Gastroenterol Hepatol. 2014;29:1470–6.

13. Shen F, Zheng RD, Mi YQ, Wang XY, Pan Q, Chen GY, et al. Controlled attenuation parameter for non-invasive assessment of hepatic steatosis in Chinese patients. World J Gastroenterol. 2014;20:4702–11.

14. Chon YE, Jung KS, Kim SU, Park JY, Park YN, Kim DY, et al. Controlled attenuation parameter (CAP) for detection of hepatic steatosis in patients with chronic liver diseases: a prospective study of a native Korean population. Liver Int. 2014;34:102–9.

15. Mi YQ, Shi QY, Xu L, Shi RF, Liu YG, Li P, et al. Controlled attenuation parameter for noninvasive assessment of hepatic steatosis using Fibroscan®: validation in chronic hepatitis B. Dig Dis Sci. 2015;60:243–51.

16. Imajo K, Kessoku T, Honda Y, Tomeno W, Ogawa Y, Mawatari H, et al. Magnetic resonance imaging more accurately classifies steatosis and fibrosis in patients with nonalcoholic fatty liver disease than transient elastography. Gastroenterology. 2016;150:626–637.e7.

17. de Lédinghen V, Wong GL, Vergniol J, Chan HL, Hiriart JB, Chan AW, et al. Controlled attenuation parameter for the diagnosis of steatosis in non-alcoholic fatty liver disease. J Gastroenterol Hepatol. 2016;31:848–55.

18. Park CC, Nguyen P, Hernandez C, Bettencourt R, Ramirez K, Fortney L, et al. Magnetic resonance elastography vs transient elastography in detection of fibrosis and noninvasive

measurement of steatosis in patients with biopsy-proven nonalcoholic fatty liver disease. Gastroenterology. 2017;152:598–607.e2.

19. Chan WK, Nik Mustapha NR, Mahadeva S, Wong VW, Cheng JY, Wong GL. Can the same controlled attenuation parameter cut-offs be used for M and XL probes for diagnosing hepatic steatosis? J Gastroenterol Hepatol. 2018;33:1787–94.

20. Garg H, Aggarwal S, Shalimar YR, Datta Gupta S, Agarwal L, et al. Utility of transient elastography (fibroscan) and impact of bariatric surgery on nonalcoholic fatty liver disease (NAFLD) in morbidly obese patients. Surg Obes Relat Dis. 2018;14:81–91.

21. Siddiqui MS, Vuppalanchi R, Van Natta ML, Hallinan E, Kowdley KV, Abdelmalek M, et al. Vibration-controlled transient elastography to assess fibrosis and steatosis in patients with nonalcoholic fatty liver disease. Clin Gastroenterol Hepatol. 2019;17:156–163.e2.

22. Eddowes PJ, Sasso M, Allison M, Tsochatzis E, Anstee QM, Sheridan D, et al. Accuracy of FibroScan controlled attenuation parameter and liver stiffness measurement in assessing steatosis and fibrosis in patients with nonalcoholic fatty liver disease. Gastroenterology. 2019;156:1717–30.

23. Karlas T, Petroff D, Sasso M, Fan JG, Mi YQ, de Lédinghen V, et al. Individual patient data meta-analysis of controlled attenuation parameter (CAP) technology for assessing steatosis. J Hepatol. 2017;66:1022–30.

24. Petroff D, Blank V, Newsome PN, Shalimar VCS, Thiele M, et al. Assessment of hepatic steatosis by controlled attenuation parameter using the M and XL probes: an individual patient data meta-analysis. Lancet. Gastroenterol Hepatol. 2021;6:185–98. https://doi.org/10.1016/S2468-1253(20)30357-5.

25. Qu Y, Song YY, Chen CW, Fu QC, Shi JP, Xu Y, et al. Diagnostic performance of FibroTouch ultrasound attenuation parameter and liver stiffness measurement in assessing hepatic steatosis and fibrosis in patients with nonalcoholic fatty liver disease. Clin Transl Gastroenterol. 2021;12:e00323. https://doi.org/10.14309/ctg.0000000000000323.

26. Zhu SH, Zheng KI, Hu DS, Gao F, Rios RS, Li G, et al. Optimal thresholds for ultrasound attenuation parameter in the evaluation of hepatic steatosis severity: evidence from a cohort of patients with biopsy-proven fatty liver disease. Eur J Gastroenterol Hepatol. 2021;33:430–5. https://doi.org/10.1097/MEG.0000000000001746.

27. Caussy C, Brissot J, Singh S, Bassirian S, Hernandez C, Bettencourt R, et al. Prospective, same-day, direct comparison of controlled attenuation parameter with the M vs the XL probe in patients with nonalcoholic fatty liver disease, using magnetic resonance imaging-proton density fat fraction as the standard. Clin Gastroenterol Hepatol. 2020;18:1842–1850.e6. https://doi.org/10.1016/j.cgh.2019.11.060.

28. Wong VWS, Petta S, Hiriart JB, Camma C, Wong GLH, Marra F, et al. Validity criteria for the diagnosis of fatty liver by M probe-based controlled attenuation parameter. J Hepatol. 2017;67:577–84. https://doi.org/10.1016/j.jhep.2017.05.005.

29. Audière S, Miette V, Fournier C, Whitehead J, Paredes A, Sandrin L, et al. Continuous CAP algorithm: reduced variability in a prospective cohort. J Hepatol. 2020;73:S436.

30. Saadeh S, Younossi ZM, Remer EM, Gramlich T, Ong JP, Hurley M, et al. The utility of radiological imaging in nonalcoholic fatty liver disease. Gastroenterology. 2002;123:745–50.

31. Sandrin L, Fourquet B, Hasquenoph JM, Yon S, Fournier C, Mal F, et al. Transient elastography: a new noninvasive method for assessment of hepatic fibrosis. Ultrasound Med Biol. 2003;29:1705–13.

32. Petta S, Wong VW, Cammà C, Hiriart JB, Wong GL, Marra F, et al. Improved noninvasive prediction of liver fibrosis by liver stiffness measurement in patients with nonalcoholic fatty liver disease accounting for controlled attenuation parameter values. Hepatology. 2017;65:1145–55.

33. Castera L, Forns X, Alberti A. Non-invasive evaluation of liver fibrosis using transient elastography. J Hepatol. 2008;48:835–47.

34. Ziol M, Handra-Luca A, Kettaneh A, Christidis C, Mal F, Kazemi F, et al. Noninvasive assessment of liver fibrosis by measurement of stiffness in patients with chronic hepatitis C. Hepatology. 2005;41:48–54.

35. Chan HL, Wong GL, Choi PC, Chan AW, Chim AM, Yiu KK, et al. Alanine aminotransferase-based algorithms of liver stiffness measurement by transient elastography (Fibroscan) for liver fibrosis in chronic hepatitis B. J Viral Hepat. 2009;16:36–44.
36. Yoneda M, Yoneda M, Mawatari H, Fujita K, Endo H, Iida H, et al. Noninvasive assessment of liver fibrosis by measurement of stiffness in patients with nonalcoholic fatty liver disease (NAFLD). Dig Liver Dis. 2008;40:371–8.
37. Yoneda M, Yoneda M, Fujita K, Inamori M, Tamano M, Hiriishi H, et al. Transient elastography in patients with non-alcoholic fatty liver disease (NAFLD). Gut. 2007;56:1330–1.
38. Wong VW, Vergniol J, Wong GL, Foucher J, Chan HL, Le Bail B, et al. Diagnosis of fibrosis and cirrhosis using liver stiffness measurement in nonalcoholic fatty liver disease. Hepatology. 2010;51:454–62.
39. Gaia S, Carenzi S, Barilli AL, Bugianesi E, Smedile A, Brunello F, et al. Reliability of transient elastography for the detection of fibrosis in non-alcoholic fatty liver disease and chronic viral hepatitis. J Hepatol. 2011;54:64–71.
40. Wong VW, Vergniol J, Wong GL, Foucher J, Chan AW, Chermak F, et al. Liver stiffness measurement using XL probe in patients with nonalcoholic fatty liver disease. Am J Gastroenterol. 2012;107:1862–71.
41. Kumar R, Rastogi A, Sharma MK, Bhatia V, Tyagi P, Sharma P, et al. Liver stiffness measurements in patients with different stages of nonalcoholic fatty liver disease: diagnostic performance and clinicopathological correlation. Dig Dis Sci. 2013;58:265–74.
42. Lee HW, Park SY, Kim SU, Jang JY, Park H, Kim JK, et al. Discrimination of nonalcoholic steatohepatitis using transient elastography in patients with nonalcoholic fatty liver disease. PLoS One. 2016;11:e0157358.
43. Fraquelli M, Rigamonti C, Casazza G, Conte D, Donato MF, Ronchi G, et al. Reproducibility of transient elastography in the evaluation of liver fibrosis in patients with chronic liver disease. Gut. 2007;56:968–73.
44. de Franchis R, Bosch J, Garcia-Tsao G, Reiberger T, Ripoll C, Baveno VII Faculty. Baveno VII—renewing consensus in portal hypertension. J Hepatol. 2022;76(4):959–74. https://doi.org/10.1016/j.jhep.2021.12.022. Epub 2021 Dec 30. Erratum in: J Hepatol. 2022 Apr 14.
45. Singh S, Fujii LL, Murad MH, Wang Z, Asrani SK, Ehman RL, et al. Liver stiffness is associated with risk of decompensation, liver cancer, and death in patients with chronic liver diseases: a systematic review and meta-analysis. Clin Gastroenterol Hepatol. 2013;11:1573–1584.e1. -e2; quiz e88-e89.
46. Pang JX, Zimmer S, Niu S, Crotty P, Tracey J, Pradhan F, et al. Liver stiffness by transient elastography predicts liver-related complications and mortality in patients with chronic liver disease. PLoS One. 2014;9:e95776.
47. Ekstedt M, Hagström H, Nasr P, Fredrikson M, Stål P, Kechagias S, et al. Fibrosis stage is the strongest predictor for disease-specific mortality in NAFLD after up to 33 years of follow-up. Hepatology. 2015;61:1547–54.
48. Kwok R, Tse YK, Wong GL, Ha Y, Lee AU, Ngu MC, et al. Systematic review with meta-analysis: non-invasive assessment of non-alcoholic fatty liver disease—the role of transient elastography and plasma cytokeratin-18 fragments. Aliment Pharmacol Ther. 2014;39:254–69.
49. Wong GL, Wong VW, Choi PC, Chan AW, Chim AM, Yiu KK, et al. On-treatment monitoring of liver fibrosis with transient elastography in chronic hepatitis B patients. Antivir Ther. 2011;16:165–72.
50. Koehler EM, Plompen EP, Schouten JN, Hansen BE, Darwish Murad S, Taimr P, et al. Presence of diabetes mellitus and steatosis is associated with liver stiffness in a general population: the Rotterdam study. Hepatology. 2016;63:138–47.
51. Kwok R, Choi KC, Wong GL, Zhang Y, Chan HL, Luk AO, et al. Screening diabetic patients for non-alcoholic fatty liver disease with controlled attenuation parameter and liver stiffness measurements: a prospective cohort study. Gut. 2016;65:1359–68.
52. Elsharkawy A, Alem SA, Fouad R, El Raziky M, El Akel W, Abdo M, et al. Changes in liver stiffness measurements and fibrosis scores following sofosbuvir based treatment regimens without interferon. J Gastroenterol Hepatol. 2017;32:1624–30.

53. Wong VW, Chan HL. Transient elastography. J Gastroenterol Hepatol. 2010;25:1726–31.
54. de Lédinghen V, Wong VW, Vergniol J, Wong GL, Foucher J, Chu SH, et al. Diagnosis of liver fibrosis and cirrhosis using liver stiffness measurement: comparison between M and XL probe of FibroScan®. J Hepatol. 2012;56:833–9.
55. Wong VW, Irles M, Wong GL, Shili S, Chan AW, Merrouche W, et al. Unified interpretation of liver stiffness measurement by M and XL probes in non-alcoholic fatty liver disease. Gut. 2019;68:2057–64.
56. Boursier J, Zarski JP, de Ledinghen V, Rousselet MC, Sturm N, Le Bail B, et al. Determination of reliability criteria for liver stiffness evaluation by transient elastography. Hepatology. 2013;57:1182–91.
57. Wong VW, Petta S, Hiriart JB, Cammà C, Wong GL, Marra F, et al. Validity criteria for the diagnosis of fatty liver by M probe-based controlled attenuation parameter. J Hepatol. 2017;67:577–84.
58. Arena U, Lupsor Platon M, Stasi C, Moscarella S, Assarat A, Bedogni G, et al. Liver stiffness is influenced by a standardized meal in patients with chronic hepatitis C virus at different stages of fibrotic evolution. Hepatology. 2013;58:65–72.
59. Wong GL, Wong VW, Choi PC, Chan AW, Chim AM, Yiu KK, et al. Increased liver stiffness measurement by transient elastography in severe acute exacerbation of chronic hepatitis B. J Gastroenterol Hepatol. 2009;24:1002–7.
60. Wong VW, Wong GL, Tsang SW, Hui AY, Chan AW, Choi PC, et al. Metabolic and histological features of non-alcoholic fatty liver disease patients with different serum alanine aminotransferase levels. Aliment Pharmacol Ther. 2009;29:387–96.
61. Petta S, Maida M, Macaluso FS, Di Marco V, Cammà C, Cabibi D, et al. The severity of steatosis influences liver stiffness measurement in patients with nonalcoholic fatty liver disease. Hepatology. 2015;62:1101–10.
62. Sasso M, Beaugrand M, de Ledinghen V, Douvin C, Marcellin P, Poupon R, et al. Controlled attenuation parameter (CAP): a novel VCTE™ guided ultrasonic attenuation measurement for the evaluation of hepatic steatosis: preliminary study and validation in a cohort of patients with chronic liver disease from various causes. Ultrasound Med Biol. 2010;36:1825–35.

The Value of Serologic Markers/Scores in the Assessment of Nonalcoholic Fatty Liver Disease

11

Carmen Preda, Mircea Manuc, and Mircea Diculescu

11.1 Introduction

Nonalcoholic fatty liver disease (NAFLD) comprises a spectrum of clinical-pathological conditions characterized histologically by hepatic steatosis, predominantly macrovesicular, which occurs in the absence of significant alcohol consumption and other etiologies of liver disease [1].

The histological spectrum of the disease can vary from simple steatosis (hepatic accumulation of triglycerides in a proportion of 5–10% of the liver weight: NAFL) to steatohepatitis (NASH: characterized by hepatic steatosis, lobular inflammation, ballooning hepatocytic degeneration, Mallory bodies, with or without fibrosis), up to liver cirrhosis (CH) [1, 2].

Based on the current knowledge, an attempt has been made to identify noninvasive serological markers that can differentiate hepatic steatosis from NASH, assess the extent of fibrosis, and monitor or predict the response after therapeutic interventions.

11.2 Serum-Based Steatosis Markers

Gholam shows that liver injury tests (aminotransferases), hyperglycemia, and markers of insulin resistance (insulinemia, HOMA-IR) can be predictors for the presence of NASH and fibrosis in patients with morbid obesity [3]. Different studies carried out so far have shown that the routine biochemical tests (considered as markers of liver damage) ALT, AST, and ALP correlate with the severity of liver damage [4].

C. Preda · M. Manuc · M. Diculescu (✉)
Gastroenterology and Hepatology Department, Carol Davila University of Medicine and Pharmacy, Clinic Fundeni Institute, Bucharest, Romania

© The Author(s), under exclusive license to Springer Nature Switzerland AG 2023
A. Trifan et al. (eds.), *Essentials of Non-Alcoholic Fatty Liver Disease*,
https://doi.org/10.1007/978-3-031-33548-8_11

Depending on the cutoff value of normal established by the laboratory, more than half of the patients with NAFLD present laboratory liver tests within normal limits; an AST/ALT ratio >1 suggests advanced fibrosis or cirrhosis. AST/ALT >2 indicates ethanol etiology, while ALT > AST indicates the presence of NASH [5, 6].

Alanine aminotransferase is by far the single most important serologic marker in the context of nonalcoholic fatty liver disease; however, recent studies have showed that ALT can be in reference limits, depending on the laboratory performing the test, in 50–79% of patients already diagnosed with nonalcoholic fatty liver disease [7], so this serum marker needs to be supplemented with others.

Since liver biopsy is an invasive method, not without risks, expensive, and with a lack of accuracy due to the inhomogeneity of the distribution of liver lesions, a series of noninvasive biochemical tests have been introduced in practice that can differentiate steatosis from NASH and liver fibrosis.

Several other markers and scores for the diagnosis of liver steatosis that have been described are the fatty liver index (FLI), hepatic steatosis index (HSI), NAFLD liver fat score (NAFLD-LFS), SteatoTest, visceral adiposity index (VAI), triglyceride × glucose (TyG) index, and lipid accumulation product (LAP) (Table 11.1).

When analyzing Table 11.1, we can see the two noninvasive tests that stand out, being the visceral adiposity index and the triglyceride/glucose index, both showing an area under the receiver characteristic of 0.92 and 0.90, respectively.

Serum biomarkers are especially useful when describing large epidemiological studies, as the European recommendation has supported [9]. One of the most recognized serum biomarkers used in diagnosing nonalcoholic fatty liver disease is the fatty liver index (FLI), also seen in Table 11.1. Bedogni et al. first proposed the fatty liver index in 2006, as an algorithm derived from the population of the Dionysos Nutrition and Liver Study [9]. The score that is derived to obtain FLI varies between 0 and 100. It includes body mass index, waist circumference, triglycerides, and GGT. A score of FLI less than 30 rules out nonalcoholic fatty liver disease, and a score of greater than or equal to 60 rules in NAFLD. Because this test includes multiple different markers and measurements, it has an accuracy of 0.84 with a 95% confidence interval [9] in detecting nonalcoholic fatty liver disease when compared to the gold standard. The fatty liver index has been proven in multiple studies, and a recent study of 2075 patients from the Regional Health Registry [9] demonstrated that the fatty liver index alone is shown to be linked to overall increased chance of cardiovascular and cancer-related 15-year mortality [9]. Furthermore, high fatty liver index scores have been shown to be associated with increased risk of type 2 DM, coronary events, and carotid atherosclerosis [15, 16].

Table 11.1 Multiple studies using different serological indices in comparing the accuracy of diagnosing NAFLD using these markers compared to the gold standard diagnostic tools (ultrasound or liver biopsy) [7]

Blood markers/algorithms	Components or formulas	AUROC	Study population (no. of participants)/ diagnostic tools
Hepatic steatosis index [8]	$8 \times ALT/AST + BMI$ (+ 2, if type 2 diabetes; + 2, if female)	0.72–0.82	Korean (10,724)/ultrasound
Fatty liver index [9]	$(e0.953 \times \ln (TG) + 0.139 \times BMI + 0.718 \times \ln (GGT) + 0.053 \times WC - 15.745)/(1 + e\ 0.953 \times \ln (TG) + 0.139 \times BMI + 0.718 \times \ln (GGT) + 0.053 \times WC - 15.745) \times 100$	0.79–0.85	Italian (496)/ultrasound
NAFLD liver fat score [10]	$- 2.89 + 1.18 \times$ metabolic syndrome (yes = 1/no = 0) + 0.45 × type 2 diabetes (yes = 2/no = 0) + 0.15 × insulin (mU/L) + 0.04 × AST − 0.94 × AST/ALT	0.78–0.87	Finish (470)/H-MRS
SteatoTest [11]	ALT, α2-macroglobulin, apolipoprotein A1, haptoglobin, total bilirubin, GGT, total cholesterol, TG, glucose, age, gender, BMI	0.72–0.86	Caucasians (2272)/liver biopsy
Lipid accumulation product (LAP) [12]	[WC (cm)–65 (male) or − 58 (female)] × [TG (mmol/L)]	0.72–0.83	Italian (588)/ultrasound
Visceral adiposity index [13]	Male: [WC/39.68 + (1.88 × BMI)] × (TG/1.03) × (1.31/HDL) Female: [WC/36.58 + (1.89 × BMI) × (TG/0.81) × (1.52/HDL)	0.92	French (324)/liver biopsy
Triglyceride/glucose index [14]	Log (TG × glucose/2)	0.90	French (324)/liver biopsy

ALT alanine aminotransferase, *AST* aspartate aminotransferase, *AUROC* area under the receiver operating characteristic, *BMI* body mass index, *GGT* gamma-glutamyl transferase, *HDL* high-density lipoprotein, *NAFLD* nonalcoholic fatty liver disease, *TG* triglycerides, *WC* waist circumference

11.3 Serum-Based Fibrosis Biomarkers

Serum noninvasive tests of liver fibrosis should accurately reflect the entire spectrum of liver fibrosis and must allow a fast and accessible screening, longitudinal tracking (reproducible), monitoring of the progression of the disease, evaluation of therapeutic effectiveness, and a prognostic evaluation.

The most widely used liver fibrosis biomarkers (APRI, FIB-4, and NAFLD fibrosis score) use routine hematological and biochemical tests and are indirect serum markers. These alterations do not necessarily reflect extracellular matrix turnover and/or fibrogenic cell changes.

Nonalcoholic fatty liver disease fibrosis score (NFS) is calculated as follows: $-1.675 + 0.037 \times$ age (years) $+ 0.094 \times$ body mass index (kg/m^2) $+ 1.13 \times$ impaired fasting glycemia or diabetes (yes $= 1$, no $= 0$) $+ 0.99 \times$ aspartate aminotransferase-to-alanine aminotransferase ratio $- 0{\cdot}013 \times$ platelet count ($\times$109/L) $- 0.66 \times$ albumin concentration (g/dL) [17]. A score of >0.675 is suggestive of advanced fibrosis; on the contrary, patients with a low risk of having an advanced fibrosis have a score of less than -1.455. However, a recent meta-analysis reported indeterminate values in 20–58% of patients [18], and thus, NFS was not able to confirm or exclude advanced fibrosis.

The fibrosis-4 (FIB-4) index for liver fibrosis is calculated using the following formula [17]:

$$\frac{\text{Age}\left(\text{years}\right) \times \text{aspartate aminotransferase concentration}\left(\text{IU}\,/\,\text{L}\right)}{\text{Platelet count}\left(\times 10^{9}\,/\,\text{L}\right) \times \left(\text{alanine aminotransferase concentration}\left[\text{IU}\,/\,\text{L}\right]\right)}.$$

The study that validated the FIB-4 score enrolled 541 patients: at a cutoff of 2.67, the PPV was 80% and the NPV was 83%, and if a cutoff of 1.3 was used, the PPV decreased to 43% but the NPV increased to 90% [19].

Fib-4 and NFS have been developed in cohorts of patients 40–50 years old. Their sensibility is low in patients younger than 35 years, and, therefore, they should not be used in this category of patients. In subjects more than 65 years of age, both FIB-4 and NFS could provide an increased rate of false-positive results; that is why some authors suggest different cutoff values in this age category [7].

APRI score or the AST/platelet ratio is calculated after the formula (AST (U/L)/ (AST upper limit of normal))/(platelet count($\times$ 109/L) $\times$ 100).

APRI was developed to predict fibrosis progression in hepatitis C, but recently, it was validated also for NAFLD patients. For a cutoff of 0.5, APRI has a sensitivity of 85% and a specificity of 71% to predict mild fibrosis (F0/F1).

The more refined markers (so-called direct serum markers) detect extracellular matrix turnover and/or fibrogenic cell changes. The enhanced liver fibrosis (ELF) test is a commercial panel of biomarkers of extracellular matrix deposits, which are characteristic in fibrotic liver, such as matrix metalloproteinase 1 (TIMP 1), HA, and PIIINP. The predictive values of ELF test were found inferior to NAFLD fibrosis score, but if we combine the two tests, we could improve the accuracy for moderate and severe fibrosis, with an AUC 0.90 vs. 0.86 and AUC 0.98 vs. 0.89, for the combination ELF-NAFLD fibrosis score vs. the ELF test, respectively [20].

ELF has this complicated formula: $2.2781 + 0.851 \times \ln [HA]$ (µg/L) $+ 10.751 \times \ln$ [P3NP] (µg/L) $+ 10.934 \times \ln$ [TIMP 1] (µg/L).

Table 11.2 describes these noninvasive fibrosis scores and their studies.

Poynard has validated a combination of 12 clinical and biochemical markers (FibroMax Test), which is a combination of five commercial different noninvasive tests: FibroTest, ActiTest, SteatoTest, NashTest, and AshTest [9].

FibroTest measures the degree of liver fibrosis (using the following parameters: haptoglobin, α2-macroglobulin, apolipoprotein A1, GGT, bilirubin, age, gender); ActiTest determines the degree of necro-inflammatory activity in patients with chronic viral hepatitis B or C; NashTest evaluates the presence of nonalcoholic steatohepatitis in obese patients, with dyslipidemia, insulin resistance, or diabetes; SteatoTest assesses the degree of steatosis liver; and AshTest measures the degree of liver damage in alcoholic patients [23].

BioPredictive tests use a combination of specific serum biomarkers to which the patient's sex, age, weight, and height are added, with all these parameters being entered into a patented calculation algorithm specific to each test.

Precautions in the interpretation of the result
- Acute hemolysis (malaria; drugs such as ribavirin and azathioprine)
- Acute viral or autoimmune hepatitis
- Acute inflammations due to bacterial or viral infections (bronchopulmonary or urinary tract infections)
- Extrahepatic cholestasis
- Chronic hemolysis, especially in patients with heart valve prostheses
- Gilbert syndrome
- HIV treatment with protease inhibitors (indinavir, atazanavir, ritonavir)

Table 11.2 Serum-based biomarkers of liver fibrosis in NAFLD (after [7])

Test	Number of NAFLD patients	AUROC/Sn/Sp/NPV/PPV
APRI [19]	145	0.67/27/89/84/37
FIB-4 [21]	1038	0.80/52/90/−/−
NFS [21]	1038	0.88/82/77/93/56
BARD [21]	1038	0.76/74/66/−/−
ELF [20]	192	0.90/80/90/94/71
FibroMeter [22]	383	0.89[a]/81[a]/84[a]/77[a]/86[a]
FibroTest [23]	267	0.81/92/71/98/33

APRI AST-to-platelet ratio index, *AUROC* area under the receiver operating characteristic, *ELF* enhanced liver fibrosis, *FIB-4* fibrosis-4 score, *NFS* nonalcoholic fatty liver disease fibrosis score, *NPV* negative predictive value, *PPV* positive predictive value
[a]Values are for prediction of significant fibrosis

The FibroMax test has a predictive value and a better benefit/risk ratio compared to liver biopsy in assessing liver fibrosis (FibroTest), steatosis (SteatoTest), and diagnosis of steatohepatitis (NashTest) in patients with nonalcoholic fatty liver disease [24].

Putting two serologic based scores together, the nonalcoholic fatty liver disease fibrosis score and the fibrosis-4 (FIB-4) index, one can determine a theoretical "diagnostic and referral pathway" for nonalcoholic fatty liver disease [25]. This pathway is important for clinicians to have in mind when suspecting a patient of having NAFLD and highlights the importance of noninvasive serological tests in the process of diagnosing NAFLD and staging the degree of fibrosis in these patients (see Fig. 11.1). Because of the high prevalence of nonalcoholic fatty liver disease, it is important for primary care physicians to have the ability to go through the diagnostic protocol when working up this disease process, as well as staging the degree of fibrosis in order to reduce overall healthcare costs. Figure 11.1 is an easy method

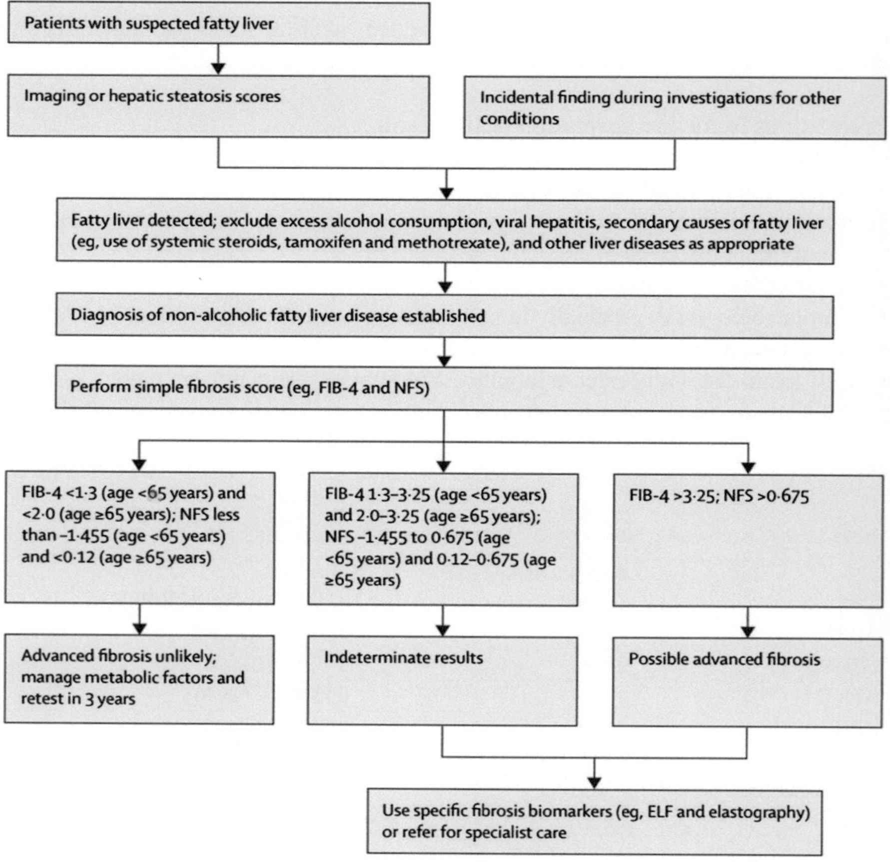

Fig. 11.1 Proposed diagnostic and referral pathway for nonalcoholic fatty liver disease in primary care (table retrieved from [25])

to follow in order to do just that, while using simple and noninvasive serologic markers and scores.

11.4 Serum Biomarkers in the Diagnosis of NASH

Unfortunately, we cannot rely on the elevated level of aminotransferases to diagnose NASH, because they present a low AUC (0.6–0.7) [17].

The risk of NASH and fibrosis is increased in patients who associate nonalcoholic fatty liver disease and metabolic syndrome.

Certain markers of inflammation (secreted by the inflammatory cells that infiltrate the adipose and liver tissue), such as elevated levels of ferritin and high sensitive CRP, correlate with the presence of NASH [26].

Due to the complexity of the pathogenesis of NASH, it has been demonstrated that adipocytokines (adiponectin, leptin, ghrelin, resistin), cytokines secreted from the adipose tissue, play an important role in the occurrence of NASH [26]. NASH patients have lower adiponectin compared with NAFL patients, while adiponectin levels have similar values in NAFL and normal individuals, according to a recent meta-analysis of 27 studies [27]. Leptin has been associated with NAFL, while higher levels may predict more advanced disease [28].

Cytokeratin 18 is a well-studied serum marker of apoptosis and hepatic necrosis, because it is a marker of hepatocyte caspase-3 activation in the apoptosis pathway. Unfortunately, the clinical utility of cytokeratin 18 in the diagnosis of NASH is limited by the low sensitivity (66–75%), despite the high specificity (82–77%), low accessibility, low reproducibility, and lack of a clear cutoff limit [29].

CK-18 was included in more complex clinical scores: for example, the NICE model, which combined CK-18, ALT, and metabolic syndrome, was able to predict NASH severity with an AUC of 0.83, sensitivity of 84%, and specificity of 86% [30]. Another example is NAFLD diagnostic panel, which used an undisclosed formula of CK-18 fragments, adiponectin, resistin, T2D, triglycerides, and gender [31].

The NashTest combines the following parameters: age, gender, and BMI; aminotransferases and lipids; as well as alpha-2 macroglobulin, ApoA1, and haptoglobin. It has low sensitivity 33%, but it can exclude NASH with a specificity of 94% and a negative predictive value (NPV) of 81% [32].

The OXNASH score incorporates AST, age, BMI, and a ratio of 13-hydroxyoctadecadienoic acid (13-HODE) to linoleic acid (LA), and it correlates with histologic features of NASH and provides AUC 0.73 [95% CI (0.637, 0.823)] for inflammation, 0.72 [95% CI (0.630, 0.816)] for ballooning, 0.705 [95% CI (0.570, 0.840)] for steatosis, and 0.673 [95% CI (0.577, 0.770)] for fibrosis [33, 81, 82].

In conclusion, even with the aid of biomarkers, the distinction between simple steatosis and nonalcoholic steatohepatitis remains a difficult task in clinical practice. Serum biomarkers are not yet fully validated to perform this. Fatty liver index (FLI) is a useful marker to screen for NAFLD in general population, and we can use NAFLD-Fib score and Fib-4 and transient elastography to predict advanced fibrosis and to select patients for whom liver biopsy is necessary.

References

1. Diculescu M, Preda CM. Boala ficatului gras non-alcoolic. In: Gastroenterologie. Manual pentru studenti. Bucuresti: Editura UMF Carol Davila; 2016.
2. Preda CM, Diculescu M. Gastroenterologie si stil de viata. Boala ficatului gras non-alcoolic. In: Medicina stilului de viata. Bucuresti: Editura Medicala; 2020.
3. Gholam PM, Flancbaum L, Machan JT, Charney DA, Kotler DP. Nonalcoholic fatty liver disease in severely obese subjects. Am J Gastroenterol. 2007;102(2):399–408. https://doi.org/10.1111/j.1572-0241.2006.01041.x.
4. Younossi ZM, Jarrar M, Nugent C, Randhawa M, Afendy M, Stepanova M, Rafiq N, Goodman Z, Chandhoke V, Baranova A. A novel diagnostic biomarker panel for obesity-related nonalcoholic steatohepatitis (NASH). Obes Surg. 2008;18(11):1430–7.
5. Araújo AR, Rosso N, Bedogni G, Tiribelli C, Bellentani S. Global epidemiology of non-alcoholic fatty liver disease/non-alcoholic steatohepatitis: what we need in the future. Liver Int. 2018;38(Suppl 1):47–51. https://doi.org/10.1111/liv.13643.
6. Nascimbeni F, Loria P, Ratziu V. Non-alcoholic fatty liver disease: diagnosis and investigation. Dig Dis. 2014;32(5):586–96. https://doi.org/10.1159/000360510.
7. Kechagias S, Ekstedt M, Simonsson C, Nasr P. Non-invasive diagnosis and staging of non-alcoholic fatty liver disease. Hormones (Athens). 2022;21(3):349–68. https://doi.org/10.1007/s42000-022-00377-8.
8. Lee JH, Kim D, Kim HJ, Lee CH, Yang JI, Kim W, Kim YJ, Yoon JH, Cho SH, Sung MW, Lee HS. Hepatic steatosis index: a simple screening tool reflecting nonalcoholic fatty liver disease. Dig Liver Dis. 2010;42(7):503–8. https://doi.org/10.1016/j.dld.2009.08.002.
9. Bedogni G, Bellentani S, Miglioli L, Masutti F, Passalacqua M, Castiglione A, Tiribelli C. The fatty liver index: a simple and accurate predictor of hepatic steatosis in the general population. BMC Gastroenterol. 2006;6:33. https://doi.org/10.1186/1471-230X-6-33.
10. Kotronen A, Peltonen M, Hakkarainen A, Sevastianova K, Bergholm R, Johansson LM, Lundbom N, Rissanen A, Ridderstråle M, Groop L, Orho-Melander M, Yki-Järvinen H. Prediction of non-alcoholic fatty liver disease and liver fat using metabolic and genetic factors. Gastroenterology. 2009;137(3):865–72. https://doi.org/10.1053/j.gastro.2009.06.005.
11. Munteanu M, Ratziu V, Morra R, Messous D, Imbert-Bismut F, Poynard T. Noninvasive biomarkers for the screening of fibrosis, steatosis and steatohepatitis in patients with metabolic risk factors: FibroTest-FibroMax experience. J Gastrointestin Liver Dis. 2008;17(2):187–91.
12. Bedogni G, Kahn HS, Bellentani S, Tiribelli C. A simple index of lipid overaccumulation is a good marker of liver steatosis. BMC Gastroenterol. 2010;10:98. https://doi.org/10.1186/1471-230X-10-98.
13. Petta S, Amato M, Cabibi D, Cammà C, Di Marco V, Giordano C, Galluzzo A, Craxì A. Visceral adiposity index is associated with histological findings and high viral load in patients with chronic hepatitis C due to genotype 1. Hepatology. 2010;52(5):1543–52. https://doi.org/10.1002/hep.23859.
14. Guerrero-Romero F, Simental-Mendía LE, González-Ortiz M, Martínez-Abundis E, Ramos-Zavala MG, Hernández-González SO, Jacques-Camarena O, Rodríguez-Morán M. The product of triglycerides and glucose, a simple measure of insulin sensitivity. Comparison with the euglycemic–hyperinsulinemic clamp. J Clin Endocrinol Metab. 2010;95(7):3347–51. https://doi.org/10.1210/jc.2010-0288.
15. Abenavoli L. Non-alcoholic fatty liver disease and cardiovascular disease: a close relationship. J Gastrointest Liver Dis. 2021;30(2):183–4. https://doi.org/10.15403/jgld-3698.
16. van Dijk AM, Schattenberg JM, Holleboom AG, Tushuizen ME. Referral care paths for non-alcoholic fatty liver disease-gearing up for an ever more prevalent and severe liver disease. United Eur Gastroenterol J. 2021;9(8):903–9. https://doi.org/10.1002/ueg2.12150.
17. Papatheodoridi M, Cholongitas E. Diagnosis of non-alcoholic fatty liver disease (NAFLD): current concepts. Curr Pharm Des. 2018;24(38):4574–86.

18. Musso G, Gambino R, Cassader M, Pagano G. Meta-analysis: natural history of non-alcoholic fatty liver disease (NAFLD) and diagnostic accuracy of non-invasive tests for liver disease severity. Ann Med. 2011;43(8):617–49.
19. McPherson S, Stewart SF, Henderson E, Burt AD, Day CP. Simple non-invasive fibrosis scoring systems can reliably exclude advanced fibrosis in patients with non-alcoholic fatty liver disease. Gut. 2010;59(9):1265–9.
20. Guha IN, Parkes J, Roderick P, Chattopadhyay D, Cross R, Harris S, Kaye P, Burt AD, Ryder SD, Aithal GP, Day CP, Rosenberg WM. Noninvasive markers of fibrosis in nonalcoholic fatty liver disease: validating the European liver fibrosis panel and exploring simple markers. Hepatology. 2008;47(2):455–60. https://doi.org/10.1002/hep.21984.
21. Sun W, Cui H, Li N, Wei Y, Lai S, Yang Y, Yin X, Chen DF. Comparison of FIB-4 index, NAFLD fibrosis score and BARD score for prediction of advanced fibrosis in adult patients with non-alcoholic fatty liver disease: a meta-analysis study. Hepatol Res. 2016;46(9):862–70. https://doi.org/10.1111/hepr.12647.
22. Calès P, Oberti F, Michalak S, Hubert-Fouchard I, Rousselet MC, Konaté A, Gallois Y, Ternisien C, Chevailler A, Lunel F. A novel panel of blood markers to assess the degree of liver fibrosis. Hepatology. 2005;42(6):1373–81. https://doi.org/10.1002/hep.20935.
23. Ratziu V, Massard J, Charlotte F, Messous D, Imbert-Bismut F, Bonyhay L, Tahiri M, Munteanu M, Thabut D, Cadranel JF, Le Bail B, de Ledinghen V, Poynard T, LIDO Study Group; CYTOL study group. Diagnostic value of biochemical markers (FibroTest–FibroSURE) for the prediction of liver fibrosis in patients with non-alcoholic fatty liver disease. BMC Gastroenterol. 2006;6:6. https://doi.org/10.1186/1471-230X-6-6.
24. Morra R, Munteanu M, Imbert-Bismut F, Messous D, Ratziu V, Poynard T. FibroMAX: towards a new universal biomarker of liver disease? Expert Rev Mol Diagn. 2007;7(5):481–90. https://doi.org/10.1586/14737159.7.5.481.
25. Powell EE, Wong VW, Rinella M. Non-alcoholic fatty liver disease. Lancet (London, England). 2021;397(10290):2212–24.
26. Sirbu A, Gologan S, Arbanas T, Copaescu C, Martin S, Albu A, Barbu C, Pirvulescu I, Fica S. Adiponectin, body mass index and hepatic steatosis are independently associated with IGF-I status in obese non-diabetic women. Growth Hormones IGF Res. 2013;23(1–2):2–7. https://doi.org/10.1016/j.ghir.2012.10.001.
27. Polyzos SA, Toulis KA, Goulis DG, Zavos C, Kountouras J. Serum total adiponectin in nonalcoholic fatty liver disease: a systematic review and meta-analysis. Metabolism. 2011;60(3):313–26.
28. Polyzos SA, Aronis KN, Kountouras J, Raptis DD, Vasiloglou MF, Mantzoros CS. Circulating leptin in non-alcoholic fatty liver disease: a systematic review and meta-analysis. Diabetologia. 2016;59(1):30–43.
29. He L, Deng L, Zhang Q, Guo J, Zhou J, Song W, Yuan F. Diagnostic value of CK-18, FGF-21, and related biomarker panel in nonalcoholic fatty liver disease: a systematic review and meta-analysis. Biomed Res Int. 2017;2017:9729107. https://doi.org/10.1155/2017/9729107.
30. Anty R, Iannelli A, Patouraux S, Bonnafous S, Lavallard VJ, Senni-Buratti M, Amor IB, Staccini-Myx A, Saint-Paul MC, Berthier F, Huet PM, Le Marchand-Brustel Y, Gugenheim J, Gual P, Tran A. A new composite model including metabolic syndrome, alanine aminotransferase and cytokeratin-18 for the diagnosis of non-alcoholic steatohepatitis in morbidly obese patients. Aliment Pharmacol Ther. 2010;32(11–12):1315–22. https://doi.org/10.1111/j.1365-2036.2010.04480.x.
31. Younossi ZM, Page S, Rafiq N, Birerdinc A, Stepanova M, Hossain N, Afendy A, Younoszai Z, Goodman Z, Baranova A. A biomarker panel for non-alcoholic steatohepatitis (NASH) and NASH-related fibrosis. Obes Surg. 2011;21(4):431–9. https://doi.org/10.1007/s11695-010-0204-1.
32. Poynard T, Ratziu V, Charlotte F, Messous D, Munteanu M, Imbert-Bismut F, Massard J, Bonyhay L, Tahiri M, Thabut D, Cadranel JF, Le Bail B, de Ledinghen V, LIDO Study Group; CYTOL Study Group. Diagnostic value of biochemical markers (NashTest) for the

prediction of non alcoholo steato hepatitis in patients with non-alcoholic fatty liver disease. BMC Gastroenterol. 2006;6:34. https://doi.org/10.1186/1471-230X-6-34.

33. Alkhouri N, Berk M, Yerian L, Lopez R, Chung YM, Zhang R, McIntyre TM, Feldstein AE, Hazen SL. OxNASH score correlates with histologic features and severity of nonalcoholic fatty liver disease. Dig Dis Sci. 2014;59(7):1617–24. https://doi.org/10.1007/s10620-014-3031-8.

Nonalcoholic Fatty Liver Disease Within Other Causes of Chronic Liver Diseases

12

Liana Gheorghe and Speranta Iacob

12.1 Introduction

Nonalcoholic fatty liver disease (NAFLD) includes a spectrum of related liver disorders [steatosis, nonalcoholic steatohepatitis (NASH), fibrosis, and cirrhosis] and represents the leading cause of chronic liver disease in Western regions [1]. NAFLD is a multisystem disease, which affects extrahepatic organs and regulatory pathways [2], with a significant impact on quality of life, morbidity, and overall mortality principally due to cardiovascular complications [3].

NAFLD is defined by the existence of hepatic steatosis (accumulation of triglycerides in >5% of hepatocytes) in the absence of other recognized causes of fatty liver (e.g., alcohol, virus, drugs, autoimmunity). NAFLD is usually found in patients with comorbidities, such as metabolic syndrome, obesity, insulin resistance, type 2 diabetes mellitus, and dyslipidemia [4, 5]. However, steatosis often occurs in association with other conditions such as alcohol abuse, HCV-infected patients, autoimmune hepatitis, celiac disease, Wilson disease, and drug- or toxin-induced hepatitis [1, 4, 6]. The hazard ratio for NAFLD liver-specific mortality is rather low [2, 6] because only a small number of patients with NAFLD progress to cirrhosis, but in the case of other diseases, coexistence, liver-related morbidity, and mortality can be increased because fibrosis stage is the most important prognostic factor. However, the great heterogeneity in the disease severity and outcome of NAFLD is multifactorial, including genetic and environmental factors.

Genome-wide association studies have contributed enormously to our understanding of the genetic contribution to NAFLD pathogenesis and variability of prognosis [7, 8].

L. Gheorghe (✉) · S. Iacob
Carol Davila University of Medicine and Pharmacy, Bucharest, Romania

Center for Digestive Diseases and Liver Transplantation, Fundeni Clinical Institute, Bucharest, Romania

© The Author(s), under exclusive license to Springer Nature Switzerland AG 2023
A. Trifan et al. (eds.), *Essentials of Non-Alcoholic Fatty Liver Disease*,
https://doi.org/10.1007/978-3-031-33548-8_12

Among the loci identified, the non-synonymous single nucleotide polymorphism (SNP) in PNPLA3 (phospholipase domain-containing 3) (rs738409) and a non-synonymous SNP in TM6SF2 (transmembrane 6 superfamily member 2) (rs58542926) have been associated with steatosis, grade of steatohepatitis, and stage of hepatic fibrosis/cirrhosis, as well as hepatocellular carcinoma (HCC).

PNPLA3 has hydrolytic activity towards triacylglycerols, diacylglycerol, and monoacylglycerol, and the I148M substitution determines a loss of function in the enzyme. This genetic variant is linked with higher liver lipid content, greater NASH activity, and enhanced risk of liver fibrosis and development of HCC [1].

A recent meta-analysis [9] pointed out that people with the CC genotype of PNPLA3 rs738409 had a 52% lower chance of developing NAFLD and those with the CG genotype had a 19% higher risk of NAFLD. People with the GG genotype were 105% more likely to evolve to NAFLD than others, while the population with CG + GG genotypes were 88% more likely to have NAFLD. In addition, these genes were also identified in the pathogenesis and progression of alcoholic liver disease (ALD).

In a representative cohort of the US population [10], the weighted allele frequency of the G (risk) allele of the rs738409 at PNPLA3 was 25.4%, and there was a significant interaction between the PNPLA3 gene G variant and alcohol consumption on hepatic steatosis; a dose-response association between alcohol consumption and hepatic steatosis among those with the GG genotype was noticed and a potential beneficial effect of moderate drinking among those with CC genotype. In patients with excess daily alcohol intake, the risk for cirrhosis is elevated by two- to three-fold in rs738409[G] carriers compared to those without this allele. In patients with NAFLD, GG homozygotes show a fivefold higher risk of HCC compared to CC homozygotes. An increased risk of HCC has also been observed in rs738409[G] carriers with alcohol-related cirrhosis [6, 11].

PNPLA3 genotype also impacts steatosis development and fibrosis progression in chronic hepatitis C and B [12, 13]. In addition, PNPLA3 SNP has been related to steatosis and fibrosis in patients with other chronic liver diseases such as Wilson disease [14], hereditary hemochromatosis [15], celiac disease [16], or autoimmune hepatitis (also linked with progression to liver transplantation or death) [17].

Lastly, the PNPLA3 (148M) variant may shortly become an important potential therapeutic target for chronic liver disease in the rs738409 allele carriers, as part of personalized medicine. For example, the PNPLA3 variant can be targeted at the RNA levels by small interfering RNA, small hairpin RNA, or antisense RNA oligo-nucleotide [18].

In 2020, a Consensus Group [19] proposed to replace the term NAFLD with MAFLD (metabolic dysfunction-associated fatty liver disease) since it does not require the elimination of alcoholic liver disease or viral hepatitis. It is a more appropriate terminology for persons with fatty liver and dysmetabolism. The new MAFLD criteria focus on the role of dysmetabolism in fat quantity in the liver, which is the most frequent driver of fatty liver injury progression. MAFLD is determined in patients when they have the liver expression of metabolic syndrome, which is diagnosed when three or more of the following settings are found: high glucose, hypertension, obesity, high triglyceride, and low high-density lipoprotein cholesterol.

In daily practice, we still use frequently only the term NAFLD, the hepatic manifestation of the metabolic syndrome, and we will refer in this chapter to the coexistence of this liver manifestation in other chronic liver diseases. From a clinical perspective, the main concerns consist of the need for further clarification and stratification of MAFLD to design decision-making and prognostic.

There is great heterogeneity in the disease severity and outcome of NAFLD/MAFLD, and there is a bidirectional linkage between fatty liver disease and all other causes of chronic liver injury (alcohol, viral, genetic, or autoimmune diseases).

12.2 Alcoholic Fatty Liver Disease (ALD) and NAFLD

Alcohol-related liver disease (ALD) and NAFLD are nowadays the leading causes of chronic liver disease. Obesity and alcohol synergistically increase the progression of fibrosis and mortality and augment hepatic carcinogenesis. One of the two conditions is often predominant, with the other acting as a cofactor of morbimortality [6].

The World Health Organization Global Status Report on Alcohol and Health estimated that 2.3 billion people are ongoing alcohol drinkers, who consume a regular of 32.8 g of pure alcohol per day [20]. Global per capita alcohol drinking increased from 1990 to 2017 and is projected to escalate further by 2030 [21]. Presently, Europe has the highest levels of alcohol drinking; however, it is projected to be exceeded by countries in the Western Pacific region by 2030. Alcohol was predicted to be linked with one-quarter of global cirrhosis deaths and one-fifth of liver cancer deaths in 2019 since it was the second fastest growing cause of liver cancer fatality from 2010 to 2019 [22].

Alcohol produces a wide spectrum of direct liver injuries ranging across steatosis, alcoholic hepatitis, cirrhosis, and hepatocellular carcinoma (HCC). However, individuals with heavy alcohol consumption (defined as consumption of >40 g of pure alcohol/day over a sustained period) will not all develop chronic liver disease, emphasizing the role of cofactors such as obesity and insulin resistance. Considering the high prevalence of overweight/obesity and alcohol use worldwide, the existence of these conditions in the same individual is frequent, and the presence of a combination of inflammatory lesions (alcoholic and nonalcoholic steatohepatitis) is highly probable [6]. Alongside the consequences to the liver, the combination of alcohol and metabolic factors is associated with an elevated risk of cardiovascular disease and cancers [23–25]. In obese patients, large alcohol consumption is associated with a higher risk (>twofold) of colorectal cancer than in obese patients with low alcohol consumption. On the other hand, NAFLD risk, as estimated by the Dallas steatosis index, is related with an increased risk of liver and non-liver gastrointestinal (esophageal, gastric, pancreatic, and colorectal) cancers. The elevated risks were similarly noted according to the history of diabetes, smoking status, and alcohol consumption and were generally stronger among men and individuals with higher body mass indexes in this very recent study [25].

The identification of patients with excess alcohol consumption and metabolic syndrome is important for the liver because it is associated not only with the incidence of steatosis, faster fibrosis progression, and higher mortality but also with less amelioration in steatosis in patients with NASH and increased liver malignancies.

Cirrhosis incidence will continue to increase by 9% over the next two decades secondary to NAFLD with an alarming rapid rise in ALD cirrhosis among young adults. NAFLD is projected to be responsible for 75% of all new cases of cirrhosis in the year 2040 across all birth cohorts in North America, in concordance with the increase in both obesity and diabetes, well-known risk factors for NAFLD. Weight loss of over 10% of total body weight is associated with fibrosis regression in patients with NAFLD and still represents the pillar of management [26]. ALD cirrhosis increased especially in those born after 1980 compared to a decrease in those born before 1946; it increased similarly in both sexes. This trend coincides with increases in binge drinking among the underaged and young adults in the United States [27].

Thus, in 2040, over 90% of all cases of cirrhosis should be, theoretically, preventable if NAFLD, ALD, and viral hepatitis can be identified and managed with lifestyle and public health interventions shown to decrease the progression of hepatic fibrosis.

The association between obesity and alcohol consumption was observed in other studies [28–30] as well: drinking more than three alcoholic drinks per day increased risks of alanine aminotransferase elevation in obese people by almost 8.9-fold; heavy drinkers and obese persons had a 5.8-fold higher risk of hepatic steatosis; binge drinking or increased weekly alcohol use (38 g/week vs. 17 g/week) was responsible for the progression of fibrosis.

However, other studies [31–33] have shown that light or modest alcohol consumption (<20 g/day or even <10 g/day) may be associated with lower rates of NAFLD, particularly in male patients or obese male patients. This positive effect seems only to be observed in wine drinkers that may buy healthier foods in comparison to beer drinkers. Any alcohol consumption, however, has been associated with increased risks (3.6-fold) of HCC in NASH patients [34].

In a study [35] that included 504,646 Korean patients, HCC incidence was associated with hepatitis B and C infection and each 20 g/day of alcohol intake increased the risk of HCC by 6%, 8%, 16%, and 30%, respectively, in subjects aged <50, 50–59, 60–69, and 70–80 years. Another European study [36] established that alcohol consumption is associated with a dose-dependent risk of advanced liver disease and neoplasia, as well as all-cause mortality. In this regard, it is not safe to recommend moderate alcohol consumption in patients with NAFLD. Also, the potential mechanism that may protect against NASH should be studied further. NASH patients have increased intestine permeability and endotoxemia, and regular drinking (<140 g/week) has been associated with lower endotoxin levels and anti-endotoxin core antibody immunoglobulin G, as well as with higher adiponectin levels and consecutive improved insulin sensitivity [37].

In clinical practice, we see patients with fatty liver diseases that have overlapping pathophysiology, frequently coexist, are rather difficult to determine the main contributing factor, and have the following features: patients with ALD that have metabolic cofactors and patients with NAFLD that drink alcohol which contributes to the disease process; in between, the great majority of patients have both conditions (NAFLD and ALD) with some showing an equal contribution of alcohol and metabolic factors (the proposed name is both alcohol and metabolic associated fatty liver disease, BAFLD) [37].

Although there is no agreement on the threshold of alcohol use that rules out NAFLD, a level of 30 g for men and 20 g daily for women, respectively, is used according to European and American guidelines [5, 38]. Light (1–9.9 g/day) or moderate (10–29.9 g/day for men and 10–19.9 g/day for women) alcohol consumption in patients with NAFLD is rather frequent. Almost two-thirds of adult patients with NAFLD in the United States drink alcohol, most of whom drink in moderation (approximately 4 drinks/week) [39]. As was already shown in the above paragraphs, there is no secure limit for alcohol consumption that should be recommended because either use can be associated with liver- or non-liver-related complications.

Recent studies are showing that MAFLD and NAFLD have similar clinical and metabolic profiles at baseline and long-term outcomes. The increased liver-related mortality among NAFLD is driven by insulin resistance, and MAFLD is primarily driven by ALD [40]. Another prospective study [41] showed that those who were excluded by the NAFLD definition and captured by the MAFLD definition seem to be at higher risk of adverse metabolic outcomes and cardiovascular events than those excluded by the MAFLD definition but captured by the NAFLD definition.

Histologically, nonalcoholic steatohepatitis (NASH) and alcohol-related steatohepatitis (ASH) are difficult to distinguish. These two entities include a certain degree of macrosteatosis, lobular inflammation, and ballooning. However, some lesions are described mainly in ASH: portal acute inflammation, presence of large numbers of neutrophils, sclerosing hyaline necrosis, and cholestasis. Other lesions such as fibro-obliterative and inflammatory lesions of the outflow veins, alcoholic foamy degeneration, and acute cholestasis are seen during ALD but have not been shown in NAFLD [6, 42].

NAFLD and ALD share common pathogenic mechanisms because obesity, metabolic syndrome, and alcohol utilization synergistically contribute to lipid dysregulation, oxidative stress, inflammation, and fibrogenesis [43]. Lipid metabolism dysregulation is a key factor in the pathogenesis of NAFLD and ALD. De novo lipogenesis and fatty acid oxidation are implicated in NAFLD pathogenesis, although lipid uptake, storage, and export may also play a role. Experimental models indicate that alcohol consumption further aggravates lipid dysregulation in metabolic syndrome. NAFLD risk factors and ethanol consumption also contribute to oxidative stress in fatty liver disease by dysregulating oxidative biochemical processes and producing reactive oxygen species (ROS). Three enzymes are decisive in the elimination of ROS: superoxide dismutase (SOD), catalase, and glutathione peroxidase. Clinical considerations illustrate that patients with NAFLD have increased SOD and glutathione peroxidase activities. Similarly, patients with ALD have upregulated SOD activity [44].

Macrophage and neutrophil activation also plays important roles in liver injury in the context of metabolic syndrome and alcohol usage. Oxidative stress, inflammation, and hepatocyte apoptosis contribute to hepatic fibrosis in NAFLD and ALD, and these pathways are mediated by hepatic stellate cells (HSCs). One significant fibrogenic mechanism in NAFLD and ALD is the TGFβ pathway. Another important signaling pathway is that of toll-like receptor 4, which responds to LPS and produces pro-inflammatory cytokines. Activated HSCs also produce tissue inhibitor of metalloproteinases, which inhibits extracellular matrix-degrading matrix metalloproteinases [42].

MicroRNAs (miRNAs), small noncoding RNAs, have been increasingly recognized as leading actors in the pathogenesis of a variety of diseases, including NAFLD and ALD, and as potential biomarkers for diagnosis or therapeutic targets. Sixteen miRNAs associated with ALD, except four (miR-199, miR-212, miR-214, and miR-497), are also proven to be related to NAFLD or lipid metabolism. On the other hand, miRNAs that are related to the pathogenesis of NAFLD (miR-122, miR-34a, and miR-155) are also clearly linked to ALD [45]. These results reflect the common mechanisms between NAFLD and ALD.

One essential point is that fibrosis is reversible in patients with ALD in a setting of prolonged abstinence as well as in NAFLD that lose weight; regressed fibrosis shares similarities in both groups and may be assessed by noninvasive methods. These findings highlight an important opportunity for public education and development of new policies and health plans surrounding alcohol and metabolic risk factors for chronic liver disease.

12.3　HCV Infection and NAFLD

Hepatic steatosis is frequently found in subjects with chronic HCV, occurring in approximately 50% of liver biopsy samples, with a reported range of 30–86%, with the highest prevalence in patients with HCV genotype 3 infections [46, 47]. Histologically, the perivenular fat distribution, ballooned hepatocytes, and pericellular fibrosis characteristic of NAFLD are usually not specific to hepatitis C, and the inflammation in hepatitis C is portal distributed [1].

Steatosis in HCV genotype 3-infected patients is associated with viral load and is therefore considered to be secondary to viral effect [48], while in non-genotype 3 patients, it is likely related to host factors (obesity, diabetes mellitus, alcohol consumption) [49]. However, a marked reduction in steatosis after weight loss has been seen in several patients infected with genotype 3, confirming that viral factors are not the single cause of fat accumulation [50].

NAFLD and HCV infection are two multisystem diseases, both leading to systemic and hepatic insulin resistance, partly mediated by the release of multiple pro-inflammatory cytokines, diabetogenic hepatocytes, and reactive oxygen species [51].

Type 2 diabetes mellitus is a prominent feature of the metabolic syndrome, which is bidirectionally associated with NAFLD, but HCV infection is also associated with specific hepatitis C-associated dysmetabolic syndrome (HCADS), which was first described by Lonardo et al. [52]. The characteristics of the HCADS are type 2 diabetes mellitus, hypertension, abdominal fat distribution, and atherogenic dyslipidemia (after HCV cure), although during active HCV infection, reversible hypocholesterolemia, hepatic steatosis (2.5- to threefold more prevalent than in other forms of hepatitis), hyperuricemia, accelerated atherogenesis, and increased risk of hepatocellular carcinoma may be acquired [51, 52].

Data from the literature suggest that improvement in NAFLD is associated with a decreased incidence of type 2 diabetes mellitus [51, 53]. Similarly, the prevention or amelioration of type 2 diabetes mellitus, as well as the reduction of cardiovascular events following HCV eradication in the era of direct-acting antiviral agents, was cited [54–57]. However, recent publications mentioned that HCV infection is positively correlated with insulin resistance, liver steatosis, metabolic syndrome, type 2 diabetes mellitus, atherosclerosis, and lipid rebound after DAA successful therapy [58, 59].

12.4 Copper and Iron Abnormalities and NAFLD

Wilson disease (WD) is a systemic disease with multiple clinical presentations, hepatic, neurological, ophthalmic, and psychiatric, that mimic other conditions. The first stage of liver disease histology in WD was considered to be steatosis [60]. This pathologic pattern mimics nonalcoholic fatty liver disease. Steatosis or nonalcoholic steatohepatitis may be present. Nuclear glycogen of hepatocytes is common. In cases with steatohepatitis, similar to NASH, large droplet steatosis, ballooning of hepatocytes, Mallory–Denk bodies, occasional acidophilic bodies, and fibrosis are seen [61].

The mechanisms linking copper to dysregulated lipid and energy metabolism in WD are not established but seem to include direct copper binding and modifications to labile proteins that impair enzymes and nuclear receptor function. Hepatic de novo lipogenesis is downregulated, and steatosis is the result of impaired mitochondrial β-oxidation, reduced very-low-density lipoprotein assembly or export, decreased utilization of lipids, and a significant downregulation in cholesterol synthesis. Altered carbohydrate metabolism may also be involved via defects in the alternating use of carbohydrates and fat as a metabolic fuel [62, 63]. On the other hand, actual evidence indicates a reciprocal connection between copper and lipid metabolism. Copper homeostasis is altered in many chronic conditions featuring dysregulation in lipid metabolism, including metabolic syndrome, obesity, and NAFLD [64, 65]. Patients with NAFLD have 50% less hepatic copper content compared to healthy subjects or patients with other liver diseases [66]. The same authors showed an inverse correlation between hepatic copper content and severity of steatosis, fasting glucose levels, insulin resistance, and presence of diabetes and metabolic syndrome.

NAFLD patients with lower serum and hepatic copper concentrations also have concomitant higher serum ferritin levels and increased hepatic iron concentrations [67].

It is universally accepted that iron overburden is common in patients with NAFLD and iron-induced lipid peroxide is one of the major contributors to NAFLD. An iron imbalance is also implicated in obesity and insulin resistance. Ferroptosis, a form of regulated cell death, is characterized by exaggerate accumulation of intracellular lipid reactive oxygen species and lipid peroxidation resulting from iron-dependent depletion of glutathione and inactivation of glutathione peroxidase 4. Ferroptosis proved to contribute to the progression of liver damage in chronic liver diseases like NAFLD. Thus, ferroptosis may be an ideal target for nonviral liver diseases [68]. Iron overload due to metabolic dysfunction (such as liver siderosis and hereditary hemochromatosis) proved to aggravate liver injury in patients with NASH [69], but the liver injury can be improved by iron removal in patients with NAFLD [68].

12.5 Celiac Disease (CD) and NAFLD

NAFLD occurrence in CD patients is considered by some authors as a coincidence rather than a true relationship, due to the high frequency of both diseases in the general population [70].

The recorded prevalence of CD in patients with NAFLD is 2–14% [71]. Although approximately 50% of treatment-naïve patients with CD had their body mass index within normal limits as expected, 8–44% of the patients were found to be overweight or obese at the time of diagnosis of CD [72, 73].

Patients with NAFLD are at increased risk for a later diagnosis of CD. On the other hand, individuals with CD seem to be at increased risk (4–6 times) of NAFLD compared to the general population. The relative risk of NAFLD development after a CD diagnosis is higher in the first 5 years but remained statistically significant even 15 years after a CD diagnosis [74].

Several studies demonstrated that gluten-free diet (GFD), although it is the treatment for CD, has potentially negative effects on nutritional and metabolic status [75, 76]. GFD can determine a higher intake of simple sugars, proteins, and saturated fat and a lower intake of complex carbohydrates and fibers. Another characteristic of gluten-free foods is represented by a higher glycemic index than that of equivalent gluten-containing foods. In patients with CD on a GFD, both the increase in nutrient absorption (as a result of the improvement of the atrophy of the gut mucosa) and the intake of higher calories, fats, and simple carbohydrates could contribute to the worsening of the metabolic status and to the increase of the prevalence of NAFLD in these patients [77]. Tortora et al. [78] reported an increase in the prevalence of metabolic syndrome from 2% at the time of diagnosis to 30% after 12 months of GFD. Thus, patients with CD on GFD should be assessed for nutritional and metabolic features at regular intervals and should be counseled about a balanced diet and sustained physical activity. This may be of great importance because GFD has become increasingly popular worldwide, with many individuals believing it to be more "healthful" and claiming that it has beneficial effects for health conditions other than CD.

12.6 Autoimmune Liver Diseases and NAFLD

Autoimmune hepatitis (AIH) and metabolic associated fatty liver disease (MAFLD) coexist rather frequently (with an overall estimated prevalence between 17 and 30%) with a potential synergistic impact on the course of both diseases and response to therapy [79].

Histologically, significant fibrosis, portal inflammation, and plasma cell infiltration were demonstrated more frequently in MAFLD/AIH compared to those with MAFLD alone [17]. Similar findings were observed in the study by Muller et al. [80] that preexisting NAFLD potentiates the severity of an autoimmune condition of the liver, such as AIH; there was an increased cellular infiltration of the liver, enhanced hepatic fibrosis, and elevated numbers of liver autoantigen-specific T cells.

An increased prevalence (20–30%) of autoantibodies is mentioned in MAFLD patients, as compared to the general population, but not all MAFLD patients with positive autoantibodies had AIH coexistence (only about 10%) [17]. Patients with NASH, who were seropositive for antinuclear antibodies (ANA), proved to have more serious fibrosis and necroinflammation in the liver than those with seronegative NASH. High titers of ANA, but not smooth muscle antibodies in NAFLD, were significantly associated with insulin resistance [81].

The impact of MAFLD on the treatment response of AIH is not extensively studied; however, it was hypothesized that the concurrent presence of MAFLD with AIH may be an explanation for the treatment failure in some patients with AIH. In a large Japanese study [82], patients with MAFLD/AIH were found to be significantly more likely to receive ursodeoxycholic acid, while they were less likely to receive prednisolone treatment compared to AIH without MAFLD. It was shown that patients with MAFLD/AIH variants could have dual mechanisms for increased risk of mortality, either hepatic or extrahepatic (non-hepatic cancers and vascular events) [17].

12.7 Drug-Induced Liver Disease and NAFLD

The relationship between DILI and NAFLD may be reciprocal: drugs can cause NAFLD by acting as steatogenic factors, and preexisting NAFLD could be a predisposing condition for certain drugs to cause DILI. Polypharmacy associated with obesity might potentiate the association between this condition and DILI [83]. There is an expanding number of clinical reports proposing that certain drugs can be more hepatotoxic in overweight patients with metabolic dysfunction-associated fatty liver disease, in contrast with the lean patient. Some of the drugs may cause more severe and/or more frequent acute liver injury in obese individuals, whereas others may trigger the transition of simple fatty liver to NASH or may worsen hepatic lipid accumulation, necroinflammation, and fibrosis [84].

Drug-induced fatty liver disease (DIFLD) is a specific form of DILI, characterized by intracellular lipid accumulation in hepatocytes with steatotic changes (macro- or microvesicular) as the predominant histopathological pattern. Although this histopathological feature is required for the diagnosis, the finding is not specific [85, 86]. DIFLD is often accompanied by inflammation and oxidative stress, which leads to the development of drug-induced steatohepatitis (DISH).

Chronic liver injury leads to hepatocyte death, followed by the activation of stellate cells, which finally results in liver tissue fibrosis. The mechanisms associated with the induction of steatosis are increased fatty acid synthesis, decreased fatty acid β-oxidation, decreased lipoprotein export, and increased mobilization and uptake of fatty acids [86, 87].

According to EASL guidelines [84, 88–91], different categories of drugs can induce the following types of liver injury
1. Acute liver injuries are caused by amiodarone, aspirin, acetaminophen, ibuprofen, isoflurane, fosinopril, halothane, vitamin A, valproate acid, tetracycline, telithromycin, piperacillin/tazobactam, nucleoside reverse transcriptase inhibitors (NRTIs), zalcitabine, losartan, omeprazole, sorafenib, ticlopidine, and troglitazone.
2. Exacerbation of preexisting fatty liver or MASH: androgenic steroids, benzbromarone, corticosteroids, irinotecan, methotrexate, tamoxifen, NRTIs, pentoxifylline, phenobarbital, rosiglitazone, and tetracycline.
3. Promoting the transition of preexisting fatty liver into MASH, fibrosis, or cirrhosis: androgenic steroids, benzbromarone, corticosteroids, irinotecan, methotrexate, and tamoxifen.

Special attention needs to be given to psychoactive drugs that are increasingly used in the long term, even beginning with early youth. This practice was even more pregnant during the COVID period, which was associated with an increased prevalence of major depressive disorder and anxiety disorders [92].

Monoamine oxidase inhibitors and tricyclic antidepressants were introduced in clinical practice in the 1950s and were often related to liver toxicity. They were replaced by safer and better tolerated new generations of antidepressants: selective serotonin reuptake inhibitors, serotonin and norepinephrine reuptake inhibitors, and serotonin antagonist and reuptake inhibitors. All these drugs demonstrate an idiosyncratic, unpredictable, and reversible hepatic injury, usually of hepatocellular type and less frequently of the cholestatic or mixed pattern [93]. However, in vitro and animal studies provided substantial evidence that various antidepressants (especially selective serotonin reuptake inhibitors: fluoxetine and fluvoxamine) have a steatogenic effect. Steatogenic effects of antipsychotics were also mentioned mainly for clozapine, risperidone, olanzapine, and aripiprazole [93].

Management of DISH usually implies stopping the offending drug.

Although the number of drugs causing DISH is a relatively small fraction of all fatty liver cases, this issue assumes a far greater significance against the background of the fast-growing metabolic NAFLD pandemic that accompanies obesity in the whole world.

In summary, NAFLD has become a relatively unknown disease to the most common cause of chronic liver disease worldwide in the last 20 years, with increased liver- and non-liver-related mortality. The prevalence of NAFLD, as well as the genetic and environmental factors that determine its associated risk, varies. NAFLD associated with other chronic liver diseases has an intertwined connection usually aggravating, but also decreasing the rate of fibrosis progression and risk of decompensated liver cirrhosis. Addressing the growing burden of NAFLD will require setting up a multidisciplinary team and collaborating to deliver a person-centered, personalized care and management of people with NAFLD. Enhanced training of the public about risk factors for chronic liver diseases (NAFLD/MAFLD, alcohol, adequate therapy of Wilson disease and celiac disease, and gluten-free diet) and actions to prevent the occurrence of cirrhosis will be essential to reduce cirrhosis burden and liver-related mortality in the future.

References

1. Chen YY, Yeh MM. Non-alcoholic fatty liver disease: a review with clinical and pathological correlation. J Formos Med Assoc. 2021;120:68–77.
2. Byrne CD, Targher G. NAFLD: a multisystem disease. J Hepatol. 2015;62:S47–64.
3. Younossi Z, Aggarwal P, Shrestha I, Fernandes J, Johansen P, Augusto M, Nair S. The burden of non-alcoholic steatohepatitis: a systematic review of health-related quality of life and patient-reported outcomes. JHEP Rep. 2022;4(9):100525.
4. Bellentani S, Saccoccio G, Masutti F, Crocè LS, Brandi G, Sasso F, et al. Prevalence of and risk factors for hepatic steatosis in Northern Italy. Ann Intern Med. 2000;132(2):112–7.
5. European Association for the Study of the Liver (EASL); European Association for the Study of Diabetes (EASD); European Association for the Study of Obesity (EASO). EASL-EASD-EASO clinical practice guidelines for the management of non-alcoholic fatty liver disease. J Hepatol. 2016;64(6):1388–402.
6. Ntandja Wandji LC, Gnemmi V, Mathurin P, Louvet A. Combined alcoholic and non-alcoholic steatohepatitis. JHEP Rep. 2020;2(3):100101.
7. Anstee QM, Day CP. The genetics of NAFLD. Nat Rev Gastroenterol Hepatol. 2013;10:645–55.
8. Anstee QM, Darlay R, Cockell S, Meroni M, Govaere O, Tiniakos D, et al. Genome-wide association study of non-alcoholic fatty liver and steatohepatitis in a histologically characterised cohort. J Hepatol. 2020;73(3):505–15.
9. Salari N, Darvishi N, Mansouri K, Ghasemi H, Hosseinian-Far M, Darvishi F, et al. Association between PNPLA3 rs738409 polymorphism and nonalcoholic fatty liver disease: a systematic review and meta-analysis. BMC Endocr Disord. 2021;21(1):125.
10. Lazo M, Bilal U, Mitchell MC, Potter J, Hernaez R, Clark JM. Interaction between alcohol consumption and *PNPLA3* variant in the prevalence of hepatic steatosis in the U.S. population. Clin Gastroenterol Hepatol. 2021;19(12):2606–2614.e4.
11. Stickel F, Hampe J, Trépo E, Datz C, Romeo S. PNPLA3 genetic variation in alcoholic steatosis and liver disease progression. Hepatobiliary Surg Nutr. 2015;4(3):152–60.
12. Trepo E, Pradat P, Potthoff A, et al. Impact of patatin-like phospholipase-3 (rs738409 C>G) polymorphism on fibrosis progression and steatosis in chronic hepatitis C. Hepatology. 2011;54:60–9.
13. Viganò M, Valenti L, Lampertico P, et al. Patatin-like phospholipase domain-containing 3 I148M affects liver steatosis in patients with chronic hepatitis B. Hepatology. 2013;58:1245–52.
14. Stättermayer AF, Traussnigg S, Dienes HP, Aigner E, Stauber R, Lackner K, et al. Hepatic steatosis in Wilson disease—role of copper and *PNPLA3* mutations. J Hepatol. 2015;63(1):156–63.

15. Valenti L, Maggioni P, Piperno A, et al. Patatin-like phospholipase domain containing-3 gene I148M polymorphism, steatosis, and liver damage in hereditary hemochromatosis. World J Gasroenterol. 2012;18:2813–20.
16. Tortora R, Rispo A, Alisi A, Imperatore N, Crudele A, Ferretti F, et al. PNPLA3 rs738409 polymorphism predicts development and severity of hepatic steatosis but not metabolic syndrome in celiac disease. Nutrients. 2018;10(9):1239.
17. Gaber Y, AbdAllah M, Salama A, Sayed M, Abdel Alem S, Nafady S. Metabolic-associated fatty liver disease and autoimmune hepatitis: an overlooked interaction. Expert Rev Gastroenterol Hepatol. 2021;15(10):1181–9.
18. Dong XC. PNPLA3—a potential therapeutic target for personalized treatment of chronic liver disease. Front Med (Lausanne). 2019;6:304.
19. Eslam M, Newsome PN, Sarin SK, Anstee QM, Targher G, Romero-Gomez M, et al. A new definition for metabolic dysfunction-associated fatty liver disease: an international expert consensus statement. J Hepatol. 2020;73(1):202–9.
20. World Health Organization. Global status report on alcohol and health 2018. WHO. https://www.who.int/publications/i/item/9789241565639.
21. Manthey J, Shield KD, Rylett M, Hasan O, Probst C, Rehm J. Global alcohol exposure between 1990 and 2017 and forecasts until 2030: a modelling study. Lancet. 2019;393(10190):2493–502.
22. Huang D, Mathurin P, Cortez-Pinto H, Rohit LR. Global epidemiology of alcohol-associated cirrhosis and HCC: trends, projections and risk factors. Nat Rev Gastroenterol Hepatol. 2022;20:37–49.
23. Massetti GM, Dietz WH, Richardson LC. Excessive weight gain, obesity, and cancer: opportunities for clinical intervention. JAMA. 2017;318(20):1975–6.
24. Targher G, Byrne CD, Tilg H. NAFLD and increased risk of cardiovascular disease: clinical associations, pathophysiological mechanisms and pharmacological implications. Gut. 2020;69(9):1691–705.
25. McHenry S, Zong X, Shi M, Fritz CDL, Pedersen KS, Peterson LR, et al. Risk of nonalcoholic fatty liver disease and associations with gastrointestinal cancers. Hepatol Commun. 2022;6(12):3299–310. https://doi.org/10.1002/hep4.2073.
26. Flemming J, Djerboua M, Groome PA, Booth C, Terrault N. NAFLD and alcohol-related liver disease will be responsible for almost all new diagnoses of cirrhosis in Canada by 2040. Hepatology. 2021;74(6):3330–44.
27. Kanny D, Naimi TS, Liu Y, Brewer RD. Trends in total binge drinks per adult who reported binge drinking—United States, 2011–2017. MMWR Morb Mortal Wkly Rep. 2020;69(2):30–4.
28. Bellentani S, Saccoccio G, Masutti F, et al. Prevalence of and risk factors for hepatic steatosis in Northern Italy. Ann Intern Med. 2000;132:112–7.
29. Loomba R, Bettencourt R, Barrett-Connor E. Synergistic association between alcohol intake and body mass index with serum alanine and aspartate aminotransferase levels in older adults: the Rancho Bernardo Study. Aliment Pharmacol Ther. 2009;30:1137–49.
30. Ekstedt M, Franzen LE, Holmqvist M, et al. Alcohol consumption is associated with progression of hepatic fibrosis in non-alcoholic fatty liver disease. Scand J Gastroenterol. 2009;44:366–74.
31. Sogabe M, Okahisa T, Taniguchi T, et al. Light alcohol consumption plays a protective role against non-alcoholic fatty liver disease in Japanese men with metabolic syndrome. Liver Int. 2015;35:1707–14.
32. Gunji T, Matsuhashi N, Sato H, et al. Light and moderate alcohol consumption significantly reduces the prevalence of fatty liver in the Japanese male population. Am J Gastroenterol. 2009;104:2189–95.
33. Dunn W, Sanyal AJ, Brunt EM, et al. Modest alcohol consumption is associated with decreased prevalence of steatohepatitis in patients with non-alcoholic fatty liver disease (NAFLD). J Hepatol. 2012;57:384–91.
34. Ascha MS, Hanouneh IA, Lopez R, et al. The incidence and risk factors of hepatocellular carcinoma in patients with nonalcoholic steatohepatitis. Hepatology. 2010;51:1972–8.

35. Yi SW, Choi JS, Yi JJ, Lee YH, Han KJ. Risk factors for hepatocellular carcinoma by age, sex, and liver disorder status: a prospective cohort study in Korea. Cancer. 2018;124:2748–57.
36. Aberg F, Puukka P, Salomaa V, Mannisto S, Lundqvist A, Valsta L, et al. Risks of light and moderate alcohol use in fatty liver disease: follow-up of population cohorts. Hepatology. 2020;71:835–48.
37. Idalsoaga F, Kulkarni AV, Mousa OY, Arrese M, Arab JP. Non-alcoholic fatty liver disease and alcohol-related liver disease: two intertwined entities. Front Med (Lausanne). 2020;7:448.
38. Chalasani N, Younossi Z, Lavine JE, Charlton M, Cusi K, Rinella M, et al. The diagnosis and management of nonalcoholic fatty liver disease: practice guidance from the American Association for the Study of Liver Diseases. Hepatology. 2018;67(1):328–57.
39. Eslam M, Sanyal AJ, George J. Toward more accurate nomenclature for fatty liver diseases. Gastroenterology. 2019;157(3):590–3.
40. Younossi ZM, Paik JM, Shabeeb RA, Golabi P, Younossi I, Henry L. Are there outcome differences between NAFLD and metabolic-associated fatty liver disease? Hepatology. 2022;76(5):1423–37.
41. Niriella M, Ediriweera DS, Kasturiratne A, De Silva ST, Dassanayaka AS, De Silva AP, et al. Outcomes of NAFLD and MAFLD: results from a community-based, prospective cohort study. PLoS One. 2021;16(2):e0245762.
42. Lackner C, Tiniakos D. Fibrosis and alcohol-related liver disease. J Hepatol. 2019;70(2):294–304.
43. Buyco DG, Martin J, Jeon S, Hooks R, Lin C, Carr R. Experimental models of metabolic and alcoholic fatty liver disease. World J Gastroenterol. 2021;27(1):1–18.
44. Robinson KE, Shah VH. Pathogenesis and pathways: nonalcoholic fatty liver disease and alcoholic liver disease. Transl Gastroenterol Hepatol. 2020;5:49.
45. Torres JL, Novo-Veleiro I, Manzanedo L, Alvela-Suárez L, Macías R, Laso FJ, Marcos M. Role of microRNAs in alcohol-induced liver disorders and non-alcoholic fatty liver disease. World J Gastroenterol. 2018;24(36):4104–18.
46. Adinolfi LE, Rinaldi L, Guerrera B, Restivo L, Marrone A, Giordano M, et al. NAFLD and NASH in HCV infection: prevalence and significance in hepatic and extrahepatic manifestations. Int J Mol Sci. 2016;17(6):1–12.
47. Ramesh S, Sanyal AJ. Hepatitis C and nonalcoholic fatty liver disease. Semin Liver Dis. 2004;24:399–413.
48. Rubbia-Brandt L, Quadri R, Abid K, Giostra E, Male P-J, Mentha G, et al. Hepatocyte steatosis is a cytopathic effect of hepatitis C virus genotype 3. J Hepatol. 2000;33(1):106–15.
49. Persico M, Iolascon A. Steatosis as a co-factor in chronic liver diseases. World J Gastroenterol. 2010;16(10):1171–6.
50. Hickman IJ, Clouston AD, Macdonald GA, Purdie DM, Prins JB, Ash S, et al. Effect of weight reduction on liver histology and biochemistry in patients with chronic hepatitis C. Gut. 2002;51:89–94.
51. Ballestri S, Nascimbeni F, Romagnoli D, Baldelli E, Targher G, Lonardo A. Type 2 diabetes in non-alcoholic fatty liver disease and hepatitis C virus infection—liver: the "musketeer" in the spotlight. Int J Mol Sci. 2016;17(3):355.
52. Lonardo A, Ballestri S, Marchesini G, Angulo P, Loria P. Nonalcoholic fatty liver disease: a precursor of the metabolic syndrome. Dig Liver Dis. 2015;47:181–90.
53. Björkström K, Stål P, Holmer M, Bengtsson B, Staaf A, Hoffstedt J, Hagström H. A personalized treatment program in persons with type 2 diabetes is associated with a reduction in liver steatosis. Eur J Gastroenterol Hepatol. 2021;33(11):1420–6.
54. Morales AL, Junga Z, Singla MB, Sjogren M, Torres D. Hepatitis C eradication with sofosbuvir leads to significant metabolic changes. World J Hepatol. 2016;8(35):1557–63.
55. Adinolfi LE, Salvatore Petta S, Fracanzani AL, Coppola C, Narciso V, Nevola R, Rinaldi L. Impact of hepatitis C virus clearance by direct-acting antiviral treatment on the incidence of major cardiovascular events: a prospective multicentre study. Atherosclerosis. 2020;296:40–7.

56. Mahmoud B, Moneim AA, Mabrouk D. The impact of HCV eradication on hyperglycemia, insulin resistance, cytokine production, and insulin receptor substrate-1 and 2 expression in patients with HCV infection. Clin Exp Med. 2022;22(4):583–93.
57. Russo FP, Zanetto A, Gambato M, Bortoluzzi I, Al Zoairy R, Franceschet E, et al. Hepatitis C virus eradication with direct-acting antiviral improves insulin resistance. J Viral Hepat. 2020;27(2):188–94.
58. Wang CC, Cheng PN, Kao JH. Systematic review: chronic viral hepatitis and metabolic derangement. Aliment Pharmacol Ther. 2020;51:216–30.
59. Iacob S, Onica M, Iacob R, Gheorghe C, Beckebaum S, Cicinnati V, Popescu I, Gheorghe L. Impact of sustained virological response on metabolic profile and kidney function in cured HCV liver transplant recipients. Surg Gastroenterol Oncol. 2021;26(2):104–10.
60. Pilloni L, Coni P, Manscou G, et al. Late onset Wilson's disease. Pathologica. 2004;96(3):105–10.
61. Guindi M. Wilson disease. Semin Diagn Pathol. 2019;36(6):415–22.
62. Mazi TA, Shibata NM, Medici V. Lipid and energy metabolism in Wilson disease. Liver Res. 2020;4(1):5–14.
63. Liggi M, Murgia D, Civolani A, Demelia E, Sorbello O, Demelia L. The relationship between copper and steatosis in Wilson's disease. Clin Res Hepatol Gastroenterol. 2013;37:36–40.
64. Saari JT. Copper deficiency and cardiovascular disease: role of peroxidation, glycation, and nitration. Can J Physiol Pharmacol. 2000;78:848–55.
65. Tang Z, Gasperkova D, Xu J, Baillie R, Lee JH, Clarke SD. Copper deficiency induces hepatic fatty acid synthase gene transcription in rats by increasing the nuclear content of mature sterol regulatory element binding protein 1. J Nutr. 2000;130:2915–21.
66. Aigner E, Strasser M, Haufe H, et al. A role for low hepatic copper concentrations in nonalcoholic fatty liver disease. Am J Gastroenterol. 2010;105:1978–85.
67. Aigner E, Theurl I, Haufe H, et al. Copper availability contributes to iron perturbations in human nonalcoholic fatty liver disease. Gastroenterology. 2008;135:680–8.
68. Jia M, Zhang H, Qin Q, Hou Y, Zhang X, Chen D, et al. Ferroptosis as a new therapeutic opportunity for nonviral liver disease. Eur J Pharmacol. 2021;908:174319.
69. Nelson JE, Wilson L, Brunt EM, Yeh MM, Kleiner DE, Unalp-Arida A, Kowdley K. Relationship between the pattern of hepatic iron deposition and histological severity in nonalcoholic fatty liver disease. Hepatology. 2011;53:448–57.
70. Freeman HJ. Hepatic manifestations of celiac disease. Clin Exp Gastroenterol. 2010;3:33–9.
71. Abenavoli L, Milic N, de Lorenzo A, Luzza F. A pathogenetic link between non-alcoholic fatty liver disease and celiac disease. Endocrine. 2013;43:65–7.
72. Singh I, Agnihotri A, Sharma A, et al. Patients with celiac disease may have normal weight or may even be overweight. Indian J Gastroenterol. 2016;35:20–4.
73. Tucker E, Rostami K, Prabhakaran S, Al Dulaimi D. Patients with coeliac disease are increasingly overweight or obese on presentation. J Gastrointest Liver Dis. 2012;21:11–5.
74. Reilly NR, Lebwohl B, Hultcrantz R, Green PHR, Ludvigsson JF. Increased risk of non-alcoholic fatty liver disease after diagnosis of celiac disease. J Hepatol. 2015;62:1405–11.
75. Agarwal A, Singh A, Mehtab W, Gupta V, Chauhan A, Rajput MS, et al. Patients with celiac disease are at high risk of developing metabolic syndrome and fatty liver. Intest Res. 2021;19:106–14.
76. Ukkola A, Mäki M, Kurppa K, Collin P, Huhtala H, Kekkonen L, Kaukinen K. Changes in body mass index on a gluten-free diet in coeliac disease: a nationwide study. Eur J Intern Med. 2012;23:384–8.
77. Valvano M, Longo S, Stefanelli G, Frieri G, Viscido A, Latella G. Celiac disease, gluten-free diet, and metabolic and liver Disorders. Nutrients. 2020;12(4):940.
78. Tortora R, Capone P, De Stefano G, et al. Metabolic syndrome in patients with coeliac disease on a gluten-free diet. Aliment Pharmacol Ther. 2015;41:352–9.
79. Dalekos GN, Gatselis NK, Zachou K, et al. NAFLD and autoimmune hepatitis: do not judge a book by its cover. Eur J Intern Med. 2020;75:1–9.

80. Müller P, Messmer M, Bayer M, Pfeilschifter JM, Hintermann E, Christen U. Non-alcoholic fatty liver disease (NAFLD) potentiates autoimmune hepatitis in the CYP2D6 mouse model. J Autoimmun. 2016;69:51–8.
81. Himoto T, Nishioka M. Autoantibodies in liver disease: important clues for the diagnosis, disease activity and prognosis. Autoimmun Highlights. 2013;4:39–53.
82. Takahashi A, Arinaga-Hino T, Ohira H, et al. Non-alcoholic fatty liver disease in patients with autoimmune hepatitis. JGH Open. 2018;2(2):54–8.
83. Bessone F, Dirchwolf M, Rodil MA, Razori MV, Roma MG. Review article: Drug-induced liver injury in the context of nonalcoholic fatty liver disease—a physiopathological and clinical integrated view. Aliment Pharmacol Ther. 2018;48(9):892–913.
84. Allard J, Le Guillou D, Begriche K, Fromenty B. Drug-induced liver injury in obesity and nonalcoholic fatty liver disease. Adv Pharmacol. 2019;85:75–107.
85. Kolaric TO, Nincevic V, Kuna L, Duspara K, Bojanic K, Vukadin S, et al. Drug-induced fatty liver disease: pathogenesis and treatment. J Clin Transl Hepatol. 2021;9(5):731–7.
86. Dash A, Figler RA, Sanyal AJ, Wamhoff BR. Drug-induced steatohepatitis. Expert Opin Drug Metab Toxicol. 2017;13(2):193–204.
87. Begriche K, Massart J, Robin MA, Borgne-Sanchez A, Fromenty B. Drug-induced toxicity on mitochondria and lipid metabolism: mechanistic diversity and deleterious consequences for the liver. J Hepatol. 2011;54(4):773–94.
88. Massart J, Begriche K, Moreau C, Fromenty B. Role of nonalcoholic fatty liver disease as risk factor for drug-induced hepatotoxicity. J Clin Transl Res. 2017;3(Suppl. 1):212–32.
89. Michaut A, Moreau C, Robin MA, Fromenty B. Acetaminophen-induced liver injury in obesity and nonalcoholic fatty liver disease. Liver Int. 2014;34:e171–9.
90. Schmajuk G, Miao Y, Yazdany J, Boscardin WJ, Daikh DI, Steinman MA. Identification of risk factors for elevated transaminases in methotrexate users through an electronic health record. Arthritis Care Res (Hoboken). 2014;66:1159–66.
91. Brennan PN, Cartlidge P, Manship T, Dillon JF. Guideline review: EASL clinical practice guidelines: drug-induced liver injury (DILI). Frontline Gastroenterol. 2021;13(4):332–6.
92. COVID-19 Mental Disorders Collaborators. Global prevalence and burden of depressive and anxiety disorders in 204 countries and territories in 2020 due to the COVID-19 pandemic. Lancet. 2021;398(10312):1700–12.
93. Vukotić NT, Đorđević J, Pejić S, Đorđević N, Pajović SB. Antidepressants- and antipsychotics-induced hepatotoxicity. Arch Toxicol. 2021;95(3):767–89.

Pathophysiology and Risk Stratification in Cardiovascular Diseases and NAFLD

13

Irina Girleanu and Stefan Chiriac

13.1 The Pathophysiological Link Between Cardiovascular Diseases and NAFLD

The heterogeneity of NAFLD is determined by the complex pathogenesis. NAFLD and cardiovascular diseases are part of a multisystem disease with complex interplay, and thus it is difficult to discern unidirectional cause-effect relationships. NAFLD and cardiovascular diseases share many risk factors such as obesity, diabetes, metabolic syndrome, and hypertension. Moreover, the key common pathophysiological factor for all of these conditions is systemic inflammation.

13.1.1 Lipid Metabolism and Dysfunctional Adipose Tissue

Nowadays, it is well known that NAFLD is associated with an atherogenic lipid profile [1]. Different pathways are involved in lipid metabolism in patients with NAFLD. The accumulation of triglycerides in the liver is a fat-balanced equation including the amounts of fatty acids produced and delivered to the liver as well as the elimination of these fatty acids by either oxidation or secretion in the form of very-low-density lipoprotein (VLDL)-triglycerides [2].

One of the main factors linking NAFLD and cardiovascular diseases is the increase in dysfunctional visceral fat situated in the pancreas and epicardial or skeletal muscles [3]. Moreover, ectopic cardiac fat plays an important role in the common pathophysiology of NAFLD and cardiovascular diseases. There are two main types of cardiac fat, with different influences on cardiovascular risk: the epicardial

I. Girleanu (✉) · S. Chiriac
"Grigore T. Popa" University of Medicine and Pharmacy, Iasi, Romania

Institute of Gastroenterology and Hepatology, "Saint Spiridon" University Hospital, Iasi, Romania

© The Author(s), under exclusive license to Springer Nature Switzerland AG 2023
A. Trifan et al. (eds.), *Essentials of Non-Alcoholic Fatty Liver Disease*,
https://doi.org/10.1007/978-3-031-33548-8_13

fat (located between the myocardium and pericardium) and the pericardial fat (surrounding the heart externally to the pericardium) [4]. The epicardial fat activates the cardiac nervous system and in healthy persons has the role of nourishing the myocardium, and also secretes anti-inflammatory and anti-fibrotic molecules [5]. In NAFLD patients, particularly in those that associate obesity, the epicardial fat decreases the release of adiponectin and increases the production of proinflammatory cytokines as interleukin (IL)-1, TNF-α, and IL-6, thus losing its protective characteristics [6, 7]. All of these changes promote coronary inflammation, myocardial fibrosis leading to heart failure with preserved ejection fraction, atrial fibrillation, as well as development of acute or chronic coronary syndrome (Fig. 13.1).

Both subcutaneous and visceral fat, and also triglycerides rich in lipoproteins, can release free fatty acids (FFAs) in the systemic circulation and the portal vein, thus delivering them to the liver. If the fatty acids are not oxidized as fuel and incorporated in triglycerides as VLDL, they accumulate in the liver [8]. In addition, circulating glucose and fructose can also stimulate fatty acid production through a mechanism known as de novo lipogenesis. The accumulation of FFA in the liver is influenced by adipokines, exosomes, secretion of insulin and glucagon, lifestyle factors, and gut microbiota [9]. It was demonstrated that the oxidation of the FFA in patients with NAFLD is the same as compared to the general population without NAFLD, although the VLDL-triglyceride (VLDL-TG) secretion rate is higher in

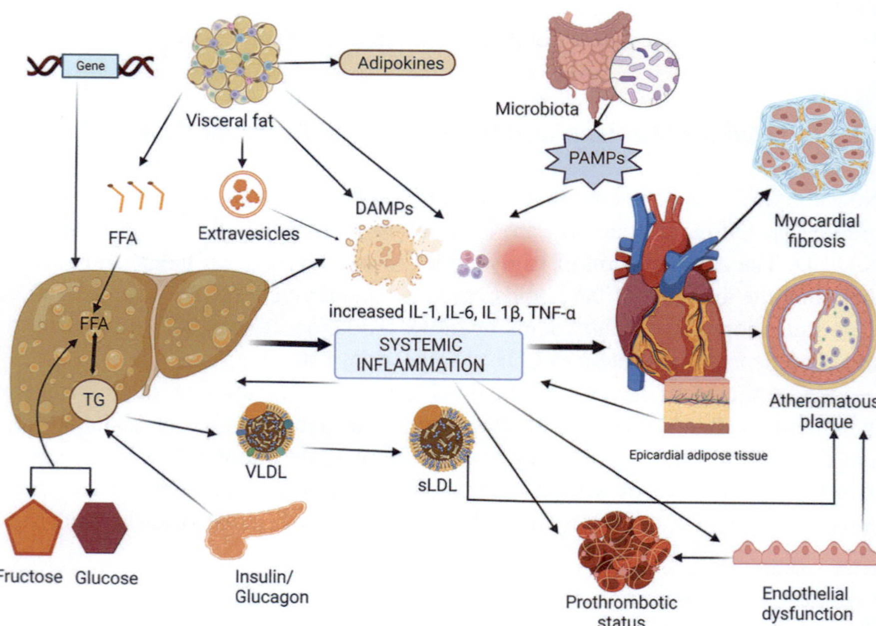

Fig. 13.1 Pathophysiology of cardiovascular diseases in patients with NAFLD. *DAMPs* damage-associated molecular patterns, *FFA* free fatty acids, *IL* interleukin, *PAMPs* pathogen-associated molecular patterns, *sLDL* small low-density lipoprotein, *TG* triglycerides, *TNF-α* tumor necrosis factor alpha, *VLDL* very-low-density lipoprotein

patients with NAFLD. VLDL-TGs either are mostly secreted by intra-abdominal fat or are a consequence of intrahepatic de novo lipogenesis. This suggests that the lipolysis of the subcutaneous fat is not contributive to the increase in VLDL-TG secretion in NAFLD patients [10, 11]. De novo hepatic lipogenesis is stimulated by glucose and insulin. The excess of FFA and other lipids induces injury of the liver cells through a variety of mechanisms including increased oxidative stress due to generation of reactive oxygen species, lipotoxicity, and endoplasmic reticulum stress. The latter usually promotes cell recovery but can lead to cell death and inflammation in some patients with nonalcoholic steatohepatitis (NASH) [12]. Also, patients with NAFLD present an increase of small low-density lipoprotein (sLDL) cholesterol particles, containing more triglycerides and less cholesterol. These are very atherogenic particles that have a higher penetrability in the vessel walls [13]. After penetrating the subendothelial vascular wall, these molecules behave as damage-associated molecular patterns (DAMPs) and stimulate the immune response by activating toll-like receptors (TLRs), especially TLR 2 and TLR 4 [14].

NAFLD is also associated with subclinical atherosclerosis and endothelial dysfunction. In a meta-analysis including 26 observational studies including a total of 29,439 NAFLD patients, it was demonstrated that NAFLD was associated with higher carotid intima-media thickness, coronary artery calcifications, and arterial stiffness and lower flow-mediated vasodilatation [15]. The atherosclerotic lesions were increased by the presence of VLDL particles presenting a high quantity of palmitic acid, a well-known characteristic of NAFLD dyslipidemia. It was demonstrated that high levels of palmitic acid were associated with increased cardiovascular morbidity and mortality [16, 17].

13.1.2 Insulin Resistance

Insulin resistance and abnormal glucose metabolism represent other mechanisms that link NAFLD to cardiovascular events. Visceral fat and systemic inflammation play an important role in the development of insulin resistance [18]. Insulin resistance determines hyperinsulinism, hepatic gluconeogenesis, and activation of de novo hepatic lipogenesis, leading to the aggravation of NAFLD lesions [19]. At the same time, insulin resistance enhances progression of the endothelial dysfunction and atherosclerotic lesions with important negative consequences on atheromatous plaque stability [20, 21].

13.1.3 Genetics

There are three genotypes associated with an increased risk of NAFLD: PNPLA3, TM6SF2, and MBOAT7, as well as one protective genotype—HSD17B13 [22]. The PNPLA3-mutated gene leads to the loss of function of triglyceride lipase and increased expression of the mutated gene along with proteasomal dysfunction. All of these changes determine the increase of proteins on the lipid droplets' surface, which allows for triglycerides to accumulate [23]. The TM6SF2 gene impairs lipid transport and determines an increased risk of cardiovascular diseases [24].

HSD17B13 rs72613567 gene variant is associated with decreased liver transaminases; reduced risk of evolution to advanced fibrosis, including liver cirrhosis in patients with NAFLD; and even protection from NAFLD development in patients with PNPLA3 gene mutation [25]. Even if genetics has a well-established influence on NAFLD development, the influence of these gene mutations on cardiovascular risk is still under debate. The majority of the studies demonstrated that PNPLA3 and TM6SF2 gene mutations were associated with cardioprotective effects for ischemic heart disease, despite NAFLD [26].

13.1.4 Inflammation

Another mechanism involved in the increase of cardiovascular risk of patients with NAFLD involves oxidative stress and systemic inflammation. The data from the Framingham study demonstrated that in patients with NAFLD, there was an increased level of IL-6, high-sensitivity C-reactive protein (hsCRP), intercellular adhesion molecule-1, P-selectin, and urine isoprostanes [27]. IL-1, IL-6, and hsCRP are activated via nucleotide oligomerization domain-like receptor (NLR) family-NLRP3 inflammasome due to an increased level of DAMPs and pathogen-associated molecular patterns (PAMPs) [28]. IL-1 induces endothelial dysfunction, elevates arterial blood pressure, promotes leukocyte-endothelium interaction, stimulates the production of other cytokines from macrophages and endothelial cells, and modulates cardiac contractility as well as myocardial metabolism [29].

Hepatokines represent other molecules recently demonstrated to be involved in the development of cardiometabolic syndrome in patients with NAFLD [30]. Of these, fetuin-A was associated with an increased cardiovascular risk [31]. Experimental studies have demonstrated that fetuin-A and free fatty acids activate inflammatory cytokines and promote atherosclerosis.

13.1.5 Endothelial Dysfunction and Procoagulant Status

Even in the absence of advanced liver fibrosis, NAFLD patients present an increased intrahepatic vascular resistance due to structural hepatic alterations consisting of hepatocyte ballooning or more importantly dynamic alterations due to the interaction between endothelium and hepatic stellate cells [32].

Endothelial dysfunction is also aggravated in patients with NAFLD due to a decrease in the hepatic breakdown of asymmetric dimethyl arginine (ADMA). ADMA, an antagonist of nitric oxide synthase (NOS), is increased in patients with NAFLD and is associated with a decreased nitric oxide (NO) bioavailability [33]. NO is also decreased by hyperhomocysteinemia, and all of these metabolic abnormalities contribute to increased vascular tone, platelet activation, and aggregation.

The extracellular vesicles could be the link between NAFLD and endothelial dysfunction [34]. A recently published study demonstrated that lipotoxic hepatocyte-derived extracellular vesicles promote monocyte adhesion to liver sinusoidal endothelial cells; they also contain integrin beta 1 with a potential link to vascular inflammation and procoagulant status [35]. The procoagulant status that links NAFLD with an increased cardiovascular risk is also promoted by the higher aggregability of thrombocytes [34]. The prothrombotic state of patients with NAFLD is complex and involves increased factor VIII, von Willebrand factor, and plasminogen-activating inhibitor-1 (PAI-1) but also decreased protein C, protein S, and anti-thrombin III [36].

13.1.6 Gut Microbiota

In addition to all of these pathophysiological mechanisms linking NAFLD with cardiovascular diseases, gut microbiota abnormalities add insult to injury and accentuate the systemic inflammation due to PAMPs derived from gut dysbiosis or DAMPs released from damaged enterocytes [37]. The increase in gut-derived endotoxins secondary to imbalanced microbiota represents one of the mechanisms that induce systemic inflammation and consequently liver fibrosis and endothelial dysfunction.

13.2 Risk Stratification in Cardiovascular Diseases and NAFLD

Patients with NAFLD have lower 10-year survival rates compared to the general population, and cardiovascular-related mortality accounts for 25% of deaths in individuals with NAFLD [38]. The question of whether NAFLD is an independent risk factor for cardiovascular diseases or if concurrent metabolic related factors lead to cardiovascular diseases remains. Risk stratification is closely related to primary prevention strategies, and together they represent the basis of a personalized approach in NAFLD patients. NAFLD shares many risk factors with cardiovascular diseases, the most important ones being insulin resistance, obesity, and dyslipidemia. Also, NAFLD influences cardiovascular diseases, as it is associated with high levels of atherogenic lipoproteins as well as inflammatory and hypercoagulable states [36, 39, 40].

Considering all the pathophysiological links and common mechanisms shared by NAFLD and cardiovascular diseases, the question arises whether NAFLD could represent an independent risk factor for cardiovascular events. In a landmark meta-analysis including 16 studies, 34,043 adult patients, and 36.3% of NAFLD patients, with a median follow-up of 6.9 years, Targher et al. demonstrated that NAFLD was independently associated with cardiovascular outcome [39]. Recently, Meyersohn et al. compared the rates of major cardiovascular events (death, myocardial infarction, unstable angina) in patients with steatosis, controlling for cardiovascular risk factors, and baseline atherosclerotic burden, using adjudicated cardiovascular outcomes [41]. The authors found that steatosis was associated with a higher prevalence of obesity, metabolic syndrome, type 2 diabetes mellitus, cardiovascular risk factor burden, and arterial calcium score. Over a median follow-up of 25.5 months, the authors identified an overall rate of major cardiovascular events of 3.1%, NAFLD at baseline being associated with a higher rate of events (4.4% vs. 2.6%, adjusted HR 1.72, $p = 0.005$) [41]. In this study, the hazard ratio was adjusted for obesity, metabolic syndrome, and baseline severity of the coronary obstruction, suggesting that NAFLD could be an independent risk factor for cardiovascular events. They also demonstrated that the presence of NAFLD was associated with an additional cardiovascular risk to the severity of the coronary obstruction. This study concluded that baseline hepatic steatosis was associated with a 70% increased risk of major adverse cardiovascular events; the risk was independent of the traditional cardiovascular risk factors and the presence or the extent of the atherosclerotic plaque.

Mantovani et al. performed a meta-analysis including 36 longitudinal studies evaluating 5,802,226 patients with 99,668 fatal and nonfatal cardiovascular events followed up for 6.5 years [42]. They demonstrated that NAFLD was independently associated with both fatal and nonfatal cardiovascular events with a pooled random effect of 1.4 and that the risk increased proportionally with the fibrosis stage.

Patients with NASH present a high risk of significant morbidity and life-threatening liver-related complications as well as of developing cardiovascular diseases, with an increased liver-specific and all-cause mortality. An important predictor of these severe outcomes is biopsy-confirmed liver fibrosis; however, liver biopsy is associated with several potential complications. The FIB-4 score and several other noninvasive scores have emerged as alternative tools to identify patients with liver fibrosis and potentially act as prognostic markers of clinical outcomes [43]. The FIB-4 score was demonstrated to be a prognostic tool both for liver and for cardiovascular events. The risk of a clinical event was also shown to be significantly higher in patients with a higher FIB-4 score after adjustment for CV risk at baseline [43].

A more recent study included 285 adults with biopsy-proven NAFLD without cardiovascular disease that were followed prospectively until either the development of the first cardiovascular incident, liver transplantation, or death. The findings indicated the incidence of cardiovascular events to be 9.1%, higher than in the general population, and the predictors of major cardiovascular events to be smoking, low albumin, and advanced liver fibrosis [44]. Steatosis, hepatocyte ballooning, lobular inflammation, or presence of steatohepatitis was not associated with a higher incidence of cardiovascular events. This study demonstrated that NAFLD fibrosis score can also predict cardiovascular events, suggesting that the noninvasive tools used for the evaluation of NAFLD could be included in the new cardiovascular risk scores.

In conclusion, as a multisystem inflammatory chronic disease, NAFLD increases the risk of cardiovascular diseases. However, the traditional and commonly used cardiovascular risk factor scoring systems may easily underestimate the cardiovascular risk burden in patients with hepatic steatosis as validated specific cardiovascular scores are not available for this population.

References

1. Deprince A, Haas JT, Staels B. Dysregulated lipid metabolism links NAFLD to cardiovascular disease. Mol Metab. 2020;42:101092.
2. Mato JM, Alonso C, Noureddin M, Lu SC. Biomarkers and subtypes of deranged lipid metabolism in non-alcoholic fatty liver disease. World J Gastroenterol. 2019;25(24):3009–20.
3. Yazıcı D, Sezer H. Insulin resistance, obesity and lipotoxicity. In: Engin AB, Engin A, editors. Obesity and lipotoxicity (Advances in experimental medicine and biology; vol. 960). Cham: Springer International Publishing; 2017. p. 277–304. https://doi.org/10.1007/978-3-319-48382-5_12.
4. Gaborit B, Ancel P, Abdullah AE, Maurice F, Abdesselam I, Calen A, et al. Effect of empagliflozin on ectopic fat stores and myocardial energetics in type 2 diabetes: the EMPACEF study. Cardiovasc Diabetol. 2021;20(1):57.
5. Lim S, Meigs JB. Links between ectopic fat and vascular disease in humans. Arterioscler Thromb Vasc Biol. 2014;34(9):1820–6.
6. Petta S, Argano C, Colomba D, Cammà C, Di Marco V, Cabibi D, et al. Epicardial fat, cardiac geometry and cardiac function in patients with non-alcoholic fatty liver disease: association with the severity of liver disease. J Hepatol. 2015;62(4):928–33.
7. Granér M, Nyman K, Siren R, Pentikäinen MO, Lundbom J, Hakkarainen A, et al. Ectopic fat depots and left ventricular function in nondiabetic men with nonalcoholic fatty liver disease. Circ Cardiovasc Imaging. 2015;8(1):e001979.
8. Alves-Bezerra M, Cohen DE. Triglyceride metabolism in the liver. In: Terjung R, editor. Comprehensive physiology. 1st ed. New York: Wiley; 2017. p. 1–22. https://doi.org/10.1002/cphy.c170012.
9. Vergani L. Fatty acids and effects on in vitro and in vivo models of liver steatosis. Curr Med Chem. 2019;26(19):3439–56.
10. Heeren J, Scheja L. Metabolic-associated fatty liver disease and lipoprotein metabolism. Mol Metab. 2021;50:101238.
11. Fabbrini E, Magkos F. Hepatic steatosis as a marker of metabolic dysfunction. Nutrients. 2015;7(6):4995–5019.
12. Rada P, González-Rodríguez Á, García-Monzón C, Valverde ÁM. Understanding lipotoxicity in NAFLD pathogenesis: is CD36 a key driver? Cell Death Dis. 2020;11(9):802.
13. Tilg H, Adolph TE, Dudek M, Knolle P. Non-alcoholic fatty liver disease: the interplay between metabolism, microbes and immunity. Nat Metab. 2021;3(12):1596–607.
14. Parlati L, Régnier M, Guillou H, Postic C. New targets for NAFLD. JHEP Rep. 2021;3(6):100346.
15. Zhou F, Zhou J, Wang W, Zhang X, Ji Y, Zhang P, et al. Unexpected rapid increase in the burden of NAFLD in China from 2008 to 2018: a systematic review and meta-analysis. Hepatology. 2019;70(4):1119–33.
16. Marra F, Svegliati-Baroni G. Lipotoxicity and the gut–liver axis in NASH pathogenesis. J Hepatol. 2018;68(2):280–95.
17. Fatima S, Hu X, Gong RH, Huang C, Chen M, Wong HLX, et al. Palmitic acid is an intracellular signaling molecule involved in disease development. Cell Mol Life Sci. 2019;76(13):2547–57.
18. Tanase DM, Gosav EM, Costea CF, Ciocoiu M, Lacatusu CM, Maranduca MA, et al. The intricate relationship between type 2 diabetes mellitus (T2DM), insulin resistance (IR), and nonalcoholic fatty liver disease (NAFLD). J Diabetes Res. 2020;2020:1–16.
19. Watt MJ, Miotto PM, De Nardo W, Montgomery MK. The liver as an endocrine organ—linking NAFLD and insulin resistance. Endocr Rev. 2019;40(5):1367–93.

20. Khan RS, Bril F, Cusi K, Newsome PN. Modulation of insulin resistance in nonalcoholic fatty liver disease. Hepatology. 2019;70(2):711–24.
21. Vairappan B. Endothelial dysfunction in cirrhosis: role of inflammation and oxidative stress. World J Hepatol. 2015;7(3):443.
22. Eslam M, Valenti L, Romeo S. Genetics and epigenetics of NAFLD and NASH: clinical impact. J Hepatol. 2018;68(2):268–79.
23. Trépo E, Valenti L. Update on NAFLD genetics: from new variants to the clinic. J Hepatol. 2020;72(6):1196–209.
24. Sharma D, Mandal P. NAFLD: genetics and its clinical implications. Clin Res Hepatol Gastroenterol. 2022;46(9):102003.
25. Vilar-Gomez E, Pirola CJ, Sookoian S, Wilson LA, Liang T, Chalasani N. The protection conferred by HSD17B13 rs72613567 polymorphism on risk of steatohepatitis and fibrosis may be limited to selected subgroups of patients with NAFLD. Clin Transl Gastroenterol. 2021;12(9):e00400.
26. Brouwers MCGJ, Simons N, Stehouwer CDA, Isaacs A. Non-alcoholic fatty liver disease and cardiovascular disease: assessing the evidence for causality. Diabetologia. 2020;63(2):253–60.
27. Fricker ZP, Pedley A, Massaro JM, Vasan RS, Hoffmann U, Benjamin EJ, et al. Liver fat is associated with markers of inflammation and oxidative stress in analysis of data from the Framingham Heart study. Clin Gastroenterol Hepatol. 2019;17(6):1157–1164.e4.
28. Park JW, Kim SE, Lee NY, Kim JH, Jung JH, Jang MK, et al. Role of microbiota-derived metabolites in alcoholic and non-alcoholic fatty liver diseases. Int J Mol Sci. 2021;23(1):426.
29. He Y, Hwang S, Ahmed YA, Feng D, Li N, Ribeiro M, et al. Immunopathobiology and therapeutic targets related to cytokines in liver diseases. Cell Mol Immunol. 2021;18(1):18–37.
30. Meex RCR, Watt MJ. Hepatokines: linking nonalcoholic fatty liver disease and insulin resistance. Nat Rev Endocrinol. 2017;13(9):509–20.
31. Stefan N, Häring HU. The role of hepatokines in metabolism. Nat Rev Endocrinol. 2013;9(3):144–52.
32. Nasiri-Ansari N, Androutsakos T, Flessa CM, Kyrou I, Siasos G, Randeva HS, et al. Endothelial cell dysfunction and nonalcoholic fatty liver disease (NAFLD): a concise review. Cell. 2022;11(16):2511.
33. Boga S, Alkim H, Koksal AR, Bayram M, Ozguven MBY, Ergun M, et al. Increased plasma levels of asymmetric dimethylarginine in nonalcoholic fatty liver disease: relation with insulin resistance, inflammation, and liver histology. J Investig Med. 2015;63(7):871–7.
34. Li D, Xie P, Zhao S, Zhao J, Yao Y, Zhao Y, et al. Hepatocytes derived increased SAA1 promotes intrahepatic platelet aggregation and aggravates liver inflammation in NAFLD. Biochem Biophys Res Commun. 2021;555:54–60.
35. Guo Q, Furuta K, Lucien F, Gutierrez Sanchez LH, Hirsova P, Krishnan A, et al. Integrin β1-enriched extracellular vesicles mediate monocyte adhesion and promote liver inflammation in murine NASH. J Hepatol. 2019;71(6):1193–205.
36. Tripodi A, Fracanzani AL, Primignani M, Chantarangkul V, Clerici M, Mannucci PM, et al. Procoagulant imbalance in patients with non-alcoholic fatty liver disease. J Hepatol. 2014;61(1):148–54.
37. Chen J, Vitetta L. Gut microbiota metabolites in NAFLD pathogenesis and therapeutic implications. Int J Mol Sci. 2020;21(15):5214.
38. Kasper P, Martin A, Lang S, Kütting F, Goeser T, Demir M, et al. NAFLD and cardiovascular diseases: a clinical review. Clin Res Cardiol. 2021;110(7):921–37.
39. Targher G, Byrne CD, Lonardo A, Zoppini G, Barbui C. Non-alcoholic fatty liver disease and risk of incident cardiovascular disease: a meta-analysis. J Hepatol. 2016;65(3):589–600.
40. Miele L, Alberelli MA, Martini M, Liguori A, Marrone G, Cocomazzi A, et al. Nonalcoholic fatty liver disease (NAFLD) severity is associated to a nonhemostatic contribution and proinflammatory phenotype of platelets. Transl Res. 2020;2020:003.
41. Meyersohn NM, Mayrhofer T, Corey KE, Bittner DO, Staziaki PV, Szilveszter B, et al. Association of hepatic steatosis with major adverse cardiovascular events, independent of coronary artery disease. Clin Gastroenterol Hepatol. 2021;19(7):1480–1488.e14.

42. Mantovani A, Csermely A, Petracca G, Beatrice G, Corey KE, Simon TG, et al. Non-alcoholic fatty liver disease and risk of fatal and non-fatal cardiovascular events: an updated systematic review and meta-analysis. Lancet Gastroenterol Hepatol. 2021;6(11):903–13.
43. Loosen S, Luedde M, Demir M, Luedde T, Kostev K, Roderburg C. An elevated FIB-4 score is not associated with cardiovascular events: a longitudinal analysis from 137,842 patients with and without chronic liver disease. Eur J Gastroenterol Hepatol. 2022;34(6):717–23.
44. Henson JB, Simon TG, Kaplan A, Osganian S, Masia R, Corey KE. Advanced fibrosis is associated with incident cardiovascular disease in patients with non-alcoholic fatty liver disease. Aliment Pharmacol Ther. 2020;51(7):728–36.

Type 2 Diabetes Mellitus and Insulin Resistance in Nonalcoholic Fatty Liver Disease

14

Catalina Mihai, Bogdan Mihai,
and Cristina Cijevschi Prelipcean

14.1 Introduction

Both nonalcoholic fatty liver disease (NAFLD) and type 2 diabetes mellitus (T2DM) are diseases with increasing incidence and prevalence, with significant morbidity and mortality, with important costs for the individual and society. NAFLD has become the most common liver disease, with a prevalence of 25–30% in the general population [1]. NAFLD includes a spectrum of diseases from simple steatosis to inflammation (nonalcoholic steatohepatitis—NASH), fibrosis, cirrhosis, or even hepatocellular carcinoma. Beyond liver complications, NAFLD is also a risk factor for heart and kidney diseases.

T2DM has a continuously increasing incidence and prevalence throughout the world; it is estimated that in 2035, there will be 592 million patients [2]. In turn, T2DM is an important risk factor for chronic kidney disease and cardiovascular diseases. The association of T2DM with NAFLD and chronic kidney disease (the "vicious triad") implies increased morbidity and mortality, being a real public health problem [3].

There is a close link between obesity, T2DM, and NAFLD. In recent years, experts have suggested the introduction of a new term: MAFLD (metabolic associated fatty liver disease). This underlines the role of insulin resistance (IR) and the metabolic syndrome in the pathogenesis of NAFLD [4].

C. Mihai (✉) · C. C. Prelipcean
"Grigore T. Popa" University of Medicine and Pharmacy, Iasi, Romania

Institute of Gastroenterology and Hepatology, "St. Spiridon" Emergency Hospital,
Iasi, Romania

B. Mihai
"Grigore T. Popa" University of Medicine and Pharmacy, Iasi, Romania

Diabetes, Nutrition and Metabolic Diseases Department, "St. Spiridon" Emergency Hospital,
Iasi, Romania

© The Author(s), under exclusive license to Springer Nature
Switzerland AG 2023
A. Trifan et al. (eds.), *Essentials of Non-Alcoholic Fatty Liver Disease*,
https://doi.org/10.1007/978-3-031-33548-8_14

14.2 Epidemiology

The prevalence of NAFLD in T2DM patients is much higher compared to the general population, reaching, according to some studies, up to 70% [3]. NAFLD is found in over 50% of patients with T2DM and in 90% of those with severe obesity [5]. 30–40% of diabetic patients have NASH and 10–15% severe fibrosis [6]. More than half of the T2DM patients will develop NAFLD in the next 3 years [7]. It is estimated that in the next 20 years, 1/3 of liver transplants will be performed in diabetic patients with NASH [6].

At the same time, multiple large population-based retrospective studies showed that the prevalence of type 2 DM is higher in patients with NAFLD compared to the general population [8]. There is a 1.6–6.8 times higher risk (variable depending on the diagnostic method used) of DM in patients with NAFLD [9]. A recent meta-analysis including over 500,000 patients from Europe, Asia, and the USA demonstrated that NAFLD doubles the risk of T2DM independent of obesity or other associated metabolic risk factors [10]. Moreover, the risk of DM is proportional to the severity of hepatic steatosis and fibrosis. There is also evidence that reducing hepatic steatosis would decrease the risk of developing DM [11]. Current guidelines recommend DM screening in all NAFLD patients.

The association of NAFLD with T2DM increases the risk of cardiovascular, renal, and oncologic diseases.

14.3 Pathophysiology

The pathogenesis of the association of NAFLD with T2DM is incompletely elucidated, but the IR is considered the main pathogenic factor. Classically, the etiopathogenesis of NAFLD is explained by the two-hit theory. The first hit is given by IR and the accumulation of fats in the hepatocytes; the second hit is represented by inflammation and damage to the hepatocytes. Currently, the theory of multiple hits is accepted, with multiple actors playing in the show: genetic factors, glucotoxicity, lipotoxicity, and intestinal microbiota (Fig. 14.1) [6].

14.3.1 Insulin Resistance

IR represents the reduction of the insulin signal in the target organs: muscle, liver, and adipose tissue. IR determines intrahepatic accumulation of lipids through multiple mechanisms: stimulation of de novo lipogenesis through insulin signaling pathway (selective IR), decrease in mitochondrial fat oxidation, and increase in the flow of fatty acids from adipocytes to the liver [11]. IR also plays an important role in the progression of fibrosis, stimulating hepatic stellate cells through both direct and indirect inflammatory mechanisms [12].

On the other hand, the relationship between IR and hepatic steatosis is bidirectional: the intrahepatic accumulation of fats (diacylglycerol, ceramides) inhibits

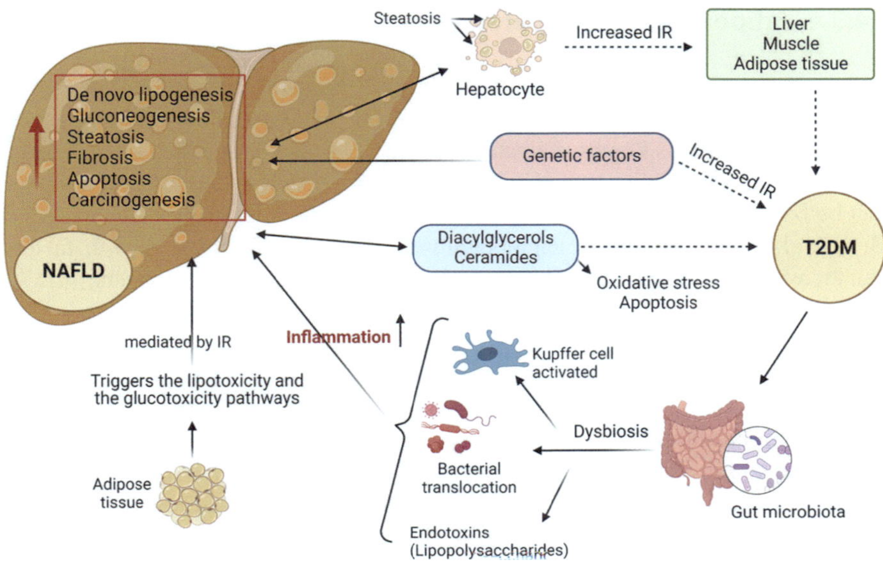

Fig. 14.1 Nonalcoholic fatty liver disease (NAFLD); insulin resistance (IR); type 2 diabetes mellitus (T2DM)

insulin signaling at the insulin receptor [12]. The increased influx of free fatty acids from adipocytes and from the diet causes hyperglycemia [13]. The accumulation of lipids in the liver is associated with an increase in IR in the liver, muscles, and adipose tissue and with an increased risk of T2DM [14].

14.3.2 Genetic Factors

Multiple genetic variants have been involved in the occurrence and progression of NASH: patatin-like phospholipase domain-containing 3 (PNPLA3), transmembrane 6 superfamily member 2 (TM6SF), glucokinase regulator (GCKR), membrane-bound O-acyltransferase domain-containing 7 (MBOAT7), and hydroxysteroid 17-dehydrogenase (HSD17B13) [13]. It is interesting that the presence of NAFLD-related genetic variants increases the risk of IR and T2DM [15].

14.3.3 Glucotoxicity

There are multiple mechanisms by which hyperglycemia can cause hepatic steatosis [6]. Advanced glycosylation end products (AGEs) cause inflammation at the level of Kupffer cells and hepatic stellate cells. Hepatic inflammation induces oxidative stress and causes lipid peroxidation. Also, glucotoxicity causes alteration of hepatic microcirculation and upregulation of genes encoding key lipogenic and glycolytic pathways.

14.3.4 Adipokines and Hepatokines

Adiponectin is a cytokine that regulates glycemic homeostasis and IR. The reduction of adiponectin leads to the impairment of fatty acid metabolism and to a pro-inflammatory status. Leptin activates stellate cells and stimulates fibrogenesis. Gremlin 1 correlates with IR and T2DM in patients with NAFLD [16]. Adipokines can be both biomarkers and therapeutic targets. In turn, hepatokines (fetuin A and B, retinol-binding protein 4, angiopoietin-like proteins, fibroblast growth factor) can increase IR, steatosis, and fibrosis and can promote hepatic carcinogenesis [17].

14.3.5 Lipotoxicity

Hyperglycemia and IR induce de novo lipogenesis through activation of the carbohydrate response element-binding protein (ChREBP) and the sterol-regulating element-binding protein 1c (SREBP1c) [16]. SREBP1c regulates cholesterol synthesis and lipid uptake and enhances triglyceride expression. At the same time, SREBP1c increases the production of diacylglycerols and ceramides. Ceramides exert harmful effects on liver cells through both direct toxic effects and inflammatory-mediated effects, leading to oxidative stress and apoptosis [18].

14.3.6 Inflammation

Lipid peroxidation will lead to oxidative stress, release of inflammatory cytokines (TNF-α, IL-1b, and IL-6), high reactive oxygen species, and reactive nitrogen species with the proliferation of stellate cells and liver fibrogenesis.

14.3.7 Intestinal Microbiota

Dysbiosis can lead to fatty acid metabolism impairment, Kupffer cell activation, inflammation, and fibrosis. DM, along with other endo- and exogenous factors, modifies the intestinal microbiota and intestinal permeability. This leads to a leaky mucosal barrier, with bacterial translocation and endotoxinemia. Endotoxins (lipopolysaccharides) increase intrahepatic accumulation of lipids, inflammation, and fibrosis [17].

14.4 Identification of Steatosis and Fibrosis in T2DM Patients

The diagnosis of NAFLD involves ultrasonography, noninvasive serological and ultrasound-based hepatic elastography tests, and magnetic resonance imaging, while liver biopsy remains the gold standard. There is currently no consensus regarding the best cost-effective, noninvasive screening method for steatosis, inflammation, and fibrosis in diabetic patients with NAFLD. The American Diabetes Association 2019 consensus recommends screening for NASH and fibrosis in all diabetic patients with elevated transaminases or fatty liver on ultrasound [19]. Lately, most authors consider that NAFLD screening and liver fibrosis stratification would be necessary in all patients with type 2 DM. It is very important to differentiate simple steatosis from steatohepatitis and to identify patients with significant fibrosis ($F \geq 2$).

Ultrasonography is the first (cheap, noninvasive, accessible) method of highlighting hepatic steatosis [20]. However, ultrasonography has many limitations (impossibility of detecting mild steatosis, interobserver variability, examination difficulties in the case of obese patients), and, moreover, it cannot quantify the degree of liver fibrosis.

Controlled attenuation parameter (CAP), which quantifies ultrasound attenuation at the center frequency of the Fibroscan probe, has become one of the steatosis evaluation methods most used in clinical practice. *Transient elastography* or *vibration-controlled transient elastography* (VCTE) and *acoustic radiation force impulse* (ARFI) quantification are elastography-based imaging techniques to assess hepatic fibrosis. VCTE (Fibroscan) tends to become "the new gold standard" in assessing fibrosis in patients with NAFLD [21]. The role of this method in the diagnosis, stratification, and monitoring of diabetic patients remains to be established.

Techniques derived from *magnetic resonance imaging* (MRI) (magnetic resonance spectroscopy and MRI-proton density fat fraction) accurately quantify hepatic triglyceride (fat) content, but they are limited by price and accessibility [14]. Magnetic resonance elastography has better performances in assessing liver fibrosis compared to VCTE [22].

Multiple *noninvasive serological scores* have been used to assess the degree of fibrosis in patients with NAFLD: fibrosis-4 (FIB-4) index, NAFLD fibrosis score (NFS), AST-to-platelet ratio index (APRI), and Hepascore. These scores can identify/exclude significant fibrosis in most patients but have limited accuracy for intermediate fibrosis [23]. It seems that in the case of diabetic patients, the fibrosis prediction scores are less accurate. Singh et al. [24] have developed a Diabetes Liver Fibrosis Score to detect advanced fibrosis in diabetics with NAFLD, based on six parameters: age, hypertension, chronic kidney disease, lipid-lowering medications, platelet count, and AST. This is difficult to calculate in practice and requires validation. Lee et al. [25] have developed another Diabetic Fibrosis Score that includes five parameters, body mass index, platelet, AST, high-density lipoprotein cholesterol, and albuminuria, and has an area under the receiver operating characteristic curve of >0.80 in fibrosis detection compared to VCTE. The Homeostatic Model Assessment of Insulin Resistance (HOMA-IR) proved to be correlated with steatosis and liver fibrosis both in patients with T2DM and in nondiabetics [13, 26].

Current recommendations propose the evaluation of NASH in two stages: one through noninvasive biological markers and, subsequently, VCTE for those at risk. However, it is not known to what extent this strategy can be applied to the diabetic population [25]. Future studies will identify the best noninvasive methods of diagnosis, as well as the cutoff values of steatosis and fibrosis in diabetic patients.

14.5   Clinical Consequences of the NAFLD–T2DM Association

The complex interrelation between T2DM and NAFLD is summarized in Fig. 14.2. On the one hand, the association of DZ with NAFLD determines the acceleration of the progression of inflammation and fibrosis, increasing the risk of liver cirrhosis and hepatocellular carcinoma. Multiple studies have demonstrated an increased prevalence of significant fibrosis and a faster progression of liver fibrosis in diabetic patients compared to nondiabetic patients [14]. In a recent study, Lomonaco et al. [27] demonstrated that one out of six patients with T2DM had associated significant liver fibrosis, evaluated by transient elastography ($F \geq 2$). There is an increased risk of hepatocellular carcinoma in patients with NAFLD; the greater, the more advanced the disease (advanced fibrosis, liver cirrhosis). The association of T2DM increases the risk of hepatocellular carcinoma more than four times in patients with NASH-cirrhosis and represents a predictive factor of mortality [13, 28].

On the other hand, the presence of NAFLD increases the progression of prediabetes to diabetes and the incidence of macro- and microvascular complications in diabetic patients [29]. In diabetic patients who have associated NAFLD, an increased risk of cardiovascular diseases, retinopathy, and diabetic nephropathy has been demonstrated [14]. The increase in mortality was also demonstrated in patients with DM type 2 and NAFLD compared to diabetics without liver damage [30].

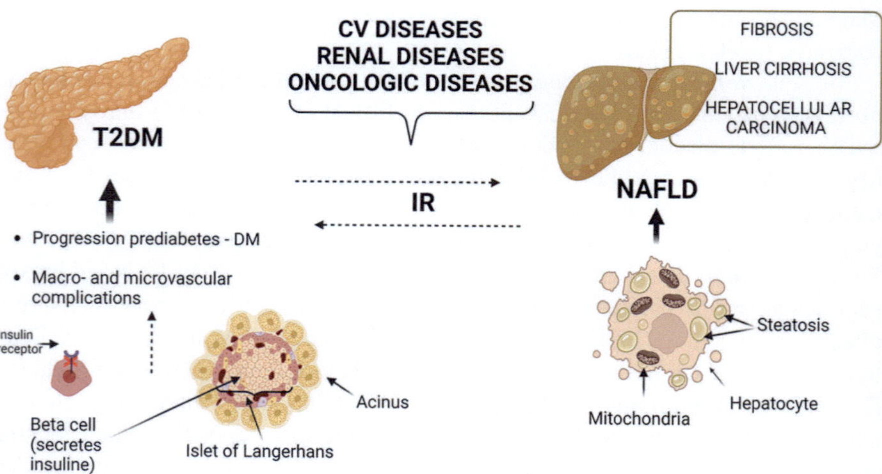

Fig. 14.2 Insulin resistance (IR); nonalcoholic fatty liver disease (NAFLD); insulin resistance (IR); type 2 diabetes mellitus (T2DM), cardiovascular (CV)

14.6   Treatment

Despite the high prevalence, morbidity, and mortality, there is no approved treatment for NAFLD. As long as the two diseases share common etiopathogenic links, the therapeutic measures address the same targets. We will review the main therapies used in the treatment of both NAFLD and T2DM.

Lifestyle change (diet, exercise) remains the central pillar of any therapy. In NAFLD, a 10% weight loss causes regression of steatosis and improvement of liver tests [20]. Both the Mediterranean-type diet and physical exercises (aerobic and resistance training) reduce the fatty load of the liver. The DiRECT Study demonstrated that weight loss in diabetic patients improves hepatic steatosis and IR [31].

It is not known whether a *good glycemic control* can determine the regression or slowing down of the evolution of steatosis and fibrosis.

Antidiabetic drugs can be beneficial in NAFLD through multiple mechanisms, from weight loss to cardio- and reno-protective effects. The American guidelines for the treatment of DM comorbidities recommend pioglitazone and glucagon-like peptide-1 receptor agonists in patients with NAFLD and T2DM [32]. The main therapies for NAFLD in diabetic patients are summarized in Table 14.1.

Table 14.1   Therapy in patients with T2DM and NAFLD

Peroxisome proliferator-activated receptor-γ (PPAR-γ) medication	Pioglitazone Elafibranor Lobeglitazone Lanifibranor	– Improve steatosis, fibrosis, IR
Glucagon-like peptide-1 receptor agonists (GLP-1 RA)	Liraglutide Exenatide Semaglutide Dulaglutide Tirzepatide	– Reduce body weight – Reduce blood glucose level and glycated hemoglobin – Reduce cardiovascular and renal complications and mortality – Reduce steatosis and inflammation
Dipeptidyl dipeptidase-4 inhibitors (DDP-4i)	Sitagliptin Vildagliptin	– No steatosis improvement – Decrease hepatic fat content
Sodium-glucose co-transporter-2 inhibitors (SGLT2i)	Ipragliflozin Canagliflozin Empagliflozin Dapagliflozin Licogliflozin	– Reduce blood glucose levels – Reduce albuminuria – Renal protective effects – Reduce steatosis, inflammation, and fibrosis
Other medication	Vitamin E Statins Metformin	– Decrease steatosis in combination with pioglitazone – Decrease the risk of hepatocellular carcinoma

14.6.1 Peroxisome Proliferator-Activated Receptor-γ (PPAR-γ) Medication

Thiazolidinediones are among the first antidiabetic drugs that have proven their effectiveness in NAFLD. Pioglitazone (not rosiglitazone) increases the level of adiponectin and reduces steatosis [33]. The study by Cusi et al. [34] has investigated the effects of pioglitazone vs. placebo in patients with prediabetes or T2DM, with a follow-up period of 36 months. The study demonstrated the improvement of steatosis, fibrosis, as well as IR. Brill et al. [35] showed that pioglitazone reduces liver fibrosis and improves IR to a greater extent in patients with T2DM compared to those with prediabetes. The improvement of liver fibrosis, especially the advanced one, was also confirmed in the meta-analysis of eight studies with pioglitazone in NASH [36]. At the same time, pioglitazone has numerous side effects: weight gain, cardiac damage, osteoporosis, and increased incidence of bladder cancer.

Newer selective peroxisome proliferator-activated receptor-γ modulators (SPPARMs) also increase adiponectin but without the side effects of thiazolidinediones (e.g., weight gain). CHRS131 is a SPPARM-γ with predominantly insulin-sensitizing actions, which has proven its effectiveness in reducing glycemia and changing the lipid profile [37]. PPAR-α/δ agonists (elafibranor, lobeglitazone) have proven their efficiency in reducing steatosis in patients with T2DM and NAFLD, without influencing liver fibrosis [38]. Lanifibranor, a pan-PPAR agonist, is a promise, proving in phase II studies its superiority compared to placebo in improving steatosis and liver fibrosis [39].

14.6.2 Glucagon-Like Peptide-1 Receptor Agonists (GLP-1 RA)

GLP-1 RA (incretin mimetics peptides) are drugs approved for the treatment of DM. They have proven their effectiveness in T2DM, reducing body weight, blood glucose level, and glycated hemoglobin, but also cardiovascular and renal complications and mortality [40]. Liraglutide demonstrated the improvement of liver tests (ALT and aspartate aminotransaminase (AST)-to-platelet ratio index—APRI) [41]. The data on the reduction of liver fat content assessed by MRI are contradictory [11]. Exenatide has shown promising results related to the reduction of IR, steatosis, and inflammation in patients with T2DM and NAFLD [42]. Semaglutide in a 72-week phase II trial demonstrated resolution of steatosis without aggravation of fibrosis in 56% of patients, compared to 20% placebo [43]. There are ongoing studies about the role of dulaglutide and tirzepatide (dual agonist of GLP1 and glucose-dependent insulinotropic polypeptides) [11].

It is not yet clear whether the effects of GLP-1 RA on hepatic steatosis are due to a direct action or are mediated by weight loss.

14.6.3 Dipeptidyl Dipeptidase-4 Inhibitors (DDP-4i)

DDP-4i are antidiabetic drugs that also act by increasing incretin. Randomized trials have failed to demonstrate favorable effects of sitagliptin on NAFLD in diabetic patients [44]. However, vildagliptin improved liver fat content (assessed by MRI) compared to placebo [11].

14.6.4 Sodium-Glucose Co-transporter-2 Inhibitors (SGLT2i)

SGLT2i inhibit the reabsorption of glucose in the proximal tubular system of the kidney, reducing blood glucose levels and macro- and microalbuminuria, with renal protective effects. Animal model studies have shown the favorable effects of SGLT2i (ipragliflozin, canagliflozin, empagliflozin) in reducing steatosis, inflammation, and liver fibrosis [3]. These effects were also confirmed in human studies that showed improvement of ALT and reduction of abdominal and liver fat in diabetic patients with NAFLD [45, 46]. Licogliflozin, a dual SGLT1–SGLT2 inhibitor, is under investigation in NASH patients.

The new classes of antidiabetic drugs, alone or in combination, seem to have complex beneficial effects, from reducing blood glycemia to reducing liver and kidney damage, with final effects on reducing cardiovascular morbidity and mortality. Combined therapies (PPAR-γ, GLP-1 RA, SGLT2i) could be the solution of the future both for the treatment of DM associated with NAFLD and for the reduction of cardiovascular and renal risk.

14.6.5 Other Medication

Vitamin E seems to have the same beneficial effects in reducing steatosis in diabetic patients, only in combination with pioglitazone [47]. Statin treatment could prevent the occurrence of hepatocarcinoma in diabetic patients with NAFLD [48]. Metformin reduces cardiovascular and hepatocellular carcinoma risk, although it has no effect on improving liver histology in patients with NAFLD and DM [49].

14.7   Future Directions and Conclusions

Evaluation of NAFLD in diabetic patients should become part of current clinical practice. Given the increased prevalence and the consequences on morbidity and mortality, NAFLD screening and fibrosis assessment should be done systematically, in all patients with T2DM, similar to other complications. The development of screening guidelines, noninvasive diagnosis, and therapeutic algorithms is imperative. Weight loss and physical exercise remain the cornerstone of any therapeutic approach. The new drugs used in the treatment of T2DM, alone or in combinations (PPAR-γ, GLP-1 RA, SGLT2i), could have the desired effects for regulating glycemia, improving steatosis and liver fibrosis, and decreasing cardiovascular risk.

References

1. Chan WK, Goh KL. Epidemiology of a fast emerging disease in the Asia-Pacific region-nonalcoholic fatty liver disease. Hepatol Int. 2013;7:65–71.
2. Guariguata L, Whiting DR, Hambleton I, et al. Global estimates of diabetes prevalence for 2013 and projections for 2035. Diabetes Res Clin Pract. 2014;103:137–49.
3. Athyros VG, Polyzos SA, Kountouras J, et al. Non-alcoholic fatty liver disease treatment in patients with type 2 diabetes mellitus; new kids on the block. Curr Vasc Pharmacol. 2020;18(2):172–81.
4. Eslam M, Sanyal A, George J. International consensus panel MAFLD: a consensus-driven proposed nomenclature for metabolic associated fatty liver disease. Gastroenterology. 2020;158:1999–2014.
5. Younossi ZM, Golabi P, de Avila L, et al. The global epidemiology of NAFLD and NASH in patients with type 2 diabetes: a systematic review and meta-analysis. J Hepatol. 2019;71:793–801.
6. Cusi K. A diabetologist's perspective of non-alcoholic steatohepatitis (NASH): knowledge gaps and future directions. Liver Int. 2020;40(Suppl 1):82–8.
7. Lee HW, Wong GL-H, Kwok R, et al. Serial transient elastography examinations to monitor patients with type 2 diabetes: a prospective cohort study. Hepatology. 2020;72:1230–41.
8. Muzica CM, Sfarti C, Trifan A, et al. Nonalcoholic fatty liver disease and type 2 diabetes mellitus: a bidirectional relationship. Can J Gastroenterol Hepatol. 2020;2020:6638306.
9. Ballestri S, Zona S, Targher G, et al. Nonalcoholic fatty liver disease is associated with an almost twofold increased risk of incident type 2 diabetes and metabolic syndrome. Evidence from a systematic review and meta-analysis. J Gastroenterol Hepatol. 2016;31:936–44.
10. Mantovani APG, Beatrice G, Tilg H, et al. Non-alcoholic fatty liver disease and risk of incident diabetes mellitus: an updated meta-analysis of 501,022 adult individuals. Gut. 2021;70:962–9.
11. Targher G, Corey KE, Byrne CD, Roden M. The complex link between NAFLD and type 2 diabetes mellitus—mechanisms and treatments. Nat Rev Gastroenterol Hepatol. 2021;18(9):599–612.
12. Finck BN. Targeting metabolism, insulin resistance, and diabetes to treat nonalcoholic steatohepatitis. Diabetes. 2018;67(12):2485–93.
13. Fujii H, Kawada N, Japan Study Group Of Nafld Jsg-Nafld. The role of insulin resistance and diabetes in nonalcoholic fatty liver disease. Int J Mol Sci. 2020;21(11):3863.
14. Lee YH, Cho Y, Lee BW, et al. Nonalcoholic fatty liver disease in diabetes. Part I: epidemiology and diagnosis. Diabetes Metab J. 2019;43(1):31–45.
15. Ziolkowska S, Binienda A, Jabłkowski M, et al. The interplay between insulin resistance, inflammation, oxidative stress, base excision repair and metabolic syndrome in nonalcoholic fatty liver disease. Int J Mol Sci. 2021;22(20):11128.
16. Tanase DM, Gosav EM, Costea CF, et al. The intricate relationship between type 2 diabetes mellitus (T2DM), insulin resistance (IR), and nonalcoholic fatty liver disease (NAFLD). J Diabetes Res. 2020;2020:3920196.
17. Kim H, Lee DS, An TH, et al. Metabolic spectrum of liver failure in type 2 diabetes and obesity: from NAFLD to NASH to HCC. Int J Mol Sci. 2021;22(9):4495.
18. Birkenfeld AL, Shulman GI. Nonalcoholic fatty liver disease, hepatic insulin resistance, and type 2 diabetes. Hepatology. 2014;59(2):713–23.
19. American Diabetes Association. 4. Comprehensive medical evaluation and assessment of comorbidities: standards of medical care in diabetes 2019. Diabetes Care. 2019;42(Suppl. 1):S34–45.

20. European Association for the Study of the Liver (EASL); European Association for the Study of Diabetes (EASD); European Association for the Study of Obesity (EASO). EASL–EASD–EASO clinical practice guidelines for the management of non-alcoholic fatty liver disease. J Hepatol. 2016;64:1388–402.
21. Cazac GD, Lăcătuşu CM, Mihai C, et al. Ultrasound-based hepatic elastography in non-alcoholic fatty liver disease: focus on patients with type 2 diabetes. Biomedicine. 2022;10:2375. https://doi.org/10.3390/biomedicines10102375.
22. Hsu C, Caussy C, Imajo K, et al. Magnetic resonance vs transient elastography analysis of patients with nonalcoholic fatty liver disease: a systematic review and pooled analysis of individual participants. Clin Gastroenterol Hepatol. 2018;17:630–7. https://doi.org/10.1016/j.cgh.2018.05.059.
23. Ciardullo S, Sala I, Perseghin G. Screening strategies for nonalcoholic fatty liver disease in type 2 diabetes: insights from NHANES 2005–2016. Diabetes Res Clin Pract. 2020;167:108358.
24. Singh A, Garg R, Lopez R, Alkhouri N. Diabetes liver fibrosis score to detect advanced fibrosis in diabetics with nonalcoholic fatty liver disease. Clin Gastroenterol Hepatol. 2022;20(3):e624–6.
25. Lee C-H, Seto W-K, Ieong K, et al. Development of a noninvasive liver fibrosis score based on transient elastography for risk stratification in patients with type 2 diabetes. Endocrinol Metab. 2021;36:134–45.
26. Gutierrez-Buey G, Núñez-Córdoba JM, Llavero-Valero M, et al. Is HOMA-IR a potential screening test for non-alcoholic fatty liver disease in adults with type 2 diabetes? Eur J Intern Med. 2017;41:74–8.
27. Lomonaco R, Godinez Leiva E, Bril F, et al. Advanced liver fibrosis is common in patients with type 2 diabetes followed in the outpatient setting: the need for systematic screening. Diabetes Care. 2021;44(2):399–406.
28. Yang JD, Ahmed F, Mara KC, et al. Diabetes is associated with increased risk of hepatocellular carcinoma in patients with cirrhosis from nonalcoholic fatty liver disease. Hepatology. 2020;71:907–16.
29. Gastaldelli A, From CK. From NASH to diabetes and from diabetes to NASH: mechanisms and treatment options. JHEP Rep. 2019;1(4):312–28.
30. Adams LA, Harmsen S, St Sauver JL, Charatcharoenwitthaya P, Enders FB, Therneau T, Angulo P. Nonalcoholic fatty liver disease increases risk of death among patients with diabetes: a community-based cohort study. Am J Gastroenterol. 2010;105:1567–73.
31. Lean ME, Leslie WS, Barnes AC, et al. Primary care-led weight management for remission of type 2 diabetes (DiRECT): an open-label, cluster-randomised trial. Lancet. 2018;391(10120):541–51.
32. American Diabetes Association. 4. Comprehensive medical evaluation and assessment of comorbidities: standards of medical care in diabetes—2022. Diabetes Care. 2022;45(Suppl 1):S46–59.
33. Polyzos SA, Mantzoros CS. Adiponectin as a target for the treatment of nonalcoholic steatohepatitis with thiazolidinediones: a systematic review. Metabolism. 2016;65:1297–306.
34. Cusi K, Orsak B, Bril F, et al. Long-term pioglitazone treatment for patients with nonalcoholic steatohepatitis and prediabetes or type 2 diabetes mellitus: a randomized trial. Ann Intern Med. 2016;165:305–15.
35. Bril F, Kalavalapalli S, Clark VC, et al. Response to pioglitazone in patients with nonalcoholic steatohepatitis with vs without type 2 diabetes. Clin Gastroenterol Hepatol. 2018;16:558–66.
36. Musso G, Cassader M, Paschetta E, et al. Thiazolidinediones and advanced liver fibrosis in nonalcoholic steatohepatitis: a meta-analysis. JAMA Intern Med. 2017;177:633–40.
37. Chiarelli F, Di Marzio D. Peroxisome proliferator-activated receptor-gamma agonists and diabetes: current evidence and future perspectives. Vasc Health Risk Manag. 2008;4:297–304.
38. Ratziu V, Harrison SA, Francque S, et al. Elafibranor, an agonist of the peroxisome proliferator-activated receptor-alpha and -delta, induces resolution of nonalcoholic steatohepatitis without fibrosis worsening. Gastroenterology. 2016;150:1147–59.

39. Francque SM, Bedossa P, Ratziu V, et al. A randomized, controlled trial of the pan-PPAR agonist Lanifibranor in NASH. N Engl J Med Overseas Ed. 2021;385:1547–58.
40. Marso SP, Daniels GH, Brown-Frandsen K, ; LEADER Steering Committee; LEADER Trial Investigators, et al Liraglutide and cardiovascular outcomes in type 2 diabetes. N Engl J Med 2016; 375:311–322.
41. Ohki T, Isogawa A, Iwamoto M, et al. The effectiveness of liraglutide in nonalcoholic fatty liver disease patients with type 2 diabetes mellitus compared to sitagliptin and pioglitazone. Sci World J. 2012;2012:496453.
42. Shao N, Kuang HY, Hao M, et al. Benefits of exenatide on obesity and non-alcoholic fatty liver disease with elevated liver enzymes in patients with type 2 diabetes. Diabetes Metab Res Rev. 2014;30:521–9.
43. Newsome PN, Buchholtz K, Cusi K, et al. A placebo-controlled trial of subcutaneous Semaglutide in nonalcoholic steatohepatitis. N Engl J Med. 2021;384:1113–24.
44. Cui J, Philo L, Nguyen P, et al. Sitagliptin vs. placebo for nonalcoholic fatty liver disease: a randomized controlled trial. J Hepatol. 2016;65:369–76.
45. Kuchay MS, Krishan S, Mishra SK, et al. Effect of empagliflozin on liver fat in patients with type 2 diabetes and nonalcoholic fatty liver disease: a randomized controlled trial (E-LIFT trial). Diabetes Care. 2018;41:1801–8.
46. Lee PCH, Gu Y, Yeung MY, et al. Dapagliflozin and empagliflozin ameliorate hepatic dysfunction among Chinese subjects with diabetes in part through glycemic improvement: a single-center, retrospective, observational study. Diabetes Ther. 2018;9:285–95.
47. Bril F, Biernacki DM, Lomonaco R, et al. Role of vitamin E for the treatment of nonalcoholic steatohepatitis in patients with type 2 diabetes: a randomized controlled trial. Diabetes Care. 2019;42:1481–8.
48. Noureddin M, Rinella ME. Nonalcoholic fatty liver disease, diabetes, obesity, and hepatocellular carcinoma. Clin Liver Dis. 2015;19:361–79.
49. Bhat A, Sebastiani G, Bhat M. Systematic review: preventive and therapeutic applications of metformin in liver disease. World J Hepatol. 2015;7(12):1652–9.

Nonalcoholic Fatty Liver Disease and Chronic Kidney Disease

15

Camelia Cojocariu, Cristina Popa, Cristina Muzica, Carol Stanciu, Tudor Cuciureanu, and Anca Trifan

15.1 Introduction

Nonalcoholic fatty liver disease (NAFLD) and chronic kidney disease (CKD) are worldwide public health problems, due to their increasing prevalence and incidence, poor outcomes, and healthcare burden [1, 2]. NAFLD is the most common chronic liver disease of our century, reaching epidemic proportions, affecting up to ~25–30% of the population worldwide [3]; CKD affects up to ~10–15% of the general adult population in many parts of the world [4, 5].

Both NAFLD and CKD are progressive chronic diseases with a wide spectrum of manifestations from benign symptoms to relatively mild disease and to severely debilitating and end-stage disease, requiring chronic dialysis or liver/kidney transplantation.

15.2 NAFLD

Nonalcoholic fatty liver disease is currently one of the most common etiologies of chronic liver disease worldwide, especially in developing countries.

C. Cojocariu (✉) · C. Muzica · T. Cuciureanu · A. Trifan
University of Medicine and Pharmacy "Grigore T. Popa", Iasi, Romania

Institute of Gastroenterology and Hepatology, St. Spiridon Emergency Hospital, Iasi, Romania

C. Popa
University of Medicine and Pharmacy "Grigore T. Popa", Iasi, Romania

Clinical Hospital CI Parhon, Iasi, Romania

C. Stanciu
Institute of Gastroenterology and Hepatology, St. Spiridon Emergency Hospital, Iasi, Romania

© The Author(s), under exclusive license to Springer Nature Switzerland AG 2023
A. Trifan et al. (eds.), *Essentials of Non-Alcoholic Fatty Liver Disease*,
https://doi.org/10.1007/978-3-031-33548-8_15

NAFLD has become a pandemic in the last decade with rising morbidity and mortality worldwide. Given the changing etiology of chronic liver disease following increased access to curative treatment for chronic hepatitis B and C, NAFLD is a major concern for hepatologists everywhere, while it is affecting one-quarter of adults worldwide [3].

The global burden of NAFLD is rising in parallel with increasing rates of obesity, type 2 diabetes mellitus (T2DM), and metabolic syndrome [6, 7]. Moreover, NAFLD is also a growing risk factor for hepatocellular carcinoma (HCC) and a leading indication for liver transplantation [8, 9] and hepatocellular cancer-related liver transplantation [10].

Statistical analyses showed that in Europe, in 2030, a timepoint we established to eradicate hepatitis C virus infection, it is estimated that the highest prevalence of NAFLD will be in Italy (29.5%) and the lowest (23.6%) in France [10]. NAFLD will be the most important challenge in hepatology in the next few years.

NAFLD includes a wide range of manifestations, from simple hepatic steatosis (a benign/silent disease with fat accumulation in liver volume more than 5%) to nonalcoholic steatohepatitis (NASH) (steatosis with inflammation) and fibrosis with high potential for progression to liver cirrhosis (and hepatocellular carcinoma), the final stage of any chronic liver disease [3, 11, 12]. The real prevalence of NASH is not known, mainly due to the asymptomatic course of the disease, but millions of people worldwide are at risk of cirrhosis associated with NAFLD [3].

As long as there is no effective treatment proven to control the disease, it is unlikely to expect a significant reduction in incidence rates in the coming years [13], but some of NAFLD extrahepatic manifestations/associated disease may be treated if they are recognized.

In the last years, several studies have focused on the association between NAFLD and CKD, regardless of the presence of known/not known risk factors for these two diseases such as obesity, arterial hypertension, type 2 diabetes mellitus (T2DM), or metabolic syndrome [14–18].

15.3 CKD

CKD is one of the important causes of mortality worldwide, and it is one of the diseases that have shown an increase in associated deaths over the past two decades. It has to emphasize that if in recent years it has been possible to reduce mortality for most diseases (cardiovascular, neoplasia, metabolic, etc.), advanced chronic liver disease is the only one in which there is an upward trend of mortality.

According to KDIGO (Kidney Disease Improving Global outcome), chronic kidney disease (CKD) is defined as abnormalities of kidney structure or function, present for more than 3 months. CKD is classified based on cause, glomerular filtration rate category (G1–G5), and albuminuria category (A1–A3). According to GFR, there are five CKD stages: stage 1—GFR more than 90 mL/min/1.73 m^2; stage 2—60–89 mL/min/1.73 m^2; stage 3—30–59 mL/min/1.73 m^2 (stage 3a, 45–59 mL/

min/1.73 m^2; stage 3b—30–44 mL/min/1.73 m^2; stage 4—15–29 mL/min/1.73 m^2; and stage 5—GFR less than 15 mL/min/1.73 m^2 [19].

The global all-age mortality associated with CKD increased by 41.5% between 1990 and 2017 [20]. Although mortality has dropped down in the last decades in patients with ESKD, the latest Global Burden of Disease (GBD) studies have shown that CKD is still an important cause of worldwide mortality [21–23]. The same report showed that the number of patients affected by CKD stages 1–5 has been increasing, affecting more than 800 million individuals worldwide in 2017 [23, 24].

CKD was the 13th leading cause of death worldwide in 2016 and the 12th in 2017 and more; it is predicted to be the fifth highest cause of years of life lost globally by 2040 [24–26], the time when hepatologists aim to eradicate/control chronic liver disease associated with viral C and B hepatitis.

In 2016, Hill et al. showed in a comprehensive systematic review and meta-analysis of 100 studies that the prevalence of CKD stages 1–5 is 13.4% worldwide (10.6% for CKD stages 3–5) and the prevalence of CKD according to the stage is variable: 8.9% (stages 1 and 2), 7.6% (stage 3), 0.4% (stage 4), and 0.1% (stage 5) [27].

The CKD prevalence has changed over time. In the United States, the prevalence of CKD stages 1–4 was 11.8% from 1988 to 1994, and it increased to 14.2% from 2015 to 2016 [23], and similarly stable prevalence of CKD stages 1–5 was reported in Norway between 1995 and 2008 [28]. In contrast, in the UK, the prevalence of CKD stages 3–5 declined significantly over 7 years [23].

The increase in the population's life expectancy could explain the high maintenance and somewhat constant prevalence of CKD. The meta-analysis of Hill et al. showed the impact of age on CKD prevalence and reported a linearly higher prevalence for CKD stages associated with advancing age, ranging from 13.7% in 30- to 40-year-old patients to 27.9% in patients aged >70–80 years [27].

Considering the rise in risk factors for CKD, such as obesity, T2DM, and metabolic disease, the prevalence of CKD is expected to increase in the next years.

15.4 NAFLD and CKD: Correlation or Causation, Pathophysiology

The nephrologists agree and preferentially use the term MAFLD for nonalcoholic fatty liver disease, a term with which hepatologists do not entirely agree.

Most of the recognized risk factors of NAFLD, i.e., visceral obesity, T2DM, arterial hypertension, atherogenic dyslipidemia, metabolic syndrome, and insulin resistance, are at the same time important risk factors for CKD [29]. In recent years, other risk factors involved in the pathogenesis of the two conditions have been analyzed (some of them confirmed): low-grade inflammatory state (increased C-reactive protein, IL-6, TNF-α levels), prothrombotic state (increased levels of factor VII, fibrinogen, tissue factor, and plasminogen activator inhibitor-1, and decreased levels of tissue plasminogen activator and other fibrinolytic factors), increased uric acid levels, low 25-hydroxy-vitamin D, decreased adiponectin levels, etc. [9, 30–33].

The pathophysiology of NAFLD is multifactorial, and not completely understood, characterized by inflammation, lipotoxicity, and fibrosis, leading to end-stage liver disease; NAFLD describes a spectrum of histological abnormalities, from steatosis to steatohepatitis, hepato-fibrosis, and cirrhosis (Fig. 15.1).

The key event of NAFLD pathophysiology is the liver's accumulation of free fatty acids (FFAs). The liver gets FFAs from three sources: (1) FFAs are taken up from the circulation with excessive mobilization of them derived from the lipolysis of adipose tissues, driven by insulin resistance (IR) (60%). (2) De novo lipogenesis (DNL) represents 26% of stored hepatic triglycerides (TGs). Excessive carbohydrates are converted to FFAs in the liver by DNL process. The rate of DNL is tightly regulated by several nuclear transcription factors (TFs), the most important being sterol regulatory element-binding protein-1c (SREBP-1c). (3) Dietary lipids constitute around 15% of TGs in the liver.

Evidence indicates that saturated FAs are more hepatotoxic than unsaturated FAs and are associated with disease progression. The mechanisms for FFA disposal in the liver are b-oxidation, in which FFAs are oxidized in mitochondria, and VLDL export, in which FFAs are re-esterified generating TGs. TGs are then assembled and secreted into the systemic circulation as a constituent of VLDLs. Hepatic steatosis occurs when the TG homeostasis is disrupted due to an increase in FA uptake and DNL and a reduction in FFA oxidation and VLDL export.

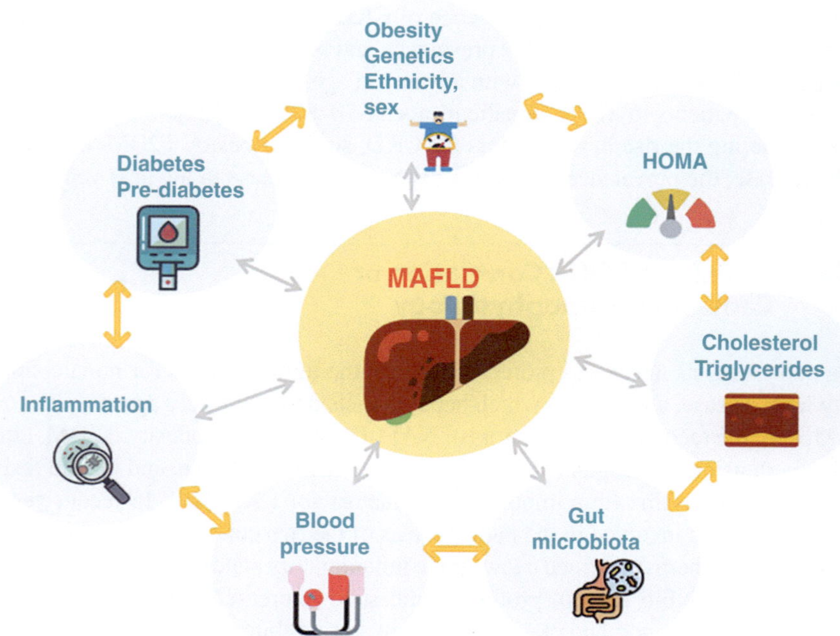

Fig. 15.1 The vicious circle in the pathophysiology of NAFLD/MAFLD

When the FFA disposal mechanisms are disrupted or overwhelmed, ROS and toxic lipid species are generated, thus triggering lipotoxicity.

Oxidative stress and inflammasome formation are the key processes that contribute to the development and progression of NASH. These processes are initiated by FFA overload and then perpetuated by several proinflammatory cells. The main intracellular sources of ROS are mitochondria, endoplasmic reticulum (ER), peroxisomes, xanthine oxidase (XO), and cytochrome P450 metabolism. Under physiological conditions, these ROS are neutralized by antioxidant mechanisms. In MASH, oxidative stress results from both increased production of oxidative species and a breakdown of antioxidant defenses. Inflammasomes are intracellular pattern recognition receptors (PRRs) that are responsible for the production of proinflammatory cytokines, such as IL-1b and IL-18. Inflammasome-mediated IL-1b secretion is initiated and then stimulated by a variety of signals. Immune dysregulation plays a crucial role in the pathogenesis of NASH. The major immune cells that contribute to NASH are Kupffer cells, monocytes, neutrophils, and T-helper (Th) and cytotoxic CD8þ T cells. Cytotoxic CD8 T cells accumulate in the liver during NAFLD, and their inhibition results in decreased steatosis, IR, inflammation, and hepatic stellate cell activation.

Activation of these cytotoxic CD8þ T cells is supported by type I IFN responses and leads to the production of the proinflammatory cytokines, IFN-γ and TNF-α. Hepatic stellate cells (HSCs) play a crucial role in MASH progression. Activation of HSC involves the transition from quiescent vitamin A-storing cells to a proliferative migratory and fibrogenic phenotype, which is characteristic of liver fibrogenesis, and free cholesterol accumulation mediates HSC activation. Fibrogenesis is a dynamic process. When there are excessive and prolonged injurious stimuli, such as lipotoxic species, profibrogenic processes predominate (HSC activation) and fibrous tissue accumulates in the liver [34].

The linking mechanisms between NAFLD and CKD are extremely complex and not fully explained. The most important studied mechanisms involved in the pathogenesis of the two diseases and that make the connection between them are represented by dysbiosis and disturbed intestinal function, dietary changes (mediating a link between NAFLD, dysbiosis, and CKD), platelet activation, T2DM and metabolic syndrome (the most studied association of NAFLD and CKD), etc.

15.4.1 Dysbiosis and Disturbed Intestinal Function, Dietary Changes

In recent years, intestinal dysbiosis has been considered an important element in the pathogenesis of most diseases (cardiovascular, neurological, degenerative, digestive, etc.); certainly, the change in the intestinal flora is responsible for many digestive symptoms and change in the quality of life, but we believe that the importance of dysbiosis in the pathogenesis of most pathologies is somewhat exaggerated.

Some experimental data suggests the role of the intestinal microbiota in the pathogenesis of both CKD and NAFLD [35, 36]. Dysbiosis may be associated with increase in gram-negative organisms, lipopolysaccharide, gut permeability, secondary bile acids (BAs), and renal toxins, which may increase the risk of development and progression of both NAFLD [36, 37] and CKD [38].

According to dysbiosis and disturbed intestinal function, dietary change is another factor that could mediate the link between NAFLD, dysbiosis, and CKD. Nowadays, the most commonly consumed sugar is fructose and its intake is associated with NASH and with increased serum uric acid concentrations in children and adolescents [39]. Although it has been thought that most of our level of fructose is due to dietary intake, Lanaspa et al. recently showed that endogenous fructose can also be generated in the liver with activation of the polyol pathway and glucose may be converted to sorbitol by aldose reductase and sorbitol is converted to fructose by sorbitol dehydrogenase [40]. Aldose reductase is an NADPH-dependent aldo-keto reductase, and in 2019, Sanchez-Lozada et al. showed that uric acid dose-dependently stimulated aldose reductase expression, and it is associated with increased endogenous fructose production and hepatic triglyceride accumulation [41]. The stimulatory mechanism is mediated by uric acid-induced oxidative stress, and the increase in uric acid concentrations leads to a further increase in endogenous fructose production by stimulating aldose reductase with the potential for uric acid-mediated kidney damage and fructose-mediated disease. Dysbiosis may also promote increased platelet activation since indoxyl sulfate activates platelets, so the following aspect stated seems logical in discussing the association between NAFLD and CKD [42].

15.4.2 T2DM, Metabolic Syndrome, NAFLD, and CKD

Numerous epidemiological data have shown that NAFLD is an independent risk factor for CKD and also that NAFLD and elements of the metabolic syndrome (MetS) intervene in the development and progression of CKD [29]. Renal damage in patients with T2DM is well known, and more than one-third of patients with NAFLD have impaired renal function. Many diabetic patients have NAFLD, and both diseases have a significant risk of kidney damage; impaired renal function in patients with NAFLD is associated with the severity of liver disease and T2DM association [43].

Considering that many times T2DM, MetS, and NAFLD coexist and share common risk factors, it is very difficult to estimate the main factor that initiates the change in renal function in these patients.

15.5 Genetic Factors

Genetic factors also play a role in the development and progression of NAFLD. The genetic variations found in NAFLD are driven by genes involved in lipid droplet biology, the most common being patatin-like phospholipase domain-containing 3 (PNPLA3) and transmembrane 6 superfamily member 2 (TM6SF2). Many other genetic factors may be involved and are yet to be discovered.

15.6 NAFLD and CKD: Correlation or Causation, Clinical Evidence of Association

When discussing the link between NAFLD and CKD, the data is controversial. On the one hand, both NAFLD and CKD share common risk factors, such as T2DM, metabolic dysregulation, and atherogenic dyslipidemia [34]. On the other hand, some studies support the fact that NAFLD is independently associated with a higher prevalence of CKD [34, 44].

There is evidence that supports the relationship between NAFLD and CKD. Three meta-analyses study the risk of CKD among NAFLD patients, and all three point towards a higher risk of incident CKD among NAFLD population, but there are some mentions. In the first meta-analysis, the results were not adjusted for common cardiorenal risk factors which can be present in both NAFLD and CKD [45]. Mantovani et al. included only observational studies and populations of Asian descent, and therefore causality cannot be proven [14]. The most recent meta-analysis shows that individuals with NAFLD have a 39% higher risk of incident CKD, irrespective of cardiorenal factors. Furthermore, the risk of CKD was higher in individuals with more severe NAFLD, and risk stratification for CKD in these patients is needed [46] (Table 15.1).

Regarding the data among MAFLD patients, there is one cross-sectional study published in 2021 that compared the prevalence of CKD among NAFLD and MAFLD patients. The study included 12,571 patients from the Third National Health and Nutrition Examination Survey 1988–1994 (NHANES III). Among the NHANES III cohort, the prevalence of MAFLD was 30.2%, whereas the prevalence of NAFLD was 36.2%. Patients with MAFLD had a higher prevalence of CKD when compared

Table 15.1 Risk of CKD among NAFLD patients

Author, year	Design	Studies included	Patients, no.	Risk of CKD in NAFLD patients
Musso et al. (2014) [45]	Meta-analysis (33 studies)	33 longitudinal and cross-sectional studies	63,902	Prevalence of CKD, pooled OR 2.12 (95% CI 1.69–2.66) Incidence of CKD: HR 1.79 (95% CI 1.65–1.95)
Mantovani et al. (2018) [14]	Meta-analysis (9 observational studies)	9 observational studies	96,595	Risk of incident CKD: HR 1.37 (95% CI 1.2–1.53)
Cai et al. (2021) [46]	Meta-analysis (11 cohort studies)	11 cohort studies	1,198,242	Unadjusted models: RR 1.54 (95% CI) of CKD Adjusted model: RR 1.39 (95% CI) Compared to non-NAFLD patients: adjusted absolute risk increase of 5.1 (95% CI 3.5–6.8) per 1000 person-years

CKD chronic kidney disease, *NAFLD* nonalcoholic fatty liver disease to NAFLD patients (29.6% versus 26.56%). Moreover, the severity of MAFLD was associated with an increased risk of prevalent CKD (1.34-fold higher risk) [47].

Although the literature available up to this point indicates an increased risk of incident CKD among NAFLD and patients, we need to take into consideration the fact that most studies included were observational and cross-sectional and a causative link is difficult to prove. However, the NHANES III points towards a higher risk of CKD among MAFLD patients, but at the same time, the subjects included were from a cohort from 1988 to 1994 and a more contemporary study is needed. Such a study exists and was published in 2021, which included 4869 patients from NHANES 2017 to 2018 and studied the association between CKD and MAFLD. Results showed that there was a higher prevalence of CKD in MAFLD patients when compared to non-MAFLD patients (22.2% versus 19.1%), but MAFLD was not independently associated with CKD [48].

A meta-analysis published in 2022 studied the association between liver stiffness and CKD in patients with NAFLD. The primary outcome of the study was CKD, defined as a composite of urinary albumin-to-creatinine ratio (UACR) $\geq$30 mg/g and estimated glomerular filtration rate (eGFR) <60 mL/min/m^2. In individuals with liver fibrosis assessed by vibration-controlled transient elastography (VCTE), the risk of CKD was higher (OR 2.49 95% CI 1.89–3.29). This suggests that elevated liver stiffness is linked to an increased risk of kidney outcomes, and screening for advanced fibrosis might also help identify patients at risk for kidney disease [49]. However, once again, the studies are cross-sectional in nature and prospective data is needed to confirm causality.

We need to take into consideration that NAFLD and CKD have common risk factors, such as obesity, decreased insulin sensitivity, T2DM, arterial hypertension, and metabolic syndrome [1]. The presence of one or more risk factors could create a vicious circle that affects both liver and kidneys, but one question remains: does NAFLD cause CKD, is it just an incident finding, or metabolic dysregulation is the sole cause of both? More prospective data are needed to define the relationship between the two entities.

Given the metabolic dysregulation in NAFLD, and the low-grade systemic inflammation, we could also speculate that NAFLD could be a new risk factor for CKD progression, but more studies involving NAFLD and CKD are needed to confirm this hypothesis.

15.7 Conclusions

However, irrespective of the causative relationship between the two, all patients with NAFLD should be screened for CKD using serum creatinine levels and urinary albumin-to-creatinine ratio to identify early kidney dysfunction. Early referral to a nephrologist and a multidisciplinary approach could be vital for the patient. Although there are no guidelines and surveillance protocols for CKD in patients with NAFLD, it is crucial to detect early renal impairment in these patients in order to prevent CKD progression, minimize complications, and improve survival.

Currently, many clinical trials are evaluating the therapeutic efficacy of new drugs for NAFLD, and regarding the association of NAFLD with CKD, it is mandatory that all future randomized controlled trials focused on testing efficient and safety treatments for NAFLD/NASH have to systematically search for CKD in patients with NAFLD.

References

1. Kiapidou S, Liava C, Kalogirou M, Akriviadis E, Sinakos E. Chronic kidney disease in patients with non-alcoholic fatty liver disease: what the hepatologist should know? Ann Hepatol. 2020;19:134–44.
2. Sesti G, Fiorentino TV, Arturi F, Perticone M, Sciacqua A, Perticone F. Association between noninvasive fibrosis markers and chronic kidney disease among adults with nonalcoholic fatty liver disease. PLoS One. 2014;9(2):e88569.
3. Younossi ZM, Koenig AB, Abdelatif D, Fazel Y, Henry L, Wymer M. Global epidemiology of nonalcoholic fatty liver disease-meta-analytic assessment of prevalence, incidence, and outcomes. Hepatology. 2016;64:73–84.
4. Couser WG, Remuzzi G, Mendis S, Tonelli M. The contribution of chronic kidney disease to the global burden of major noncommunicable diseases. Kidney Int. 2011;80:1258–70.
5. Eckardt KU, Coresh J, Devuyst O, Johnson RJ, Kottgen A, Levey AS, et al. Evolving importance of kidney disease: from subspecialty to global health burden. Lancet. 2013;382:158–69.
6. Takalkar UV, Nageshwar DR. Non-alcoholic fatty liver disease-hepatic manifestation of obesity. Austin J Obes Metab Syndr. 2018;3:1–3.
7. Williamson RM, Price JF, Glancy S, Perry E, Nee LD, Hayes PC, Frier BM, Van Look LAF, Johnston GI, Reynolds RM, et al. Prevalence of and risk factors for hepatic steatosis and nonalcoholic fatty liver disease in people with type 2 diabetes: the Edinburgh type 2 diabetes study. Diabetes Care. 2011;34:1139–44.
8. Wong RJ, Aguilar M, Cheung R, et al. Nonalcoholic steatohepatitis is the second leading etiology of liver disease among adults awaiting liver transplantation in the United States. Gastroenterology. 2015;148:547–55.
9. Younossi ZM, Loomba R, Anstee QM, et al. Diagnostic modalities for nonalcoholic fatty liver disease, nonalcoholic steatohepatitis, and associated fibrosis. Hepatology. 2018;68:349–60.
10. Younossi Z, Stepanova M, Ong JP, et al. Nonalcoholic steatohepatitis is the fastest growing cause of hepatocellular carcinoma in liver transplant candidates. Clin Gastroenterol Hepatol. 2019;17:748–755.e3.
11. Rinella ME, Loomba R, Caldwell SH, et al. Controversies in the diagnosis and management of NAFLD and NASH. Gastroenterol Hepatol. 2014;10(4):219–27.
12. Singh S, Allen AM, Wang Z, et al. Fibrosis progression in nonalcoholic fatty liver vs nonalcoholic steatohepatitis: a systematic review and meta-analysis of paired-biopsy studies. Clin Gastroenterol Hepatol. 2015;13:643–54.
13. Raza S, Rajak S, Upadhyay A, et al. Current treatment paradigms and emerging therapies for NAFLD/NASH. Front Biosci (Landmark Ed). 2021;26:206–37.
14. Mantovani A, Zaza G, Byrne CD, Lonardo A, Zoppini G, Bonora E, et al. Nonalcoholic fatty liver disease increases risk of incident chronic kidney disease: a systematic review and meta-analysis. Metabolism. 2018;79:64–76.
15. Sirota JC, McFann K, Targher G, et al. Association between non-alcoholic liver disease and chronic kidney disease: an ultrasound analysis from NHANES 1988–1994. Am J Nephrol. 2012;36(5):466–71.
16. Chang Y, Ryu S, Sung E, et al. Nonalcoholic fatty liver disease predicts chronic kidney disease in nonhypertensive and nondiabetic Korean men. Metabolism. 2008;57(4):569–76.

17. Zhang M, Lin S, Wang M, Huang J, et al. Association between NAFLD and risk of prevalent chronic kidney disease: why there is a difference between east and west? BMC Gastroenterol. 2020;20(1):139.

18. Armstrong M, Adams L, Canbay A, et al. Extrahepatic complications of nonalcoholic fatty liver disease. Hepatology. 2014;59:1174–97.

19. de Boer IH, Caramori ML, et al. Executive summary of the 2020 KDIGO diabetes management in CKD guideline: evidence-based advances in monitoring and treatment. Kidney Int. 2020;98(4):839–48. https://doi.org/10.1016/j.kint.2020.06.024.

20. GBD Chronic Kidney Disease Collaboration. Global, regional, and national burden of chronic kidney disease, 1990–2017: a systematic analysis for the Global Burden of Disease Study 2017. Lancet. 2020;395:709–33.

21. Saran R, Robinson B, Abbott KC, et al. US Renal Data System 2019 annual data report: epidemiology of kidney disease in the United States. Am J Kidney Dis. 2020;75:A6–7.

22. GBD Mortality Causes of Death Collaborators. Global, regional, and national age-sex specific all-cause and cause-specific mortality for 240 causes of death, 1990–2013: a systematic analysis for the Global Burden of Disease Study 2013. Lancet. 2015;385:117–71.

23. Kovesdy CP. Epidemiology of chronic kidney disease: an update 2022. Kidney Int Suppl (2011). 2022;12(1):7–11.

24. Jager KJ, Kovesdy C, Langham R, et al. A single number for advocacy and communication-worldwide more than 850 million individuals have kidney diseases. Kidney Int. 2019;96:1048–50.

25. GBD Causes of Death Collaborators. Global, regional, and national age-sex specific mortality for 264 causes of death, 1980–2016: a systematic analysis for the Global Burden of Disease Study 2016. Lancet. 2017;390:1151–210.

26. Foreman KJ, Marquez N, Dolgert A, et al. Forecasting life expectancy, years of life lost, and all-cause and cause-specific mortality for 250 causes of death: reference and alternative scenarios for 2016–2040 for 195 countries and territories. Lancet. 2018;392:2052–90.

27. Hill NR, Fatoba ST, Oke JL, et al. Global prevalence of chronic kidney disease-a systematic review and meta-analysis. PLoS One. 2016;11:e0158765.

28. Hallan SI, Ovrehus MA, Romundstad S, et al. Long-term trends in the prevalence of chronic kidney disease and the influence of cardiovascular risk factors in Norway. Kidney Int. 2016;90:665–73.

29. Byrne DC, Targher G. NAFLD as a driver of chronic kidney disease. J Hepatol. 2020;72:785–801.

30. Lonardo A, Bellentani S, Argo CK, Ballestri S, Byrne CD, Caldwell SH, et al. Epidemiological modifiers of non-alcoholic fatty liver disease: focus high-risk groups. Dig Liver Dis. 2015;47:997–1006.

31. Kendrick J, Chonchol MB. Nontraditional risk factors for cardiovascular disease in patients with chronic kidney disease. Nat Clin Pract Nephrol. 2008;4:672–81.

32. Kronenberg F. Emerging risk factors and markers of chronic kidney disease progression. Nat Rev Nephrol. 2009;5:677–89.

33. Targher G, Byrne CD. Non-alcoholic fatty liver disease: an emerging driving force in chronic kidney disease. Nat Rev Nephrol. 2017;13(5):297–310. https://doi.org/10.1038/nrneph.2017.16.

34. Kuchay MS, Choudhary NS, Mishra SK. Pathophysiological mechanisms underlying MAFLD. Diabetes Metab Syndr. 2020;14(6):1875–87. https://doi.org/10.1016/j.dsx.2020.09.026.

35. Marcuccilli M, Chonchol M. NAFLD and chronic kidney disease. Int J Mol Sci. 2016;17:562.

36. Briskey D, Tucker P, Johnson DW, Coombes JS. The role of the gastrointestinal tract and microbiota on uremic toxins and chronic kidney disease development. Clin Exp Nephrol. 2017;21:7–15.

37. Kim HN, Joo EJ, Cheong HS, Kim Y, Kim HL, Shin H, et al. Gut microbiota and risk of persistent nonalcoholic fatty liver diseases. J Clin Med. 2019;8:E1089.

38. Wieland A, Frank DN, Harnke B, Bambha K. Systematic review: microbial dysbiosis and nonalcoholic fatty liver disease. Aliment Pharmacol Ther. 2015;42:1051–63.
39. Mosca A, Nobili V, De Vito R, Crudele A, Scorletti E, Villani A, et al. Serum uric acid concentrations and fructose consumption are independently associated with NASH in children and adolescents. J Hepatol. 2017;66:1031–6.
40. Lanaspa MA, Ishimoto T, Li N, Cicerchi C, Orlicky DJ, Ruzycki P, et al. Endogenous fructose production and metabolism in the liver contributes to the development of metabolic syndrome. Nat Commun. 2013;4:2434.
41. Sanchez-Lozada LG, Andres-Hernando A, Garcia-Arroyo FE, Cicerchi C, Li N, Kuwabara M, et al. Uric acid activates aldose reductase and the polyol pathway for endogenous fructose and fat production causing the development of fatty liver in rats. J Biol Chem. 2019;294:4272–81.
42. Chen PC, Kao WY, Cheng YL, Wang YJ, Hou MC, Wu JC, et al. The correlation between fatty liver disease and chronic kidney disease. J Formos Med Assoc. 2020;119(1 Pt 1):42–50.
43. Kaya E, Yilmaz Y. Metabolic-associated fatty liver disease (MAFLD): a multi-systemic disease beyond the liver. J Clin Transl Hepatol. 2022;10(2):329–38. https://doi.org/10.14218/JCTH.2021.00178.
44. Yang K, Du C, Wang X, Li F, Xu Y, Wang S, et al. Indoxyl sulfate induces platelet hyperactivity and contributes to chronic kidney disease-associated thrombosis in mice. Blood. 2017;129:2667–79.
45. Musso G, Cassader M, Cohney S, De Michieli F, Pinach S, Saba F, et al. Fatty liver and chronic kidney disease: novel mechanistic insights and therapeutic opportunities. Diabetes Care. 2016;39:1830–45.
46. Cai X, Sun L, Liu X, Zhu H, Zhang Y, Zheng S, Huang Y. Non-alcoholic fatty liver disease is associated with increased risk of chronic kidney disease. Ther Adv Chronic Dis. 2021;12:20406223211024361. https://doi.org/10.1177/20406223211024361.
47. Sun DQ, Jin Y, Wang TY, Zheng KI, et al. MAFLD and risk of CKD. Metabolism. 2021;115:154433. https://doi.org/10.1016/j.metabol.2020.154433.
48. Deng Y, Zhao Q, Gong R. Association between metabolic associated fatty liver disease and chronic kidney disease: a cross-sectional study from NHANES 2017–2018. Diabetes Metab Syndr Obes. 2021;14:1751–61. https://doi.org/10.2147/DMSO.S292926.
49. Ciardullo S, Ballabeni C, Trevisan R, Perseghin G. Liver stiffness, albuminuria and chronic kidney disease in patients with NAFLD: a systematic review and meta-analysis. Biomol Ther. 2022;12(1):105. https://doi.org/10.3390/biom12010105.

Endocrinopathies in Nonalcoholic Fatty Liver Disease

16

Ana Maria Singeap and Laura Huiban

16.1 Introduction

Nonalcoholic fatty liver disease (NAFLD) represents one of the main causes of chronic liver disease, which includes a wide spectrum from simple steatosis to advanced fibrosis, cirrhosis, and, eventually, even hepatocellular carcinoma. Evidence so far sustains a clear relationship between various endocrine dysfunctions and nonalcoholic fatty liver disease (Fig. 16.1). Endocrinopathies may be involved in the development and progression of NAFLD. Awareness, early diagnosis, appropriate surveillance, and treatment are mandatory for optimal patients' approach.

A. M. Singeap (✉) · L. Huiban
Gastroenterology Department, Grigore T. Popa University of Medicine and Pharmacy, Iasi, Romania

Institute of Gastroenterology and Hepatology, St. Spiridon Emergency Hospital, Iasi, Romania

A. Trifan et al. (eds.), *Essentials of Non-Alcoholic Fatty Liver Disease*, https://doi.org/10.1007/978-3-031-33548-8_16

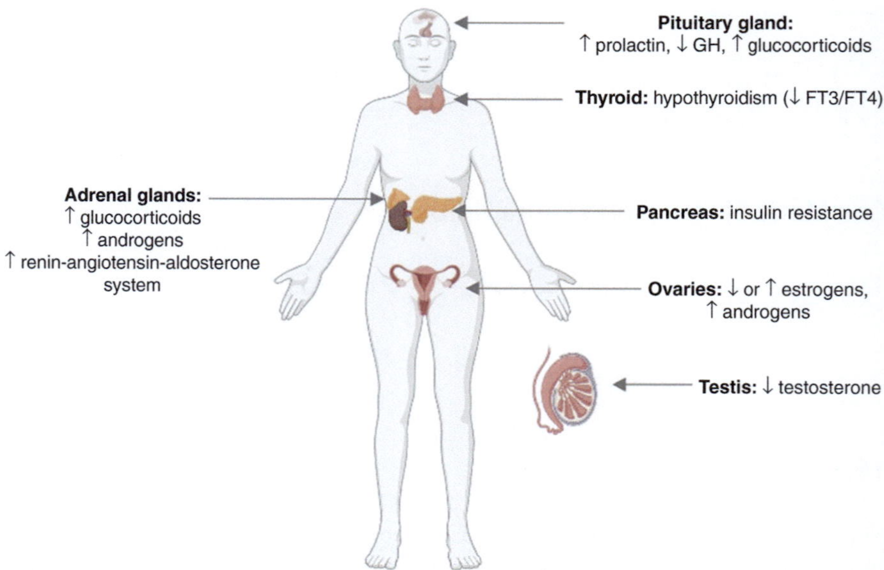

Fig. 16.1 Endocrine disorders associated with nonalcoholic fatty liver diseases (*created with* BioRender.com)

16.2 NAFLD and Hypothyroidism

The thyroid gland has a dominant role in the control of many metabolic processes. Thyroid dysfunction, represented by thyroid hormone level disorders, either clinically overt or subclinical, may cause insulin resistance, hyperlipidemia, and obesity, viewed as acknowledged risk factors for NAFLD development [1]. Thyroid hormones modulate cholesterol synthesis, transformation, and clearance [2]. Thyroid-stimulating hormone (TSH) has as direct result an increase of liver gluconeogenesis, at the same time decreasing 3-hydroxy-3-methylglutaryl coenzyme A (HMG-CoA) reductase phosphorylation, causing hypercholesterolemia [3]. In addition, a common pathophysiological pathway for hypothyroidism and NAFLD is represented by oxidative stress [4].

Association between thyroid abnormalities and NAFLD has been extensively debated in time, with initial conflicting results; however, growing evidence is showing that hypothyroidism may be a risk factor for NAFLD. While the prevalence of hypothyroidism in the population of the United States was found to be 3.7% [5], a systematic review performed in 2014 and including 11 articles showed a hypothyroidism prevalence between 15.2 and 36.3% among NAFLD patients [6]; NAFLD was diagnosed in five studies by liver biopsy, while in the other six studies, ultrasonographic criteria were used. Another systematic review and meta-analysis on more than 40,000 patients included in 13 studies showed a significant correlation between NAFLD and hypothyroidism, sustaining by epidemiological arguments the risk for NAFLD in patients with hypothyroidism, in comparison with persons with euthyroidism [7]. Overt hypothyroidism, understood as elevated TSH and decreased free thyroxine 4 (FT4), was more significantly associated with NAFLD than subclinical hypothyroidism, defined as high TSH and normal FT4, the probable explanation being the combined concomitant effects of thyroid hormones and TSH-level variations [7]. Similar results were showed by another recent systematic review and meta-analysis performed on a total of 51,407 hypothyroidism patients, where hypothyroidism was positively associated with the risk of NAFLD [8]. In this study, the elevated concentrations of TSH levels and low FT4 were significantly correlated with the risk of NAFLD, while free triiodothyronine (FT3) was not significantly linked to the risk of NAFLD [8]. Subclinical hypothyroidism was associated with NAFLD in a dose-dependent relationship even in the presence of normal TSH range, and association with NAFLD was proved even if other metabolic issues were concomitantly present or absent [9]. In addition, "low-normal" thyroid was incriminated as a contributing factor to advanced fibrosis [10].

Recently, the connection of hypothyroidism with liver fibrosis was suggested. Even if it is still incompletely understood if or how thyroid dysfunction accelerates NAFLD progression to steatohepatitis and, furthermore, to advanced fibrosis, there are some evidences in this regard. Thus, the thyroid hormone receptor might have a role in the activation of hepatic stellate cell [11]. At the same time, in hypothyroidism patients, higher levels of serum leptin were remarked, which not only increases hepatic insulin resistance but also promotes synthesis of collagen in the liver [12]. Moreover, hypothyroidism appears to be related to elevated plasma levels of fibroblast growth factor-21, independently of body mass index, or lipid or glucose metabolism [13]. In real-world setting, studies showed that among NAFLD patients, increased TSH levels were significantly associated with higher risk of liver fibrosis, estimated either on transient elastography as liver stiffness ≥ 8.0 kPa [14] or by fibrosis-4 (FIB-4) index value of ≥ 2.6 [15], advocating that TSH levels might be a marker for liver fibrosis in NAFLD patients.

In the light of the assumed causal relationship between hypothyroidism and NAFLD, the question of a potential benefit on NAFLD following the hypothyroidism treatment appears as a challenging and attractive topic. Data so far showed that the replacement treatment with thyroid hormones is followed by a significant reduction of serum lipids and has a favorable effect on obesity or overweight [16], acting against risk factors for NAFLD. More specific results were shown by an interventional study where levothyroxine therapy for a period of 1 year and 3 months in patients diagnosed with subclinical hypothyroidism had a favorable effect on serological hepatic tests and ultrasound liver appearance in terms of steatosis features [17]. Moreover, decrease of liver fat, quantified by magnetic resonance spectroscopy, was documented after administration of levothyroxine for a 4-month period in patients with type 2 diabetes, normal thyroid function, and NAFLD [18]. At the same time, administration of an FGF-21 analogue in NASH patients leads to reducing liver fat content [19].

Evidences so far suggest that hypothyroidism may have an important role in the development and progression of NAFLD, and hypothyroidism-induced NAFLD may be already regarded as a definite entity. As subsequent advice for the clinical practice, it appears as mandatory that thyroid function must be evaluated in NAFLD patients and vice versa. Hypothyroidism is a modifiable risk factor, and even if there are still aspects to clarify, there is hope that thyroid replacement therapy NAFLD patients might have a benefit on the disease status and might prevent progression.

16.3　NAFLD and Hypopituitarism

The adenohypophysis, represented by the anterior pituitary part, is responsible for secreting into the circulation various hormones: thyroid-stimulating hormone (TSH), somatotropin; growth hormone (GH), corticotropin; or adrenocorticotropic hormone (ACTH), gonadotropins and prolactin.

Classically, the association between hypopituitarism, metabolic syndrome, and NAFLD is linked to lipid disequilibrium and liver fat accumulation. In hypopituitarism, modifications of lipid levels were described, the most important being the reduction of high-density lipoprotein cholesterol and the elevation of the proportion of low-density/high-density lipoprotein [20]. High prevalence of both NAFLD and metabolic syndrome was evidenced in hypopituitarism, with cardiac morbidity being significantly higher and higher associated premature mortality [21]. Moreover, leptin resistance associated with hypopituitarism may contribute to NAFLD pathogenesis, by the route of insulin resistance, overeating, and obesity [22].

Hypopituitarism may be linked to rapidly progressive NAFLD, as showed by a study reporting young patients with fast deterioration towards cirrhosis [23], and represents a risk factor for cardiovascular diseases, as demonstrated by a cohort cross-sectional study where non-treated female patients with hypopituitarism presented a twofold increase in cardiovascular mortality versus general population [23]. A recent study analyzing retrospectively surgical and nonsurgical hypopituitarism patients found that hepatic fibrosis rapidly progresses in the cases of NAFLD patients undergoing cranial surgery, in correlation with leptin, body mass index, and diabetes mellitus [24].

16.4　NAFLD and Growth Hormone Deficiency

Growth hormone (GH), secreted primarily by pituitary gland, exercises its effects through insulin-like growth factor-1 (IGF-1) synthetized in the liver, having as a consequence the stimulation of lipolysis, increase of free fatty acids, inhibition of glucose oxidation, and impairment of insulin sensitivity [25]. In adults, GH deficiency is correlated with decreased use of lipids as an energy source, decreased lipolysis and visceral adiposity, and insulin resistance; consequently, NAFLD is increasingly recognized as part of the metabolic complications related to adult GH deficiency [26]. Moreover, leptin resistance associated with hypopituitarism may contribute to NAFLD pathogenesis, via insulin resistance, hyperphagia, and obesity [22].

An observational study analyzing 69 patients diagnosed with hypopituitarism with no hormonal replacement treatment showed a 77% prevalence of NAFLD—diagnosed by ultrasound, significantly higher than in controls, where NAFLD prevalence was 12% [27]. Among patients with NAFLD proved by liver biopsy, reduced GH levels were correlated to higher grade of steatosis, while low IGF-1 was linked to higher grade of fibrosis and histologic features of NASH [28]. Restoration of GH levels is followed by improvement of lipid profile, increase of lean body mass, and decrease of body fat [29]. Moreover, several studies demonstrated an improvement in the liver function after GH administration, as well as after a synthetic form of GH-releasing hormone (tesamorelin), resulting in the reduction of the liver fat fraction [30, 31].

In every adult patient with hypothalamic and pituitary disorders, GH levels must be assessed; if GH deficiency is confirmed, replacement treatment must be initiated, in order to avoid progression of NAFLD to NASH and cirrhosis. Because GH deficiency is concomitantly associated with insulin resistance and type 2 diabetes, as well as with visceral obesity and dyslipidemia, early identification is necessary for a complete treatment strategy.

Thus, proper screening and early interventions consisting of diet measures and hormone replacement therapy appear as not only useful, but also mandatory for ensuring the prevention of a progressive hepatic disease.

16.5 NAFLD and Hyperprolactinemia

Prolactin is a multifunctional polypeptide with various metabolic effects. Apart from its main roles related to pregnancy and lactation, prolactin takes part in general homeostasis processes, related especially to body weight control, adipose tissue function, and adrenal response to stress [32]. Moreover, recent data showed that prolactin is implicated in the occurrence and progression of NAFLD [33].

Thus, hyperprolactinemia induces adipogenesis and favors obesity, hyperinsulinemia, and insulin resistance, while administration of dopamine antagonists aiming at normalization of prolactin levels is followed by body weight control, insulin sensitivity, and improving of lipid metabolism [34]. Experimental studies in animal models showed that triglyceride liver concentrations increase after prolactin administration [35]. As prolactin appears to regulate hepatic triglyceride accumulation, ablation of prolactin receptors might be a newer therapeutic solution for NAFLD [36].

16.6 NAFLD and Hypercortisolism

Increased levels of circulating glucocorticoids (GCs) promote hepatic gluconeogenesis and reduce insulin sensitivity, favoring accumulation of visceral and hepatic fat, dyslipidemia, diabetes, and arterial hypertension. However, rather locally available GCs appear to be most responsible for the metabolic syndrome components than high-circulating free corticoid levels [37]. As proof, as showed by a study assessing the prevalence of steatosis in patients with Cushing's syndrome (CS), only 20% of patients had liver steatosis on computed tomography findings [38]. Moreover, in NAFLD, no evidence for concomitant Cushing-like syndrome was found, despite proofs concerning increased urinary free cortisol levels and decreased dexamethasone suppression of serum cortisol [39]. Thus, a key role was attributed to the specific pre-receptor enzyme 11β-hydroxysteroid dehydrogenase-1 (11β-HSD 1), which catalyzes the conversion of inert cortisone in cortisol (the active form of cortisone), in visceral fat tissue and in the liver.

In addition, an interesting adaptive mechanism was stipulated in cortisol metabolism, in relationship to progressive NAFLD. During the stage of simple steatosis, there are local decreased levels of cortisol due to a higher clearance, restricting lipid accumulation, while in NASH stages, there is an increased activity of 11β-HSD 1, limiting hepatic inflammation [40]. In therapeutic implications terms, 11β-HSD 1 inhibition might be beneficial in early stages, by deduction of local cortisol levels, while if NASH is already present, the inflammatory response might be worsened [37].

16.7   NAFLD and Polycystic Ovarian Syndrome

Polycystic ovary syndrome (PCOS) is one of the most common endocrine, reproductive, and metabolic disorders in women characterized by hyperandrogenism, polycystic ovaries, and anovulation [41]. Clinically, PCOS is manifested by infertility, anovulatory menstrual cycles, and hirsutism. The prevalence of NAFLD is significantly higher in women with PCOS, and its pathogenesis can be associated with risk factors such as hyperandrogenemia, obesity, chronic low-grade inflammation, insulin resistance, and genetic factors [42].

PCOS has been linked to many complications such as metabolic syndrome, cardiovascular disease, and obstetric and psychological disorders. Lately, many studies have shown that there is a connection between PCOS and nonalcoholic fatty liver disease, especially since the risk factors of NAFLD are also comorbidities found in PCOS [43]. For the first time, Brown et al. described NAFLD after liver biopsy in a 24-year-old female patient with PCOS, obesity, no diabetes, no known liver disease or alcohol drinking, and persistently elevated transaminases [44].

Many studies showed an NAFLD prevalence of 35–70% in women with PCOS, indifferent of the concomitance of obesity, compared to 20–30% in age- and body mass index (BMI)-matched control women [45]. In 2007, it was stated that women with NAFLD of reproductive age should be investigated for PCOS, which necessitated liver evaluation [46]. A little later, a prospective study showed that 10 of 14 women with NAFLD of reproductive age (half with NAFLD demonstrated by liver biopsy) had associated PCOS according to the Rotterdam criteria [47].

Currently, there is no clearly established management of NAFLD in PCOS. Studies on the treatment of NAFLD in PCOS mainly include lifestyle modification, pharmacological therapy, and bariatric surgery [48]. The main treatment for PCOS and NAFLD is lifestyle modification, which includes diet control and regular exercise to achieve weight loss. By changing the lifestyle, it is possible to reduce weight, decrease hyperandrogenism, and increase insulin sensitivity in women with PCOS [49]. A 6-week study on dietary modification for 18 women with anovulatory PCOS demonstrated that dietary restriction led to a decrease in body fat, regulation of menstrual cycles, and a decrease in alanine aminotransferase (ALT) levels in women with PCOS [49].

The main pharmacological treatments identified in clinical trials are represented by metformin, thiazolidinediones, GLP1 receptor agonists, spironolactone, and nutritional supplements (omega-3 fatty acids, vitamin E supplements). It has been shown to improve liver function and histological appearance, the main common mechanism to reduce lipid aggregation in PCOS [50].

Metformin acts by activating the AMP-activated protein kinase (AMPK), resulting in the inhibition of glucose, lipid, and protein synthesis, as well as cell growth, on the one hand, and the stimulation of fatty acid oxidation and glucose absorption on the other hand [51]. Thiazolidinediones, as PPARγ agonists, have been widely accepted in the treatment of NASH because they increase hepatic insulin sensitivity, improve ALT and GGT levels, and decrease hepatocyte histological damage and fibrosis. However, the use of thiazolidinedione in women with PCOS is limited by its cardiovascular and weight gain side effects [52]. Liraglutide, the main GLP1 receptor agonist, improves insulin resistance, reduces free testosterone levels, and improves menstrual cycle and ovarian function in women with PCOS. At the same time, liraglutide reduced liver fat content by 44%, visceral adipose tissue by 18%, and prevalence of NAFLD by two-thirds in these patients [53]. Spironolactone reduces serum free fatty acid levels in PCOS, reduces hepatic triglyceride accumulation, and causes attenuation of lesions in NAFLD [54]. Bariatric surgery has proven useful in the management of obese women with PCOS because it can reduce body weight and improve glucose metabolism and dyslipidemia in obese PCOS patients [55].

In conclusion, there is ample evidence that PCOS may increase the prevalence of NAFLD. Therefore, screening for NAFLD should be implemented in PCOS patients, especially those with an insulin resistance profile.

16.8 NAFLD and Hypogonadism

Hypogonadism is defined as an inherited or acquired pathological state characterized, in both male and female subjects, by lower reproductive function [56]. Hypogonadism can be of primary or secondary cause. Primary or peripheral, gonadal hypogonadism (hypergonadotropic) is defined by an inadequate response of the gonads to gonadotropins, which results in a decrease in the level of sex hormones and an increase in the level of gonadotropins [follicle-stimulating hormone (FSH) and luteinizing hormone (LH)]. Secondary or central hypogonadism (hypogonadotropic) is defined by the inability of the pituitary gland or hypothalamus to produce enough LH and FSH, which causes low concentrations of sex hormones [57].

Currently, many studies have demonstrated a bidirectional relationship between hypogonadism and NAFLD in both sexes. A cross-sectional study that included nonalcoholic male patients reported a significantly lower serum testosterone level in those with NAFLD compared to patients without NAFLD [58].

At the same time, it was shown that men with hypogonadism who received hormone replacement therapy had an improvement in NAFLD status and patients with prostate neoplasm and hypogonadism secondary to androgen deprivation therapy have a higher risk of NAFLD [59].

Similarly, in female patients with hypogonadism, it has been shown that there is an increased prevalence of NAFLD manifested biologically by the permanent increase of liver enzymes [60].

In recent studies, estrogen deficiency in hypogonadism or postmenopausal women was associated with an elevated NAFLD prevalence [61]. Long-term estrogen deficiency was proved to be a risk factor for advanced hepatic fibrosis [62].

The mechanisms that explain the presence of NAFLD in patients with hypogonadism are complex. Recent data showed that visceral adiposity, estrogen deficiency, reduced dehydroepiandrosterone levels, decreased insulin resistance, and microbiota disorders leading to lower androgen hormones are factors involved in the NAFLD development and the progression of liver lesions [63]. General therapeutic measures consist of changing the lifestyle, which includes a balanced diet and regular physical exercises. The specific treatment consists of the administration of testosterone for men with hypogonadism, and estrogen replacement therapy in the case of women.

In conclusion, there is a complex relationship between androgens and NAFLD, and understanding the molecular mechanism of androgens in the liver can help to discover therapies that are based on the mechanisms found in the occurrence of NAFLD.

References

1. Chung GE, Kim D, Kim W, Yim JY, Park MJ, Kim YJ, Yoon JH, et al. Non-alcoholic fatty liver disease across the spectrum of hypothyroidism. J Hepatol. 2012;57:150–6.
2. Su X, Peng H, Chen X, Wu X, Wang B. Hyperlipidemia and hypothyroidism. Clin Chim Acta. 2022;527:61–70. https://doi.org/10.1016/j.cca.2022.01.006.
3. Li Y, Wang L, Zhou L, Song Y, Ma S, Yu C, Zhao J, Xu C, Gao L. Thyroid stimulating hormone increases hepatic gluconeogenesis via CRTC2. Mol Cell Endocrinol. 2017;5(446):70–80.
4. Koroglu E, Canbakan B, Atay K, Hatemi I, Tuncer M, Dobrucali A, et al. Role of oxidative stress and insulin resistance in disease severity of non-alcoholic fatty liver disease. Turk J Gastroenterol. 2016;27(4):361–6.
5. Aoki Y, Belin RM, Clickner R, Jeffries R, Phillips L, Mahaffey KR. Serum TSH and total T4 in the United States population and their association with participant characteristics: National Health and Nutrition Examination Survey (NHANES 1999–2002). Thyroid. 2007;17:1211–23.
6. Eshraghian A, Hamidian JA. Non-alcoholic fatty liver disease and thyroid dysfunction: a systematic review. World J Gastroenterol. 2014;20:8102–9.
7. He W, An X, Li L, et al. Relationship between hypothyroidism and non-alcoholic fatty liver disease: a systematic review and meta-analysis. Front Endocrinol (Lausanne). 2017;8:335.
8. Zeng X, Li B, Zou Y. The relationship between non-alcoholic fatty liver disease and hypothyroidism: a systematic review and meta-analysis. Medicine (Baltimore). 2021;100(17):e25738. https://doi.org/10.1097/MD.0000000000025738.

9. Kim D, Kim W, Joo SK, Bae JM, Kim JH, Ahmed A. Subclinical hypothyroidism and low-normal thyroid function are associated with nonalcoholic steatohepatitis and fibrosis. Clin Gastroenterol Hepatol. 2018;16:123–31.

10. Kim D, Yoo ER, Li AA, et al. Low-normal thyroid function is associated with advanced fibrosis among adults in the United States. Clin Gastroenterol Hepatol. 2019;17:2379–81.

11. Manka PP, Coombes JD, Bechmann LP, et al. Thyroid hormone receptor regulates hepatic stellate cell activation. J Hepatol. 2017;66(1 Suppl):S582.

12. Saxena NK, Ikeda K, Rockey DC, Friedman SL, Anania FA. Leptin in hepatic fibrosis: evidence for increased collagen production in stellate cells and lean littermates of ob/ob mice. Hepatology. 2002;35(4):762–71. https://doi.org/10.1053/jhep.2002.32029.

13. Lee Y, Park YJ, Ahn HY, Lim JA, Park KU, Choi SH, Park DJ, Oh BC, Jang HC, Yi KH. Plasma FGF21 levels are increased in patients with hypothyroidism independently of lipid profile. Endocr J. 2013;60(8):977–83. https://doi.org/10.1507/endocrj.ej12-0427.

14. Bano A, Chaker L, Plompen EP, Hofman A, Dehghan A, Franco OH, Janssen HL, Darwish Murad S, Peeters RP. Thyroid function and the risk of nonalcoholic fatty liver disease: the Rotterdam study. J Clin Endocrinol Metab. 2016;101(8):3204–11. https://doi.org/10.1210/jc.2016-1300.

15. Tahara K, Akahane T, Namisaki T, Moriya K, Kawaratani H, Kaji K, Takaya H, Sawada Y, Shimozato N, Sato S, Saikawa S, Nakanishi K, Kubo T, Fujinaga Y, Furukawa M, Kitagawa K, Ozutsumi T, Tsuji Y, Kaya D, Ogawa H, Takagi H, Ishida K, Mitoro A, Yoshiji H. Thyroid-stimulating hormone is an independent risk factor of non-alcoholic fatty liver disease. JGH Open. 2019;4(3):400–4. https://doi.org/10.1002/jgh3.12264.

16. Chaker L, Bianco AC, Jonklaas J, Peeters RP. Hypothyroidism. Lancet. 2017;390(10101):1550–62.

17. Liu L, Yu Y, Zhao M, Zheng D, Zhang X, Guan Q, Xu C, Gao L, Zhao J, Zhang H. Benefits of levothyroxine replacement therapy on nonalcoholic fatty liver disease in subclinical hypothyroidism patients. Int J Endocrinol. 2017;2017:5753039.

18. Bruinstroop E, Dalan R, Cao Y, Bee YM, Chandran K, Cho LW, Soh SB, Teo EK, Toh SA, Leow MKS, Sinha RA, Sadananthan SA, Michael N, Stapleton HM, Leung C, Angus PW, Patel SK, Burrell LM, Lim SC, Sum CF, Velan SS, Yen PM. Low-dose levothyroxine reduces intrahepatic lipid content in patients with type 2 diabetes mellitus and NAFLD. J Clin Endocrinol Metab. 2018;103(7):2698–706.

19. Sanyal A, Charles ED, Neuschwander-Tetri BA, Loomba R, Harrison SA, Abdelmalek MF, Lawitz EJ, Halegoua-DeMarzio D, Kundu S, Noviello S, Luo Y, Christian R. Pegbelfermin (BMS-986036), a PEGylated fibroblast growth factor 21 analogue, in patients with non-alcoholic steatohepatitis: a randomised, double-blind, placebo-controlled, phase 2a trial. Lancet. 2019;392(10165):2705–17. https://doi.org/10.1016/S0140-6736(18)31785-9.

20. Bulow B, Hagmar L, Eskilsson J, Erfurth EM. Hypopituitary females have a high incidence of cardiovascular morbidity and an increased prevalence of cardiovascular risk factors. J Clin Endocrinol Metab. 2000;85(2):574–84.

21. Rose T, Bengstsson BA. Premature mortality due to cardiovascular disease in hypopituitarism. Lancet. 1990;336:285–8.

22. Nyenwe EA, Williamson-Baddorf S, Waters B, Wan JY, Solomon SS. Nonalcoholic fatty liver disease and metabolic syndrome in hypopituitary patients. Am J Med Sci. 2009;338(3):190–5.

23. Yang Y, Qi ZR, Zhang TT, Kang YJ, Wang X. Rapidly progressive non-alcoholic fatty liver disease due to hypopituitarism. Report of 5 cases. Neuro Endocrinol Lett. 2018;39(2):99–104.

24. Kodama K, Ichihara A, Seki Y, et al. Characteristics of NAFLD based on hypopituitarism. Can J Gastroenterol Hepatol. 2020;2020:8814435.

25. Vijayakumar A, Yakar S, Leroith D. The intricate role of growth hormone in metabolism. Front Endocrinol (Lausanne). 2011;2:32. https://doi.org/10.3389/fendo.2011.00032.

26. Doycheva I, Erickson D, Watt KD. Growth hormone deficiency and NAFLD: an overlooked and underrecognized link. Hepatol Commun. 2022;6(9):2227–37. https://doi.org/10.1002/hep4.1953.

27. Nishizawa H, Iguchi G, Murawaki A, Fukuoka H, Hayashi Y, Kaji H, Yamamoto M, Suda K, Takahashi M, Seo Y, et al. Nonalcoholic fatty liver disease in adult hypopituitary patients with GH deficiency and the impact of GH replacement therapy. Eur J Endocrinol. 2012;167:67–74.

28. Dichtel LE, Corey KE, Misdraji J, Bredella MA, Schorr M, Osganian SA, Young BJ, Sung JC, Miller KK. The association between IGF-1 levels and the histologic severity of nonalcoholic fatty liver disease. Clin Transl Gastroenterol. 2017;8(1):e217. https://doi.org/10.1038/ctg.2016.72.

29. Newman CB, Carmichael JD, Kleinberg DL. Effects of low dose versus high dose human growth hormone on body composition and lipids in adults with GH deficiency: a meta-analysis of placebo-controlled randomized trials. Pituitary. 2015;18(3):297–305. https://doi.org/10.1007/s11102-014-0571-z.

30. Rufinatscha K, Ress C, Folie S, Haas S, Salzmann K, Moser P, Dobner J, Weiss G, Iruzubieta P, Arias-Loste MT, Crespo J, Tilg H, Kaser S. Metabolic effects of reduced growth hormone action in fatty liver disease. Hepatol Int. 2018;12(5):474–81. https://doi.org/10.1007/s12072-018-9893-7.

31. Stanley TL, Fourman LT, Feldpausch MN, Purdy J, Zheng I, Pan CS, Aepfelbacher J, Buckless C, Tsao A, Kellogg A, Branch K, Lee H, Liu CY, Corey KE, Chung RT, Torriani M, Kleiner DE, Hadigan CM, Grinspoon SK. Effects of tesamorelin on non-alcoholic fatty liver disease in HIV: a randomised, double-blind, multicentre trial. Lancet HIV. 2019;6(12):e821–30. https://doi.org/10.1016/S2352-3018(19)30338-8.

32. Bernard V, Young J, Binart N. Prolactin—a pleiotropic factor in health and disease. Nat Rev Endocrinol. 2019;15(6):356–65. https://doi.org/10.1038/s41574-019-0194-6.

33. Zhang P, Feng W, Chu X, et al. A newly noninvasive model for prediction of non-alcoholic fatty liver disease: utility of serum prolactin levels. BMC Gastroenterol. 2019;19:202.

34. dos Santos Silva CM, Barbosa FR, Lima GA, Warszawski L, Fontes R, Domingues RC, Gadelha MR. BMI and metabolic profile in patients with prolactinoma before and after treatment with dopamine agonists. Obesity (Silver Spring). 2011;19(4):800–5. https://doi.org/10.1038/oby.2010.150.

35. Park S, Kim DS, Daily JW, Kim SH. Serum prolactin concentrations determine whether they improve or impair β-cell function and insulin sensitivity in diabetic rats. Diabetes Metab Res Rev. 2011;27(6):564–74. https://doi.org/10.1002/dmrr.1215.

36. Shao S, Yao Z, Lu J, Song Y, He Z, Yu C, Zhou X, Zhao L, Zhao J, Gao L. Ablation of prolactin receptor increases hepatic triglyceride accumulation. Biochem Biophys Res Commun. 2018;498(3):693–9. https://doi.org/10.1016/j.bbrc.2018.03.048.

37. Von-Hafe M, Borges-Canha M, Vale C, Leite AR, Sérgio Neves J, Carvalho D, Leite-Moreira A. Nonalcoholic fatty liver disease and endocrine axes—a scoping review. Metabolites. 2022;12(4):298. https://doi.org/10.3390/metabo12040298.

38. Rockall AG, Sohaib SA, Evans D, Kaltsas G, Isidori AM, Monson JP, Besser GM, Grossman AB, Reznek RH. Hepatic steatosis in Cushing's syndrome: a radiological assessment using computed tomography. Eur J Endocrinol. 2003;149:543–8.

39. Hazlehurst JM, Tomlinson JW. Non-alcoholic fatty liver disease in common endocrine disorders. Eur J Endocrinol. 2013;169(2):R27–37. https://doi.org/10.1530/EJE-13-0296.

40. Ahmed A, Rabbitt E, Brady T, Brown C, Guest P, Bujalska IJ, Doig C, Newsome PN, Hubscher S, Elias E, Adams DH, Tomlinson JW, Stewart PM. A switch in hepatic cortisol metabolism across the spectrum of nonalcoholic fatty liver disease. PLoS One. 2012;7(2):e29531. https://doi.org/10.1371/journal.pone.0029531.

41. Wang D, He B. Current perspectives on nonalcoholic fatty liver disease in women with polycystic ovary syndrome. Diabetes Metab Syndr Obes. 2022;15:1281–91. https://doi.org/10.2147/DMSO.S362424.

42. Vassilatou E. Nonalcoholic fatty liver disease and polycystic ovary syndrome. World J Gastroenterol. 2014;20(26):8351–63. https://doi.org/10.3748/wjg.v20.i26.8351.

43. Cardoso AC, de Figueiredo-Mendes C. Current management of NAFLD/NASH. Liver Int. 2021;41(Suppl 1):89–94. https://doi.org/10.1111/liv.14869.

44. Brown AJ, Tendler DA, McMurray RG, Setji TL. Polycystic ovary syndrome and severe non-alcoholic steatohepatitis: beneficial effect of modest weight loss and exercise on liver biopsy findings. Endocr Pract. 2005;11:319–24.

45. Falzarano C, Lofton T, Osei-Ntansah A, Oliver T, Southward T, Stewart S, Andrisse S. Nonalcoholic fatty liver disease in women and girls with polycystic ovary syndrome. J Clin Endocrinol Metab. 2022;107(1):258–72. https://doi.org/10.1210/clinem/dgab658.
46. Carmina E. Need for liver evaluation in polycystic ovary syndrome. J Hepatol. 2007;47:313–5.
47. Brzozowska MM, Ostapowicz G, Weltman MD. An association between non-alcoholic fatty liver disease and polycystic ovarian syndrome. J Gastroenterol Hepatol. 2009;24:243–7.
48. Mundi MS, Velapati S, Patel J, et al. Evolution of NAFLD and its management. Nutr Clin Pract. 2020;35(1):72–84. https://doi.org/10.1002/ncp.10449.
49. Li C, Xing C, Zhang J, et al. Eight-hour time-restricted feeding improves endocrine and metabolic profiles in women with an ovulatory polycystic ovary syndrome. J Transl Med. 2021;19(1):148. https://doi.org/10.1186/s12967-021-02817-2.
50. Lim SS, Hutchison SK, Van Ryswyk E, et al. Lifestyle changes in women with polycystic ovary syndrome. Cochrane Database Syst Rev. 2019;3(3):CD007506. https://doi.org/10.1002/14651858.CD007506.pub4.
51. Guan Y, Wang D, Bu H, et al. The effect of metformin on polycystic ovary syndrome in overweight women: a systematic review and meta-analysis of randomized controlled trials. Int J Endocrinol. 2020;2020:5150684. https://doi.org/10.1155/2020/5150684.
52. Xu Y, Wu Y, Huang Q. Comparison of the effect between pioglitazone and metformin in treating patients with PCOS: a meta-analysis. Arch Gynecol Obstet. 2017;296(4):661–77. https://doi.org/10.1007/s00404-017-4480-z.
53. Tian D, Chen W, Xu Q, et al. Liraglutide monotherapy and add on therapy on obese women with polycystic ovarian syndromes: a systematic review and meta-analysis. Minerva Med. 2021;113:542–50. https://doi.org/10.23736/S0026-4806.21.07085-3.
54. Adeyanju OA, Falodun TO, Michael OS, et al. Spironolactone reversed hepato-ovarian triglyceride accumulation caused by letrozole-induced polycystic ovarian syndrome: tissue uric acid—a familiar foe. Naunyn Schmiedebergs Arch Pharmacol. 2020;393(6):1055–66. https://doi.org/10.1007/s00210-020-01809-1.
55. Ezzat RS, Abdallah W, Elsayed M, et al. Impact of bariatric surgery on androgen profile and ovarian volume in obese polycystic ovary syndrome patients with infertility. Saudi J Biol Sci. 2021;28(9):5048–52. https://doi.org/10.1016/j.sjbs.2021.05.022.
56. Lonardo A, Mantovani A, Lugari S, Targher G. NAFLD in some common endocrine diseases: prevalence, pathophysiology, and principles of diagnosis and management. Int J Mol Sci. 2019;20:11–2841.
57. Song MJ, Choi JY. Androgen dysfunction in non-alcoholic fatty liver disease: role of sex hormone binding globulin. Front Endocrinol (Lausanne). 2022;13:1053709. https://doi.org/10.3389/fendo.2022.1053709.
58. Eslam M, Newsome PN, Sarin SK, Anstee QM, Targher G, Romero-Gomez M, et al. A new definition for metabolic dysfunction-associated fatty liver disease: an international expert consensus statement. J Hepatol. 2020;73:202–9. https://doi.org/10.1016/j.jhep.2020.03.039.
59. Gild P, Cole AP, Krasnova A, et al. Liver disease in men undergoing androgen deprivation therapy for prostate cancer. J Urol. 2018;200(3):573–81.
60. Polyzos SA, Mousiolis A, Mintziori G, Goulis DG. Nonalcoholic fatty liver disease in males with low testosterone concentrations. Diabetes Metab Syndr Clin Res Rev. 2020;14(5):1571–7.
61. Singeap AM, Stanciu C, Huiban L, Muzica CM, Cuciureanu T, Girleanu I, Chiriac S, Zenovia S, Nastasa R, Sfarti C, Cojocariu C, Trifan A. Association between nonalcoholic fatty liver disease and endocrinopathies: clinical implications. Can J Gastroenterol Hepatol. 2021;2021:6678142. https://doi.org/10.1155/2021/6678142.
62. Arefhosseini S, Ebrahimi-Mameghani M, Najafipour F, Tutunchi H. Non-alcoholic fatty liver disease across endocrinopathies: interaction with sex hormones. Front Endocrinol (Lausanne). 2022;13:1032361. https://doi.org/10.3389/fendo.2022.1032361.
63. Yuan S, Chen J, Li X, Fan R, Arsenault B, Gill D, Giovannucci EL, Zheng JS, Larsson SC. Lifestyle and metabolic factors for nonalcoholic fatty liver disease: Mendelian randomization study. Eur J Epidemiol. 2022;37(7):723–33. https://doi.org/10.1007/s10654-022-00868-3.

Nonalcoholic Fatty Liver Disease and Extrahepatic Malignancies

17

Tudor Cuciureanu, Anca Trifan, and Carol Stanciu

17.1 Introduction

Nonalcoholic fatty liver disease (NAFLD) is a common cause for diagnosis of chronic liver disease, characterized by rapid accumulation of fat in the hepatocytes. Nowadays, we assist at an increasing number of patients diagnosed with this pathology; its prevalence reaches 25% in adults and about 10% in children. It is found that NAFLD can be present even in nonobese patients, and its prevalence can vary from 25 to 50% in some countries [1].

NAFLD affects the function and structure of the liver, and it is associated with liver failure, cirrhosis, and hepatocellular carcinoma. The burden of NAFLD is not confined only to the liver complication; it is also associated with extrahepatic malignant complications such as colorectal cancer (CRC); esophageal, gastric, pancreatic, and kidney cancer in men; and breast cancer in women [2, 3].

17.2 Mechanism of NAFLD

The presence of steatosis has two basic mechanisms that take place in the hepatocyte. Increased accumulation of fatty acids from adipose tissue is a major contributor to fat storage, accelerated lipogenesis, and free fat accumulation

T. Cuciureanu (✉) · A. Trifan
Gastroenterology Department, Grigore T. Popa University of Medicine and Pharmacy, Iasi, Romania

Institute of Gastroenterology and Hepatology, St. Spiridon Emergency Hospital, Iasi, Romania

C. Stanciu
Institute of Gastroenterology and Hepatology, St. Spiridon Emergency Hospital, Iasi, Romania

A. Trifan et al. (eds.), *Essentials of Non-Alcoholic Fatty Liver Disease*, https://doi.org/10.1007/978-3-031-33548-8_17

from outsource dietary regime and reduced output due to decrees in fat oxidation are the main psychopathological mechanisms. Obesity, insulin resistance, and type 2 diabetes are major contributors to NAFLD. The key mechanism that ignites the inflammation in the hepatocyte that contributes to conversion from simple steatosis to steatohepatitis is still controversial. Many authors consider that there is a direct relation between insulin resistance and NAFLD, in obese or nonobese patients [4, 5]. A recent meta-analysis presents a different point of view, wherein NAFLD is associated with twofold higher risk in developing type 2 diabetes [6].

Current evidence suggests that hyperinsulinemia is a process that is initiated first in obese patients. It is considered a normal response in order to maintain normal glycemic levels in blood. High levels of insulin can be found years before the onset of diabetes mellitus [7]. Initial storage of fat is in the adipose tissue, predominantly subcutaneous, and excess will be deposited and form visceral adipose tissue in the liver [7].

17.3   NAFLD and Colorectal Cancer

NAFLD is associated with the presence of metabolic syndrome, insulin resistance, and even type 2 diabetes. Obesity is frequently associated with NAFLD, and it is well known that obese people have higher risk for digestive malignancies such as CRC [1].

According to the GLOBOCAN data, CRC is the third leading cause of death, with 1.9 million new CRC cases and 930,000 deaths estimated in 2020 [8].

In the interrelation between NAFLD and obesity, the mechanism is partially known and systemic changes are related to obesity, including insulin levels, adiponectin, adipokines, and circulating free fatty acids, which increase hepatocyte lipid storage. Some underlying conditions such as inflammatory bowel disease, diet consisting of low vegetable and increased red meat consumption, obesity, and family history of colorectal malignancies represent additional risk factors for CRC. NAFLD was associated with the presence of colorectal adenomas, which can be considered premalignant lesions [9].

The first data showing an interrelation between NAFLD and an increased risk for adenomatous polyps appeared with Hwang et al.'s study. A cohort of 2917 patients were included and examined by colonoscopy, abdominal ultrasound, and liver tests. The group was divided into two (patients with adenomatous polyps 559, and normal group 2361 patients). The result was remarkable showing that 41.5% of the patients with adenomatous polyps had also been diagnosed with NAFLD. On the opposite side in the normal group, NAFLD had a prevalence of 30.2%. This study highlighted that NAFLD was associated with a greater risk of colorectal adenomas [10].

Interest for finding a relation between patients with NAFLD and CRC increased, and as a confirmation of Hwang study, a larger cohort of Korean women were screened for NAFLD and adenomatous polyps. A total of 5.517 women were included in the study. The result shows that the incidence of adenomas and CCR was two times higher in the NAFLD group compared with controls [11].

Emerging from the definition of NAFLD, the presence of histological nonalcoholic steatohepatitis (NASH) can relate to an increased incidence in colorectal adenomas. It is proven that NASH patients have a higher incidence of CRC compared to those with simple steatosis (51.0% vs. 25.6% and 34.7% vs. 14.0%) [12]. Contrasting results can be found in other studies. Two studies have showed lack of association between NAFLD and colorectal adenomas. One study did not find a higher incidence of colorectal adenomas in the NAFLD patients enrolled; on the other hand, CRC was correlated with the presence of insulin resistance in some patients [13]. The other observational study enrolled 233 patients who underwent screening colonoscopy. Patients were stratified in those with NASH and those with steatosis, based on a previous liver biopsy. After colonoscopy evaluation, comparing the findings with a control group without NAFLD, the researcher observes no difference in colonic adenomas when compared with NAFLD group [14]. Results of several studies showing association between NAFLD and adenomas of CCR are summarized in Table 17.1.

Table 17.1 Studies that associated nonalcoholic fatty liver disease with adenomas or colorectal cancer

Author, year of publication	Study design	Patients enrolled	Diagnosis of NAFLD	Results
Lin et al. [15]	Retrospective	263 NAFLD vs. 2052 non-NAFLD	Ultrasonography	Adenomatous polyps' prevalence: 32% vs. 21%
Lee et al. [11]	Retrospective	5517 women 831 NAFLD vs. 4686 non-NAFLD	Ultrasonography and liver biopsy	Adenomas prevalence: 24.4% vs. 25.1%
Huang et al. [16]	Retrospective	216 with colorectal adenoma vs. 1306 without colorectal adenoma	Ultrasonography	Prevalence: 55.6% vs. 38.8%; $p < 0.05$
Hwang et al. [16]	Cross-sectional	2917 patients who underwent routine colonoscopy (556 with polyps vs. 2361 without polyps)	Ultrasonography	NAFLD prevalence: 41.5% vs. 30.2%
Ahn et al. [17]	Retrospective	26,540 subjects evaluated by colonoscopy	Ultrasonography	NAFLD was associated with colorectal neoplasia (adjusted OR, 1.10; 95% CI 1.03–1.17)

17.4 Gastric and Esophageal Cancer and NAFLD

Gastric cancer is the fifth deadliest cancer worldwide according to GLOBOCAN updated in 2020. It accounted for 1,000,000 new cases and 769,000 deaths worldwide. It follows only lung cancer and CRC in overall mortality, and it is considered in many cases as a preventable form of cancer due to its risk factors [18].

It is more prevalent in males compared to females and has a higher incidence in developed countries. In some regions on the globe, it is the number one cancer diagnosed in males. Mortality rates associated with gastric cancer are higher in males and in the regions with high incidence such as Asia and Latin America. Due to limited treatment options, preventing gastric cancer still remains the solution for reducing mortality rates [19].

Gastric cancer can be classified into two forms due to anatomic localization of the neoplasia and its risk factors. Smoking and obesity, which are well-known risk factors, are attributed to cardia form of gastric cancer. *Helicobacter pylori* and obesity remain the risk factors for noncardia forms [20, 21].

Despite the fact that a direct link between NAFLD and gastric cancer cannot be established, obesity as a component of the metabolic syndrome has been attributed along time to a higher incidence in stomach neoplasia. A total of 22 studies were included in a meta-analysis conducted by Turati et al. The results showed a total of 8000 cases with esophageal and gastric adenocarcinoma. Body mass index (BMI) was a correlating factor for cases with the diagnosis of esophageal and gastric adenocarcinoma. The overall relative risk (RR) was 1.71 for BMI between 25 and 30. Patients found with this neoplasia and BMI over 30 had RR of 2.34 (95% CI 1.95–2.81) [22].

Taking into consideration the influence of the metabolic syndrome and obesity as carcinogenic risk factors, there should be a connection between NAFLD and occurrence of gastric cancer. An interest for setting a connection between NAFLD and gastric cancer was seen in a Turkish study. A total of 1840 patients were included. All the patients underwent upper gastrointestinal endoscopy. A total of 14 cases of distal gastric cancer were found. The results showed that a higher incidence of NAFLD was found in the gastric cancer patients, compared with the average incidence in the Turkish population [23].

Esophageal cancer is the sixth deadliest cancer worldwide accounting for 604,000 deaths in 2020. It is predominant in men with a threefold difference in incidence between genders. Although some regions in the world such as Eastern Asia have a higher incidence compared to other regions, the question remains as regards if there are new risk factors that can be attributed to esophageal cancer [18].

One-third of the cases of esophageal cancer are represented by adenocarcinoma. Among dietary risk factors for esophageal adenocarcinoma, obesity was associated with a higher prevalence of esophagus neoplasia. In high-income countries, because of dietary habits and excess trans-fat food, gastroesophageal reflux, and obesity, a higher incidence of esophageal adenocarcinoma is diagnosed [24, 25].

A potential link between NAFLD and esophageal cancer was set by Lee et al. who investigated a possible association between NAFLD and gastrointestinal tract cancers. The study design was retrospective and enrolled using the National Health Care database, 8,120,674 patients. Out of all, 11.5% had NAFLD. Fatty liver index greater than 60 was associated with esophageal (HR 2.10, 95% CI 1.88–2.35), stomach (HR 1.18, 95% CI 1.14–1.22), and colon cancer (HR 1.23, 95% CI 1.19–1.26) after multivariable adjustment. All-cause mortality was increased in patients with NAFLD and fatty liver index greater than 60 [26].

17.5 NAFLD and Pancreatic Cancer

Pancreatic cancer is a worldwide health burden, the seventh leading cause of global cancer mortality, mostly in developed countries. The statistics issued by GLOBOCAN 2020 estimate that pancreatic cancer is the 11th most common cancer in the world, with 456,918 new cases each year and a total of 432,242 deaths worldwide. The etiology of pancreatic cancer is not well known, although some risk factors such as age over 50 years, male gender, ethnicity, diabetes mellitus, genetics, and smoking can represent causes for diagnosing this neoplasia [19].

In 2007, the World Cancer Research Fund Panel study showed that increased BMI can represent a modifiable risk factor for pancreatic neoplasia [27]. Obesity, depending on the severity, can represent an additional risk factor for pancreatic cancer. A meta-analysis showed a correlation between waist circumference and incidence of pancreatic cancer. An RR of 1.11 was found for every 10 cm above normal waist circumference (95% Cl 1.05–1.18) [28].

Chang and collaborators showed in an observational study that NAFLD can be considered an independent risk factor for pancreatic cancer. Patients without NAFLD had longer survival rates compared with non-NAFLD patients [29]. Further studies are needed to highlight the relation between NAFLD and pancreatic cancer.

17.6 NAFLD and Breast Cancer

Out of all malignancies, breast cancer is the most common cancer in women, and it is a leading cause of death-related malignancies in women. According to the latest statistics, 5-year survival rate in advanced forms with metastasis is less than 30%, despite the advanced new chemotherapy [30].

International Agency for Research on Cancer reported over 2.3 million new cases from 185 countries, an aspect that reveals that this malignancy is a worldwide health burden. It has a higher incidence in developed countries compared to low-income areas (Kashyap 2022).

Several risk factors have been associated with breast cancer in women and in men. Early puberty and menarche, late childbirth, lactation failure, and hereditary causes are the main risk factors of breast cancer onset in women. Other risk factors common in both genders are smoking, obesity, lack of physical exercise, and alcohol consumption [31].

The interrelation between obesity and diagnosis of NAFLD in these patients started a general concern linking NAFLD to extrahepatic malignancies such as breast cancer. Therefore, several studies investigated this association between NAFLD and breast cancer in both genders, regardless of the higher incidence in women.

Kwak and Collaborators conducted a case-control study in order to investigate the interrelation between NAFLD and breast cancer in women. A total of 540 patients were included, out of which 270 women were diagnosed with breast cancer and 270 were controls. The results revealed that 81 cancer patients and 54 controls had NAFLD. When obesity was correlated with NAFLD, the multivariate analysis ($p = 0.046$) showed a strong association with breast cancer cases. Also, NAFLD was associated with breast cancer and nonobese cases. The study highlighted that NAFLD can be considered an important risk factor for breast cancer in obese and nonobese women [32].

NAFLD can also be considered a bad predictor for long-term survival in patients with breast cancer after they received curative treatment. Lee et al. persuade this idea in a recent study, which enrolled 1587 patients with breast cancer between 2007 and 2017 and a control healthy group ($n = 123$). Prevalence of NAFLD in the breast cancer group was 15.8% (251/1587), compared with controls 8.9% (11/123). NAFLD was considered a good predictor for poor prognosis in breast cancer recurrence after hormonal or surgical treatment [33].

17.7 NAFLD and Kidney Cancer

Besides traditional risk factors such as smoking and dietary habits, some components of the metabolic syndrome may be responsible for the occurrence of kidney cancer.

Kidney cancer is an insidious neoplastic, responsible for more than 2% of the oncological cases worldwide. It has a higher incidence in developed countries, and the number of cases doubled in the latest years. Under 10% of the cases are diagnosed after they present clinical symptoms such as pain, hematuria, and weight loss. Most of the cases are diagnosed after routine computed tomography or magnetic resonance [34].

In the latest guidelines, two of the metabolic components, obesity and hypertension, are stated as risk factors.

Recent studies tried to verify if metabolic syndrome and NAFLD are major contributors to kidney cancer. A European study tried to set a direct relationship between metabolic risk and renal cancer. The metabolic score based on BMI, hypertension, triglycerides, and glucose was associated with a higher risk of kidney cancer [27].

Few studies in the literature have researched the link between NAFLD and renal cancer. A breakthrough was in 2003 when a Danish study made on the Danish population associated a higher risk for kidney cancer in patients with NAFLD. In 2020, Wang and Collaborators tried to verify if NAFLD can be considered an independent risk factor for kidney cancer. Out of 54,187 men enrolled in the study, 32.3% had

NAFLD. A significant correlation was seen between men with NAFLD and kidney cancer without diabetes mellitus, HR of 1.57 (1.03–2.40, $P = 0.04$). Patients without diabetes and NAFLD had an additional risk for kidney cancer probably because of obesity-related disorders. In the group with diabetes, insulin resistance and inflammation are also etiological factors for renal cancer [35].

References

1. Amalou K, Rekab R, Fadel S, et al. Nonalcoholic fatty liver disease (NAFLD) and extra hepatic malignancies. Am J Biomed Sci Res. 2021;14(6):2060.
2. Angulo P. Long-term mortality in nonalcoholic fatty liver disease: is liver histology of any prognostic significance? Hepatology. 2010;51:373–5.
3. Tilg H, Moschen AR. Mechanisms behind the link between obesity and gastrointestinal cancers. Best Pract Res Clin Gastroenterol. 2014;28:599–610.
4. Chakravarthy MV, Neuschwander-Tetri BA. The metabolic basis of nonalcoholic steatohepatitis. Endocrinol Diabetes Metab. 2020;3(4):e00112.
5. Roeb E, Weiskirchen R. Fructose and non-alcoholic steatohepatitis. Front Pharmacol. 2021;12:634344.
6. Mantovani A, Petracca G, Beatrice G, Tilg H, Byrne CD, Targher G. Non-alcoholic fatty liver disease and risk of incident diabetes mellitus: an updated meta-analysis of 501,022 adult individuals. Gut. 2021;70:962–9.
7. Venniyoor A, Al Farsi AA, Al Bahrani B. The troubling link between non-alcoholic fatty liver disease (NAFLD) and extrahepatic cancers (EHC). Cureus. 2021;13(8):e17320.
8. Morgan E, Arnold M, Gini A, et al. Global burden of colorectal cancer in 2020 and 2040: incidence and mortality estimate from GLOBOCAN. Gut. 2022;72:338–44.
9. Johnson CM, Wei C, Ensor JE, et al. Meta-analyses of colorectal cancer risk factors. Cancer Causes Control. 2013;24:1207–22.
10. Hwang ST, Cho YK, Park JH, Kim HJ, Park DI, et al. Relationship of non-alcoholic fatty liver disease to colorectal adenomatous polyps. J Gastroenterol Hepatol. 2010;25(3):562–7.
11. Lee YI, Lim YS, Park HS. Colorectal neoplasms in relation to non-alcoholic fatty liver disease in Korean women: a retrospective cohort study. J Gastroenterol Hepatol. 2012;27(1):91–5.
12. Wong VWS, Wong GLH, Tsang SWC, Fan T, Chu WCW, et al. High prevalence of colorectal neoplasm in patients with non-alcoholic steatohepatitis. Gut. 2011;60(6):829–36.
13. Basyigit S, Uzman M, Kefeli A, et al. Absence of non-alcoholic fatty liver disease in the presence of insulin resistance is a strong predictor for colorectal carcinoma. Int J Clin Exp Med. 2015;8(10):18601–10.
14. Touzin NT, Bush KNV, Williams CD, Harrison SA. Prevalence of colonic adenomas in patients with nonalcoholic fatty liver disease. Ther Adv Gastroenterol. 2011;4(3):169–76.
15. Lin XF, Shi KQ, You J, et al. Increased risk of colorectal malignant neoplasm in patients with nonalcoholic fatty liver disease: a large study. Mol Biol Rep. 2014;41(5):2989–97.
16. Huang KW, Leu HB, Wang YJ, et al. Patients with nonalcoholic fatty liver disease have higher risk of colorectal adenoma after negative baseline colonoscopy. Color Dis. 2013;15(7):830–5.
17. Ahn JS, Sinn DH, Min YW, Hong SN, Kim HS, et al. Non-alcoholic fatty liver diseases and risk of colorectal neoplasia. Aliment Pharmacol Ther. 2017;45(2):345–53.
18. Sung H, Ferlay J, Siegel RL, et al. Global cancer statistics 2020: GLOBOCAN estimates of incidence and mortality worldwide for 36 cancers in 185 countries. CA Cancer J Clin. 2021;71:209–49.
19. Rawla P, Barsouk A. Epidemiology of gastric cancer: global trends, risk factors and prevention. Prz Gastroenterol. 2019;14(1):26–38.
20. Karimi P, Islami F, Anandasabapathy S, Freedman ND, Kamangar F. Gastric cancer: descriptive epidemiology, risk factors, screening, and prevention. Cancer Epidemiol Biomark Prev. 2014;23(5):700–13.

21. Thrift AP, El Serag HB. Burden of gastric cancer. Clin Gastroenterol Hepatol. 2020;18(3):534–42.
22. Turati F, Tramacere I, La Vecchia C, Negri E. A meta-analysis of body mass index and esophageal and gastric cardia adenocarcinoma. Ann Oncol. 2013;24(3):609–17.
23. Uzel M, Sahiner Z, Filik L. Non-alcoholic fatty liver disease, metabolic syndrome and gastric cancer: single center experience. J BUON. 2015;20:662.
24. Blot WJ, Tarone RE, Thun M, et al. Esophageal cancer. In: Cancer epidemiology and prevention. 4th ed. Oxford: Oxford University Press; 2018. p. 579–93.
25. Arnold M, Laversanne M, Brown LM, Devesa SS, Bray F. Predicting the future burden of esophageal cancer by histological subtype: international trends in incidence up to 2030. Am J Gastroenterol. 2017;112:1247–55.
26. Lee HS, Chang SW, Lee CU, et al. Underlying nonalcoholic fatty liver disease is a significant factor for breast cancer recurrence after curative surgery. Medicine (Baltimore). 2019;98(39):e17277.
27. Sanna C, Rosso C, Marietti M, Bugianesi E. Non-alcoholic fatty liver disease and extra-hepatic cancers. Int J Mol Sci. 2016;17(5):717.
28. Aune D, Greenwood DC, Chan DSM, et al. Body mass index, abdominal fatness, and pancreatic cancer risk: a systematic review and non-linear dose-response meta-analysis of prospective studies. Ann Oncol. 2012;23(4):843–52.
29. Chang CF, Tseng YC, Huang HH, Shih YL, Hsieh TY, Lin HH. Exploring the relationship between nonalcoholic fatty liver disease and pancreatic cancer by computed tomographic survey. Int Emerg Med. 2018;13:191–7.
30. Riggio AI, Varley KE, Welm AL. The lingering mysteries of metastatic recurrence in breast cancer. Br J Cancer. 2021;124:13–26.
31. Kashyap D, Pal D, Sharma R, et al. Global increase in breast cancer incidence: risk factors and preventive measures. Biomed Res Int. 2022;2022:e9605439.
32. Kwak MS, Yim JY, Yi A, et al. Nonalcoholic fatty liver disease is associated with breast cancer in nonobese women. Dig Liver Dis. 2019;51(7):1030–5.
33. Lee YS, Lee HS, Chang SW, et al. Underlying nonalcoholic fatty liver disease is a significant factor for breast cancer recurrence after curative surgery. Medicine (Baltimore). 2019;98(39):e17277.
34. Padala SA, Barsouk A, Thandra KC, et al. Epidemiology of renal cell carcinoma. World J Oncol. 2020;11(3):79–87.
35. Wang Z, Zhao X, Chen S, et al. Associations between nonalcoholic fatty liver disease and cancers in a large cohort in China. Clin Gastroenterol Hepatol. 2021;19(4):788–796.e4.

Psychological Burden of NAFLD and Psychiatric Disorders as Extrahepatic Manifestations

18

Oana Petrea, Gabriela Stefanescu, and Cristinel Stefanescu

18.1 Introduction

Nonalcoholic fatty liver disease (NAFLD) represents an important global health issue with a prevalence of approximately 25–30% worldwide with variability depending on the studied population or diagnostic criteria used [1]. This prevalence is intended to increase in addition to the rising incidence rates of metabolic syndrome (MetS) and obesity [2, 3]. The prevalence of NAFLD-related advanced hepatic fibrosis, which leads to increased mortality risk due to liver cirrhosis complications, is also steadily increasing [4]. Therefore, NAFLD could become the most frequent indication for liver transplantation in the near future [1].

Nonalcoholic fatty liver disease is characterized by excessive hepatic fat accumulation. This is defined as the presence of steatosis in >5% of hepatocytes according to histological criteria [5]. It is associated with insulin resistance, and along with abdominal obesity, high blood pressure, hyperglycemia, elevated triglycerides, and low high-density lipoprotein cholesterol play a major role in high-risk mortality associated with MetS [5]. In addition, recent studies demonstrated a significant association between major psychiatric disorders, such as bipolar disorder, depressive disorder, or schizophrenia, and MetS, partly due to specific psychotropic medication used and an unhealthy style of living [6].

O. Petrea (✉) · G. Stefanescu
Gastroenterology Department, Grigore T. Popa University of Medicine and Pharmacy, Iasi, Romania

Institute of Gastroenterology and Hepatology, St. Spiridon Emergency Hospital, Iasi, Romania

C. Stefanescu
Psychiatry Department, Grigore T. Popa University of Medicine and Pharmacy, Iasi, Romania

Socola Institute of Psychiatry, Iasi, Romania

A. Trifan et al. (eds.), *Essentials of Non-Alcoholic Fatty Liver Disease*,
https://doi.org/10.1007/978-3-031-33548-8_18

On the other hand, more and more evidence indicates that depression is associated with increased risk of mortality, as well as different multiple diseases, especially obesity, hypertension, diabetes, and stroke. These entities are also frequently associated with NAFLD [7, 8]. Still, the real and veridical relationship between psychiatric disorders and NAFLD remains uncertain. According to previous studies, the reported results were contrasting [9, 10].

In agreement with recent data, it seems that there is a complex, bidirectional relationship between NAFLD and metabolic diseases, a relationship that could be extrapolated to cognitive disorders also [11]. Some peculiarities of the MetS as inflammation, endothelial dysfunction, and atherosclerosis, have frequently been related to cognitive disturbances, which has given birth to the notion of the metabolic cognitive syndrome [12]. These are all characteristics also related with NAFLD, but it is unsettled if NAFLD itself generates cognitive dysfunction.

Because of the strong associations between metabolic syndrome and NAFLD, the full spectrum of risk factors and the underlying mechanisms that relate them are currently under continuous research [13, 14].

Despite the above-noted associations, and although high prevalence rates of such mental disorders have been identified among patients with NAFLD, less work has focused on the potential relationship between NAFLD and mental health [14, 15]. Given the aforementioned close links between NAFLD and metabolic syndrome, the potential bidirectional associations between NAFLD and common mental health disorders that may coexist in patients with NAFLD are worth further analysis. In this context, this review aims to discuss the main mechanisms involved in NAFLD and psychiatric disorders, by emphasizing the presence of a bidirectional relationship that links the two entities.

18.2　Epidemiology of NAFLD in Psychiatric Patients

Nonalcoholic fatty liver disease (NAFLD) remains an important worldwide health problem with a prevalence estimated at 25–30%, but it is variable across countries and depending on diagnostic tools used. Currently, it is considered to develop in 24% of the general population in Europe and the USA, 30% in South America, 32% in the Middle East, and 27% in Asia [16].

Epidemiologic data regarding the prevalence of NAFLD in patients diagnosed with psychiatric illnesses are contrasting. First of all, there are some studies that reported an increased prevalence of depression/anxiety in patients with NAFLD/NASH [17]. Secondly, there is a much greater evidence regarding the incidence of NAFLD in patients with mental disorders. In this regard, Weinstein et al. identified a higher prevalence of NAFLD/NASH in patients with depression, compared to general population and patients with viral hepatitis B [18].

On the other hand, both NAFLD and NASH were reported as having a higher prevalence among patients diagnosed with bipolar disorders and schizophrenia [19]. In the study published by Fuller et al. patients with schizophrenia had a higher prevalence of NAFLD. The main risk factors for NAFLD were hypertriglyceridemia (OR = 2.07) and presence of schizophrenia itself (OR = 4.93) [20].

Likewise, Yan et al. in a large cross-sectional study comparing young males with schizophrenia with young males from the general population without schizophrenia, demonstrated a significantly higher prevalence of NAFLD of up to 49.5% in the study group compared to 20.1% in the control group. The risk factors linked to NAFLD were triglyceride serum levels, BMI, medication, and drug dosage [21].

Evidence data suggest that NAFLD/NASH are more prevalent among males. As a matter of fact, gender differences were also reported in most psychiatric disturbances, such as schizophrenia, which is more common in males [22].

Regarding the connection between NAFLD and various mental disturbances, numerous studies pointed to an important relation among patients with NAFLD and memory impairment [23, 24]. As such, Seo et al. after analyzing data from the National Health and Nutrition Examination Survey that included 874 NAFLD patients, reported a clear association between NAFLD and impaired memory and attention, along with alteration of psychomotor function [23]. However, Weinstein et al. identified no independent association of NAFLD with cognitive dysfunction after evaluating cognitive function in 378 patients with NAFLD [24].

While the total prevalence of chronic liver diseases in patients with mental illnesses is not fully known [25], the prevalence of MetS in schizophrenic or bipolar patients is very high, ranging from 22 to 42%, compared to nonpsychiatric population control group. Thus, the existing literature evidence warrants further research aiming to clarify the potential associations and relationship between psychiatric disorders and NAFLD [16].

18.3 Pathophysiology of NAFLD and Psychiatric Disorders

NAFLD is considered a multisystemic disease and, along with diabetes mellitus type 2 and obesity as part of MetS, shares some similar and common risk factors and pathophysiological mechanisms. As such, there is more and more evidence regarding bidirectional relationship between NAFLD and psychiatric disorders, with some common factors like genetics, intestinal dysbiosis, inflammation with mitochondrial dysfunction, chronic stress, and psychological and lifestyle factors [16].

18.3.1 Genetic Common Factors

Genome-wide association studies have identified a few genetic loci linked to regulation of lipid metabolism, inflammation, and oxidative stress. Among them, adiponutrin plays a significant role in regulating glucose and fatty acid metabolism, being associated with bipolar disorder and NAFLD, according to Kenneson et al. [26]. Likewise, it seems that microRNA has an important role in signaling cellular stress, and it was positively related to NAFLD evolution. In fact, microRNA is responsible for regulating hepatic lipogenesis, and it was found to be elevated in serum patients with NAFLD. Obviously, the same microRNA was found to have higher levels in patients with bipolar disturbances, suggesting that there is an important link between NAFLD and psychiatric disorder pathogenesis [27].

18.3.2 Inflammation and Mitochondrial Dysfunction

Mitochondria are considered the area responsible for free fatty acid oxidation, thus playing a significant protective role against fatty acid accumulation. Due to the pro-inflammatory state of patients with NAFLD/NASH, mitochondria suffer a metabolism dysregulation, responsible for the development of excessive oxidative species [16]. Similarly, mitochondria dysfunction, chronic inflammation, and oxidative stress (Fig. 18.1) are considered involved in the pathogenesis of psychiatric disorders like schizophrenia, depression, and autism [28].

18.3.3 Chronic Stress and Hypothalamic–Pituitary–Adrenal Axis

Multiple studies highlighted the fact that chronic stress can determine a hyperactivation of the hypothalamic–pituitary–adrenal axis (HPA) with close association with obesity and MetS, respectively. HPA axis is responsible for stress regulation, by releasing or not glucocorticoids. It is a well-known fact that glucocorticoids can

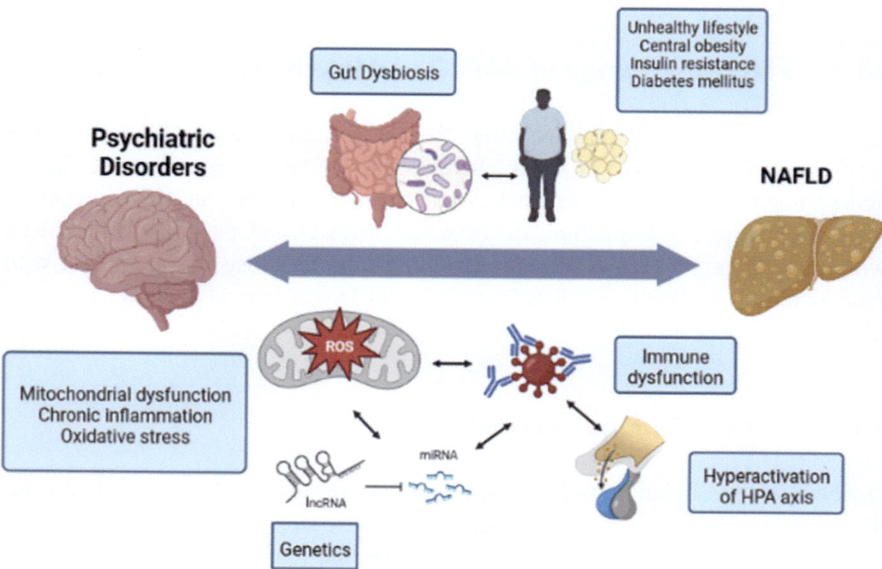

Fig. 18.1 Bidirectional pathophysiological relations between NAFLD and psychiatric disorders. *miRNA* microRNAs, *NAFLD* nonalcoholic fatty liver disease, *HPA* hypothalamic–pituitary–adrenal. (*Created with* Biorender.com, *adapted from Soto-Angona* et al. [16])

increase hepatic gluconeogenesis and lipolysis, thus promoting visceral fat accumulation. As such, these constant metabolic effects are associated in time with central obesity, insulin resistance, and also development and advancement of NAFLD [17].

18.3.4 Gut Microbiota Dysbiosis

There is a lot of evidence regarding the association of gut microbiome with the development of neuropsychiatric and psychological disturbances, especially with dementia and depression, through an inflammatory dysregulation mediated by bacterial fragments [29]. Similarly, the gut microbiome is influenced by lifestyle factors like diet, which can determine dysbiosis and an inflammatory process with a greater impact on mental and physical health, by promoting obesity. In this regard, gut dysbiosis in obesity-related metabolic diseases may be involved in the pathogenesis between NAFLD and mental disorders like depression, anxiety, cognitive impairments, and chronic stress [30].

18.3.5 Lifestyle Factors

Unhealthy lifestyle habits, like having diets rich in complex carbohydrates and saturated fats, and drug use, along with a lack of physical exercise, have a greater impact on physiological and mental health, by being associated with an elevated risk of NAFLD/NASH. The other way around, patients with psychiatric disorders can have behavior disturbances associated with the risk of developing NAFLD. According to Stewart et al. low consciousness and high neuroticism were associated with weight gain and higher risk for NAFLD [31].

18.4   NAFLD and Psychiatric Disorders

As previously mentioned, strong scientific evidence is now available demonstrating the increased risk of metabolic syndrome in patients with mental disorders. Because NAFLD is the hepatic manifestation of metabolic syndrome, it is expected that NAFLD is more common among people with mental disorders [32].

In the following, aspects related to the most studied associations between NAFLD and psychiatric conditions (depression, anxiety, and cognitive disorders) are briefly presented.

18.4.1 The Relationship Between Metabolic Syndrome (MetS) and Depressive/Anxiety Disorders

It is known that patients with depressive and/or anxiety disorder frequently have metabolic syndrome and are at increased risk of developing cardiovascular disease.

A potential bidirectional causal relationship can be suspected because depression can promote metabolic syndrome, while factors related to metabolic syndrome (psychological factors: obesity-related stigma, and biological factors: increased activation of pro-inflammatory pathways), can lead to depression [33, 34].

It is possible that one of the important risk factors in this association is excessive alcohol consumption, commonly found in patients with depression/anxiety along with other unhealthy eating habits and sedentary lifestyle [35].

At the same time, there are numerous studies that have demonstrated positive associations between metabolic syndrome and anxiety, indicating that, in addition to depression, anxiety is significantly more prevalent in people with metabolic syndrome compared to the general population [36, 37].

18.4.2 Depression/Anxiety and NAFLD

In a study by Youssef et al. the potential association between depression/anxiety and histological features of NAFLD was studied. Subclinical depression was identified in 53% of these patients, and overt depression was observed in 14%. Similarly, subclinical and clinical anxiety were observed in 45% and 25% of these patients, respectively. Furthermore, this study identified a positive association between the degree of steatosis and depression in patients with NAFLD [38].

Although the exact mechanisms underlying these associations remain unclear, it is noteworthy that clinical and lifestyle variables (including BMI, diabetes, and female gender), and hypertension were associated with both depression and anxiety severity [38].

An important point for clinical practice is that depressive disorders can have a significant impact on treatment outcomes in patients with NAFLD. This was reported by Tomeno et al. who looked at the effects of a lifestyle intervention in NAFLD patients with and without major depressive disorder (MDD). Patients with NAFLD and MDD showed a poor response with less effective treatment outcomes. The poor adherence/outcomes seen in these patients could be due to psychological factors related to depression, including effects on memory. This suggests that more complex individualized lifestyle modification programs may be needed in patients presenting with both NAFLD and MDD [39].

In summary, the abovementioned aspects argue for a bidirectional association of depression/anxiety with the occurrence and severity of NAFLD.

18.4.3 The Relationship Between Cognitive Impairment and NAFLD

In recent years, cognitive impairment has been increasingly interpreted as a complication of NAFLD. Memory, attention, concentration, and confusion problems have been identified in 70% of patients with nonalcoholic fatty liver disease [15, 40].

In a few small studies, the relationship between the severity of liver disease and the degree of cognitive impairment has been investigated, and it has been shown that there is a directly proportional relationship between them [23, 24]. In this sense, Felipo et al. showed that no cognitive impairment was found in patients with simple steatosis. In contrast, NASH patients in pre-cirrhotic stages, but with systemic inflammation and hyperammonemia, performed poorly on all subtests of the test used for the diagnosis of portosystemic encephalopathy (PSE) [41]. These findings suggest that simple steatosis per se is not an independent risk factor for cognitive dysfunction and the factors associated with more severe forms of the disease (e.g., hyperammonemia and systemic inflammation), are involved in the pathogenesis of cognitive impairment [41]. Systemic inflammation, vascular damage, and atherosclerosis are components of the metabolic syndrome and are characteristics of NAFLD. At the same time, they are closely associated with cognitive impairment, which justifies the term *metabolic cognitive syndrome* [12].

In addition, NAFLD patients also show disruption of gut microbiota and hepatic urea synthesis, leading to ammonia accumulation even in pre-cirrhotic stages [42]. These aspects, in the context of systemic inflammation, are the main changes at the level of the brain–intestinal axis and represent the most important mechanisms involved in hepatic encephalopathy that occurs in severe liver disease [43]. On the other hand, diabetes and obesity as independent factors, and mainly the metabolic syndrome, are currently considered as important risk factors for mild cognitive disorders but also for the onset of dementia [44, 45].

Another link between nonalcoholic fatty liver and cognitive impairment is through other mental disorders. As mentioned above, anxiety and depression are frequently associated with dysmetabolic liver disease while affecting cognitive processes (memory, attention, and executive function) [46, 47].

All these mechanisms involved both in the pathogenesis of nonalcoholic fatty liver disease and in cognitive impairment justify the hypothesis that the two conditions are independently associated. In this context, the increased prevalence of NAFLD and the potential negative impact on cognitive function may generate significant social and economic costs.

18.5 Diagnosis

Due to the increased prevalence of NAFLD and NASH among patients with psychiatric disorders, this pathology needs to be considered when evaluating such patients, and their specific impact needs to be further investigated. Diagnosis is currently based on imaging (liver ultrasound, MRI ultrasound, elastography, etc.) and histology.

Figure 18.2 shows a diagnostic algorithm for NAFLD in patients with psychiatric pathology based on the guidelines of the American Association for the Study of Liver Diseases (AASLD).

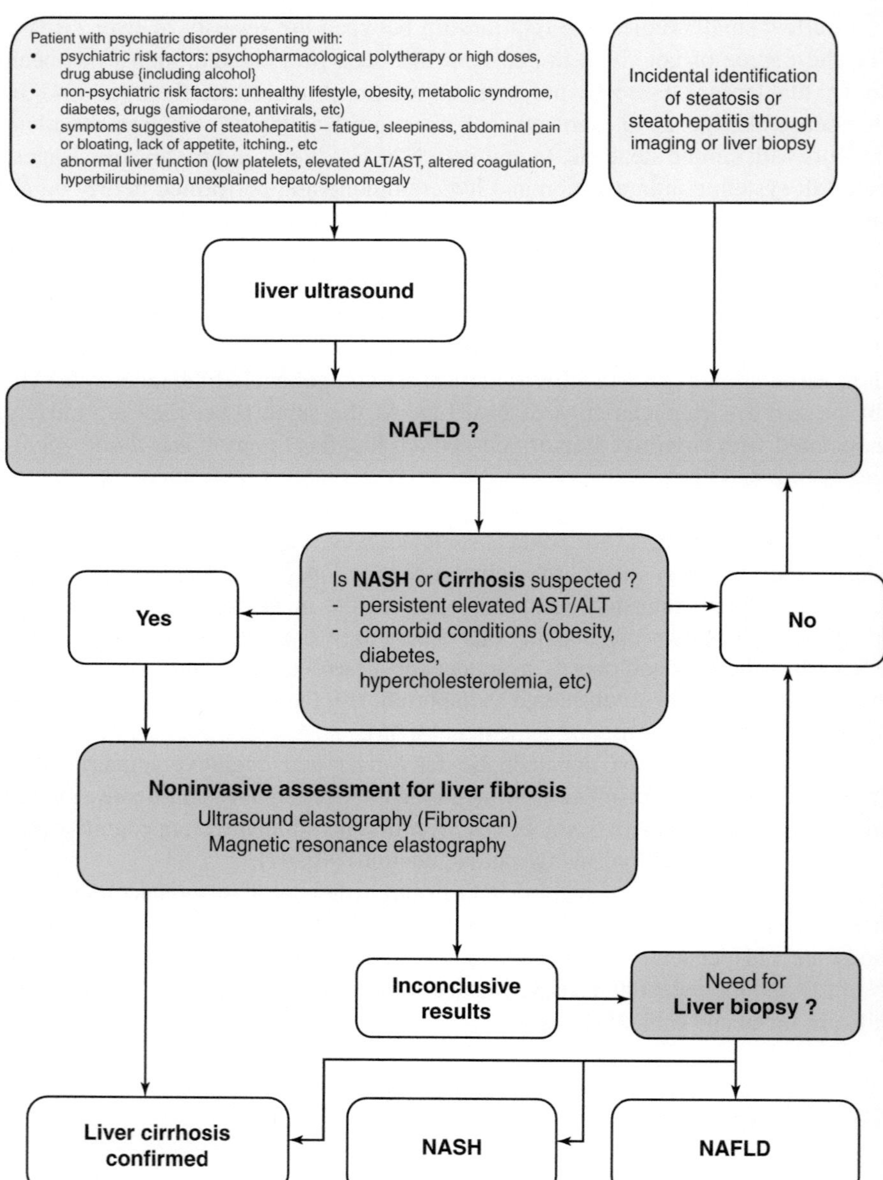

Fig. 18.2 Diagnostic algorithm for NAFLD and NASH in the psychiatric population. (Adapted from Soto Angona [16])

18.6 Therapeutic Principles in Patients with NAFLD and Associated Psychiatric Pathology

The first line of treatment in NAFLD and NASH is lifestyle change (healthy diet, weight loss, and physical activity). That is why NAFLD/NASH has been proposed as a cognitive-behavioral disorder [47]. However, in more advanced stages of liver disease, pharmacological treatment is also required, mainly insulin sensitizers or even more aggressive approaches such as bariatric surgery.

On the other hand, physical exercise, healthy diet, and weight loss substantially improve the course of many psychiatric diseases, improving cognitive functioning, negative symptoms, depression, or anxiety [47].

Another important aspect in the therapeutic management of patients with psychiatric disorders is the fact that, even if the impairment of liver function is not severe, many psychotropic drugs are metabolized by the liver and, as a result, their half-life, side effects, and metabolism could be altered.

On another note, given the previously mentioned common pathophysiological mechanisms, some therapeutic approaches proposed to correct the metabolic imbalance underlying NAFLD might also be beneficial for psychiatric disorders. For example, a new insulin sensitizer that targets the newly identified mitochondrial pyruvate carrier could improve the metabolic pathways that lead to type 2 diabetes, inflammation, and oxidative stress and therefore could be helpful in both pathologies [48].

Vitamin E, through its antioxidant effect, has recently been tested as a treatment with promising results for both NAFLD and some psychiatric conditions [49]. Also based on the correlation between unhealthy lifestyle and depressive symptoms, antidepressants could be used in the treatment of NAFLD, although they may have side effects that affect metabolism [50].

Statins are also an interesting therapeutic option for treating both NAFLD and psychiatric diseases. They have a role in lowering free cholesterol and have been found to protect against histological injury [51]. Because they have anti-inflammatory and antioxidant effects, they have also been proposed as adjunctive therapies for a number of psychiatric disorders [52].

Another interesting example of a common treatment is the cannabinoid receptor 1, which modulates hepatic energy metabolism. The role of cannabinoid receptors in the development of psychiatric disorders is also widely studied, although evidence remains limited and caution is advised [53].

Numerous studies are currently underway with various substances, some of which also have anti-inflammatory, neurotrophic, or neuroprotective properties [e.g., glucagon-like peptide-1 (GLP-1) analogs and peroxisome proliferator-activated receptor (PPAR) agonists]. In the future, these could be therapeutic options for patients with NAFLD [54].

All the previously presented aspects suggest a direct or indirect relationship of NAFLD with a number of mental health problems (depression, anxiety, cognitive dysfunctions), thus expanding the spectrum of its potential pathophysiological associations.

Mental disorders and cognitive impairment in patients with NAFLD are frequent and have a significant socio-psycho-economic impact by decreasing the quality of life and by the costs involved in the decrease in work productivity and the need for medical care. In this context, efforts must be made to identify and treat them early, even in patients who are not in advanced stages of liver disease.

References

1. Maurice J, Manousou P. Non-alcoholic fatty liver disease. Clin Med (Lond). 2018;18(3):245–50. https://doi.org/10.7861/clinmedicine.18-3-245.
2. Neuschwander-Tetri BA. Non-alcoholic fatty liver disease. BMC Med. 2017;15:45. https://doi.org/10.1186/s12916-017-0806-8.
3. Rinella ME. Nonalcoholic fatty liver disease: a systematic review. JAMA. 2015;313:2263–73. https://doi.org/10.1001/jama.2015.5370.
4. Kim D, Kim W, Adejumo AC, Cholankeril G, Tighe SP, Wong RJ, et al. Race/ethnicity-based temporal changes in prevalence of NAFLD-related advanced fibrosis in the United States, 2005–2016. Hepatol Int. 2019;13(2):205–13. https://doi.org/10.1007/s12072-018-09926-z.
5. Chalasani N, Younossi Z, Lavine JE, et al. The diagnosis and management of nonalcoholic fatty liver disease: practice guidance from the American Association for the Study of Liver Diseases. Hepatology. 2018;67(1):328–57. https://doi.org/10.1002/hep.29367.
6. Penninx BWJH, Lange SMM. Metabolic syndrome in psychiatric patients: overview, mechanisms, and implications. Dialog Clin Neurosci. 2018;20(1):63–73. https://doi.org/10.31887/DCNS.2018.20.1/bpenninx.
7. Dong JY, Zhang YH, Tong J, Qin LQ. Depression and risk of stroke: a meta-analysis of prospective studies. Stroke. 2012;43(1):32–7. https://doi.org/10.1161/STROKEAHA.111.630871.
8. Cuijpers P, Vogelzangs N, Twisk J, Kleiboer A, Li J, Penninx BW. Comprehensive meta-analysis of excess mortality in depression in the general community versus patients with specific illnesses. Am J Psychiatry. 2014;171(4):453–62. https://doi.org/10.1176/appi.ajp.2013.13030325.
9. Jung JY, Park SK, Oh CM, Chung PW, Ryoo JH. Non-alcoholic fatty liver disease and its association with depression in Korean general population. J Korean Med Sci. 2019;34(30):e199. https://doi.org/10.3346/jkms.2019.34.e199.
10. Surdea-Blaga T, Dumitraşcu DL. Depression and anxiety in nonalcoholic steatohepatitis: is there any association? Rom J Intern Med. 2011;49(4):273–80.
11. Lonardo A, Nascimbeni F, Mantovani A, Targher G. Hypertension, diabetes, atherosclerosis and NASH: cause or consequence? J Hepatol. 2018;68(2):335–52. https://doi.org/10.1016/j.jhep.2017.09.021.
12. Frisardi V, Solfrizzi V, Seripa D, Capurso C, Santamato A, Sancarlo D, et al. Metabolic-cognitive syndrome: a cross-talk between metabolic syndrome and Alzheimer's disease. Ageing Res Rev. 2010;9:399–417. https://doi.org/10.1016/j.arr.2010.04.007.
13. Wang HH, Lee DK, Liu M, Portincasa P, Wang DQ. Novel insights into the pathogenesis and management of the metabolic syndrome. Pediatr Gastroenterol Hepatol Nutr. 2020;23:189–230. https://doi.org/10.5223/pghn.2020.23.3.189.
14. Zafar U, Khaliq S, Ahmad HU, Manzoor S, Lone KP. Metabolic syndrome: an update on diagnostic criteria, pathogenesis, and genetic links. Hormones. 2018;17:299–313. https://doi.org/10.1007/s42000-018-0051-3.
15. Colognesi M, Gabbia D, De Martin S. Depression and cognitive impairment-extrahepatic manifestations of NAFLD and NASH. Biomedicine. 2020;8:229. https://doi.org/10.3390/biomedicines8070229.
16. Soto-Angona Ó, Anmella G, Valdés-Florido MJ, De Uribe-Viloria N, Carvalho AF, Penninx BWJH, Berk M. Non-alcoholic fatty liver disease (NAFLD) as a neglected metabolic com-

panion of psychiatric disorders: common pathways and future approaches. BMC Med. 2020;18(1):261. https://doi.org/10.1186/s12916-020-01713-8.

17. Elwing JE, Lustman PJ, Wang HL, Clouse RE. Depression, anxiety, and nonalcoholic steatohepatitis. Psychosom Med. 2006;68(4):563–9. https://doi.org/10.1097/01.psy.0000221276.17823.df.

18. Weinstein AA, Kallman Price J, Stepanova M, et al. Depression in patients with nonalcoholic fatty liver disease and chronic viral hepatitis B and C. Psychosomatics. 2011;52(2):127–32. https://doi.org/10.1016/j.psym.2010.12.019.

19. Hsu JH, Chien IC, Lin CH. Increased risk of chronic liver disease in patients with bipolar disorder: a population-based study. Gen Hosp Psychiatry. 2016;42:54–9. https://doi.org/10.1016/j.genhosppsych.2016.07.006.

20. Fuller BE, Rodriguez VL, Linke A, Sikirica M, Dirani R, Hauser P. Prevalence of liver disease in veterans with bipolar disorder or schizophrenia. Gen Hosp Psychiatry. 2011;33(3):232–7. https://doi.org/10.1016/j.genhosppsych.2011.03.006.

21. Yan J, Hou C, Liang Y. The prevalence and risk factors of young male schizophrenics with non-alcoholic fatty liver disease. Neuropsychiatr Dis Treat. 2017;13:1493–8. https://doi.org/10.2147/NDT.S137183.

22. Riecher-Rössler A, Butler S, Kulkarni J. Sex and gender differences in schizophrenic psychoses—a critical review. Arch Womens Ment Health. 2018;21(6):627–48. https://doi.org/10.1007/s00737-018-0847-9.

23. Seo SW, Gottesman RF, Clark JM, Hernaez R, Chang Y, Kim C, et al. Nonalcoholic fatty liver disease is associated with cognitive function in adults. Neurology. 2016;86:1136–42. https://doi.org/10.1212/WNL.0000000000002498.

24. Weinstein G, Davis-Plourde K, Himali JJ, Zelber-Sagi S, Beiser AS, Seshadri S. Nonalcoholic fatty liver disease, liver fibrosis score and cognitive function in middle-aged adults: the Framingham study. Liver Int. 2019;39:1713–21. https://doi.org/10.1111/liv.14161.

25. Carrier P, Debette-Gratien M, Girard M, Jacques J, Nubukpo P, Loustaud-Ratti V. Liver illness and psychiatric patients. Hepat Mon. 2016;16(12):1–9. https://doi.org/10.5812/hepatmon.41564.

26. Kenneson A, Funderburk JS. Patatin-like phospholipase domain-containing protein 3 (PNPLA3): a potential role in the association between liver disease and bipolar disorder. J Affect Disord. 2017;209:93–6. https://doi.org/10.1016/j.jad.2016.11.035.

27. Sermin AB, Genc SJH. Diagnostic and therapeutic potential of microRNAs in neuropsychiatric disorders: past, present, and future. Prog Neuropsychopharmacol Biol Psychiatry. 2017;73:87–103. https://doi.org/10.1016/j.pnpbp.2016.03.010.

28. Czarny P, Wigner P, Galecki P, Sliwinski T. The interplay between inflammation, oxidative stress, DNA damage, DNA repair and mitochondrial dysfunction in depression. Prog Neuropsychopharmacol Biol Psychiatry. 2018;80:309–21. https://doi.org/10.1016/j.pnpbp.2017.06.036.

29. Fung TC, Olson CA, Hsiao EY. Interactions between the microbiota, immune and nervous systems in health and disease. Nat Neurosci. 2017;20(2):145–55. https://doi.org/10.1038/nn.4476.Interactions.

30. Barber TM, Valsamakis G, Mastorakos G, Hanson P, Kyrou I, Randeva HS, et al. Dietary influences on the microbiota–gut–brain axis. Int J Mol Sci. 2021;22:3502. https://doi.org/10.3390/ijms22073502.

31. Oni ET, Kalathiya R, Aneni EC, et al. Relation of physical activity to prevalence of nonalcoholic fatty liver disease independent of cardiometabolic risk. Am J Cardiol. 2015;115(1):34–9. https://doi.org/10.1016/j.amjcard.2014.09.044.

32. Ma Q, Yang F, Ma B, et al. Prevalence of nonalcoholic fatty liver disease in mental disorder inpatients in China: an observational study. Hepatol Int. 2021;15:127–36. https://doi.org/10.1007/s12072-020-10132-z.

33. Gheshlagh R, Parizad N, Sayehmiri K. The relationship between depression and metabolic syndrome: systematic review and meta-analysis study. Iran Red Crescent Med J. 2016;18:e26523. https://doi.org/10.5812/ircmj.26523.

34. Tsigos C, Kyrou I, Kassi E, Chrousos GP. Stress: endocrine physiology and pathophysiology. In: Feingold KR, Anawalt B, Boyce A, Chrousos G, de Herder WW, Dhatariya K, Dungan K, Grossman A, Hershman JM, Hofland J, et al., editors. Endotext. South Dartmouth: MDText. com, Inc.; 2020.

35. Bica T, Castello R, Toussaint LL, Monteso-Curto P. Depression as a risk factor of organic diseases: an international integrative review. J Nurs Scholarsh. 2017;49:389–99. https://doi. org/10.1111/jnu.12303.

36. Butnoriene J, Steibliene V, Saudargiene A, Bunevicius A. Does presence of metabolic syndrome impact anxiety and depressive disorder screening results in middle aged and elderly individuals? A population based study. BMC Psychiatry. 2018;18:5. https://doi.org/10.1186/s12888-017-1576-8.

37. Shinkov A, Borissova AM, Kovatcheva R, Vlahov J, Dakovska L, Atanassova I, Petkova P. Increased prevalence of depression and anxiety among subjects with metabolic syndrome and known type 2 diabetes mellitus—a population-based study. Postgrad Med. 2018;130:251–7. https://doi.org/10.1080/00325481.2018.1410054.

38. Youssef NA, Abdelmalek MF, Binks M, Guy CD, Omenetti A, Smith AD, Diehl AM, Suzuki A. Associations of depression, anxiety and antidepressants with histological severity of non-alcoholic fatty liver disease. Liver Int. 2013;33:1062–70. https://doi.org/10.1111/liv.12165.

39. Tomeno W, Kawashima K, Yoneda M, Saito S, Ogawa Y, Honda Y, Kessoku T, Imajo K, Mawatari H, Fujita K, et al. Non-alcoholic fatty liver disease comorbid with major depressive disorder: the pathological features and poor therapeutic efficacy. J Gastroenterol Hepatol. 2015;30:1009–14. https://doi.org/10.1111/jgh.12897.

40. Kjærgaard K, Mikkelsen AC, Wernberg CW, Grønkjær LL, Eriksen PL, Damholdt MF, et al. Cognitive dysfunction in non-alcoholic fatty liver disease—current knowledge, mechanisms and perspectives. J Clin Med. 2021;10:673. https://doi.org/10.3390/jcm10040673.

41. Felipo V, Urios A, Montesinos E, Molina I, Garcia-Torres ML, Civera M, et al. Contribution of hyperammonemia and inflammatory factors to cognitive impairment in minimal hepatic encephalopathy. Metab Brain Dis. 2012;27:51–8. https://doi.org/10.1007/s11011-011-9269-3.

42. Lykke Eriksen P, Sorensen M, Gronbaek H, Hamilton-Dutoit S, Vilstrup H, Thomsen KL. Non-alcoholic fatty liver disease causes dissociated changes in metabolic liver functions. Clin Res Hepatol Gastroenterol. 2019;43:551–60. https://doi.org/10.1016/j.clinre.2019.01.001.

43. Rose CF, Amodio P, Bajaj JS, et al. Hepatic encephalopathy: novel insights into classification, pathophysiology and therapy. J Hepatol. 2020;73:1526–47. https://doi.org/10.1016/j.jhep.2020.07.013.

44. Ng TP, Feng L, Nyunt MS, et al. Metabolic syndrome and the risk of mild cognitive impairment and progression to dementia: follow-up of the Singapore longitudinal ageing study cohort. JAMA Neurol. 2016;73:456–63. https://doi.org/10.1001/jamaneurol.2015.4899.

45. Atti AR, Valente S, Iodice A, et al. Metabolic syndrome, mild cognitive impairment, and dementia: a meta-analysis of longitudinal studies. Am J Geriatr Psychiatry. 2019;27:625–37. https://doi.org/10.1016/j.jagp.2019.01.214.

46. Labenz C, Huber Y, Michel M, Nagel M, Galle PR, Kostev K, Schattenberg JM. Nonalcoholic fatty liver disease increases the risk of anxiety and depression. Hepatol Commun. 2020;4:1293–301. https://doi.org/10.1002/hep4.1541.

47. Macavei B, Baban A, Dumitrascu DL. Psychological factors associated with NAFLD/NASH: a systematic review. Eur Rev Med Pharmacol Sci. 2016;20:5081–97.

48. Colca J. NASH (nonalcoholic steatohepatitis), diabetes, and macrovascular disease: multiple chronic conditions and a potential treatment at the metabolic root. Expert Opin Investig Drugs. 2020;29(2):191–19. https://doi.org/10.1080/13543784.2020.1715940.

49. Armstrong MJ, Houlihan DD, Rowe IA. Pioglitazone, vitamin E, or placebo for nonalcoholic steatohepatitis. N Engl J Med. 2010;363(12):1185–6. https://doi.org/10.1056/NEJMc1006581.

50. Lonardo A, Ballestri S. Perspectives of nonalcoholic fatty liver disease research: a personal point of view. Explor Med. 2020;2020:7. https://doi.org/10.37349/emed.2020.00007.

51. Dongiovanni P, Petta S, Mannisto V, et al. Statin use and non-alcoholic steatohepatitis in at risk individuals. J Hepatol. 2015;63(3):705–12. https://doi.org/10.1016/j.jhep.2015.05.006.

52. Kim SW, Kang HJ, Jhon M, et al. Statins and inflammation: new therapeutic opportunities in psychiatry. Front Psychiatry. 2019;10:103. https://doi.org/10.3389/fpsyt.2019.00103.
53. Black N, Stockings E, Campbell G, et al. Cannabinoids for the treatment of mental disorders and symptoms of mental disorders: a systematic review and meta-analysis. Lancet Psychiatry. 2019;6(12):995–1010. https://doi.org/10.1016/S2215-0366(19)30401-8.
54. Grieco M, Giorgi A, Gentile MC, D'Erme M, Morano S, Maras B, Filardi T. Glucagon-like peptide-1: a focus on neurodegenerative diseases. Front Neurosci. 2019;13:1112. https://doi.org/10.3389/fnins.2019.01112.

Obstructive Sleep Apnea Syndrome and Nonalcoholic Fatty Liver Disease

19

Robert Nastasa, Carol Stanciu, Roxana Nemteanu, and Anca Trifan

19.1 Introduction

Obstructive sleep apnea syndrome (OSAS) is a common disorder among patients with various conditions of the metabolic syndrome, such as hypertension, atherosclerosis, alteration of carbohydrate, or lipid metabolism (decrease in LDL cholesterol, increase in HDL cholesterol, hypertriglyceridemia) [1]. OSAS has an estimated prevalence of 3–7%, but in obese patients, the rates are higher, reaching 48% in men and 38% in women, indicating a slight difference in favor of the male sex [2, 3].

19.2 Epidemiology

According to the recent WHO reports, it is estimated that about 2 billion adults are overweight, while 650 million are obese worldwide [4]. If current trends continue, it is expected that 2.7 billion adults will be overweight, over 1 billion affected by obesity, and 177 million adults severely affected by obesity by 2025 [5]. By 2030, it is predicted that 1 in 5 women and 1 in 7 men will be living with obesity [6]. As this silent epidemic extends globally, so does the prevalence of obesity-related chronic diseases, NAFLD and OSA, respectively. NAFLD is the fastest-growing obesity-related noncommunicable disease and a strong predictor of liver and cardiovascular mortality [7]. The worldwide prevalence is currently estimated at 32.4%, and it is significantly higher in men compared to women (39.7% vs. 25.6%). The incidence

R. Nastasa (✉) · C. Stanciu · R. Nemteanu · A. Trifan
Gastroenterology Department, Grigore T. Popa University of Medicine and Pharmacy, Iasi, Romania

Institute of Gastroenterology and Hepatology, St. Spiridon Emergency Hospital, Iasi, Romania

A. Trifan et al. (eds.), *Essentials of Non-Alcoholic Fatty Liver Disease*, https://doi.org/10.1007/978-3-031-33548-8_19

217

is estimated to be 46.9 cases per 1000 person-years [8]. About one-third of the European adult population has NAFLD [9]. Nevertheless, as obesity and metabolic syndrome are strongly associated with NAFLD, it is likely that its prevalence will continue to grow substantially over the next decade.

While OSA has multiple etiologic determinants, obesity remains its strongest phenotypic risk factor [10]. However, recent reports showed a strong association between steatosis and OSA severity, and 26% of patients with severe OSA patients have fibrosis [11]. OSA is estimated to affect 20–50% of ethnic populations worldwide and up to 48–70% of obese populations [12]. In addition to being comorbid diseases of obesity, some observational studies have reported that OSA is independently related to NAFLD [13]. Lu et al. found that among patients with NAFLD, 64–87% have OSA with a prevalence of liver steatosis in the OSA cohort of 73.9% [14].

19.3 Pathophysiology

OSAS is characterized by chronic intermittent hypoxia that occurs during sleep, being induced by partial or complete airway obstruction, which occurs repeatedly [2]. This type of nocturnal hypoxia can vary considerably among subjects with OSA. Among those diagnosed with OSAS, some patients may have a high apnea-hypopnea index (AHI) with relatively mild desaturations, while others may have few but more frequent intermittent hypoxic events, resulting in a marked hypoxemia [1]. The apnea-hypopnea index (AHI) represents the average number of periods of sleep apnea and hypopnea per hour and determines the severity of OSA.

It can be considered to be mild when between 5 and 14 events occur, moderate when between 15 and 29 events occur, and severe when more than 30 sleep apnea and hypopnea episodes occur per hour. Moreover, other factors, such as oxyhemoglobin desaturation and percentage of time desaturation persists during sleep, also influence the severity of OSAS [14].

Numerous data from the literature presented in recent years have suggested that both OSAS and chronic intermittent hypoxia are independent risk factors for liver injury [2, 3]. This type of hypoxia leads to oxidative stress, lipid peroxidation, endothelial dysfunction, insulin resistance, metabolic dysregulation, and production of proinflammatory cytokines, which promote the progression of liver fibrosis by targeting hepatocytes, hepatic stellate cells, and Kupffer cells [15].

At the same time, in the pathogenesis of OSAS, in addition to chronic hypoxia, other pathophysiological mechanisms play an extremely important role [16]
- Oscillations of intrathoracic pressure: The negative intrathoracic pressure during inspiration can be greatly accentuated in the presence of apnea, as the patient has multiple failed attempts to inhale against a collapsed oropharynx [16].
- Fragmentation of sleep: OSAS occurs mainly during the REM phase of sleep, in which there is muscle atony, facilitating upper airway obstruction, and most apnea events culminate in an awakening or microarousal that leads to recovery of

muscle tone and cessation of obstruction. Given the disordered respiratory events during wakefulness, evidence of transient awakening from sleep was observed over time via electroencephalography. Consequently, sleep fragmentation is thus generated [16].

- Hypercapnia: With each respiratory-altering event, there may be an increase in the partial pressure of carbon dioxide ($PaCO_2$). CO_2 monitoring in OSA is not routinely performed but can generally be performed by means of transcutaneous $PaCO_2$ measuring devices or by determination of end-tidal CO_2 (end-tidal CO_2). The increase in CO_2 level may be higher in patients with underlying lung conditions, such as chronic obstructive pulmonary disease, pulmonary fibrosis, as well as various interstitial pneumonias [16].

- Airway edema and surface tension: Accumulation of edematous fluid even in small quantities (100–200 mL) enlarges upper airway soft-tissue structures in OSA patients determining snoring and therefore sleep-disordered breathing [17]. Surface tension plays a role in modulating upper airway patency, and the therapy with instillation of surfactant may decrease the OSAS severity [18].

- Obesity, leptin, and inflammation: Central, or visceral, obesity is associated with the greatest risk for OSA because of reduction in lung volumes due to increased abdominal fat mass in the supine position [16]. Leptin acts like a respiratory stimulant, and in obese patients, leptin resistance or leptin deficiency may cause a hypoventilation syndrome [19]. Humoral factors including classical proinflammatory cytokines such as tumor necrosis factor-α (TNF-α) and interleukin (IL)-6 are elevated in OSAS patients contributing to the patency of upper airways [20].

Chronic intermittent hypoxia plays a key role in the pathophysiology of OSAS, the intricate mechanism likely being similar to that in ischemia-reperfusion injury. Moreover, in patients with OSA, some oxidative stress markers are increased and could play an essential role in the development and progression of inflammation, endothelial dysfunction, and atherosclerosis [21]. Over time, the effects of hypoxia on metabolic pathways and mechanisms of hepatocellular injury in patients with NAFLD have been determined. Savransky et al. showed that intermittent hypoxia induces hyperglycemia and hepatic lipid peroxidation, but also enhances the activity of nuclear factor kappa B (NF-κB), a master regulator of the inflammatory response. Thus, there is a significant increase in glycogen accumulation in hepatocytes, suggesting that intermittent hypoxia can independently lead to mild hepatic injury in the absence of obesity-inducing risk factors [22].

19.4 Risk Factors of Obstructive Sleep Apnea Syndrome

There are many risk factors that are associated with the occurrence of OSAS, among which we can list the following [16, 17]

- Anatomical changes: contribute to the reduction of the oropharyngeal space. Thus, obese people with increased neck circumference and craniofacial changes such as the growth of the base of the tongue and hypertrophy of the tonsil and uvula, but also people with maxillomandibular deficiencies present a greater risk of apnea, because there is a reduction in the lumen of the upper airways.

- The supine position during sleep: facilitates the occurrence of apnea due to the posterior repositioning of the tongue by gravitational effect. The use of substances with a sedative or muscle relaxant effect aggravates this effect of posterior repositioning of the tongue by muscle relaxation both at the base of the tongue and at the level of the posterior pharyngeal wall.
- Smoking: it is also considered a risk factor for contributing to upper airway dysfunction during sleep, as it tends to promote relaxation of the respiratory muscles due to the neural reflexes caused by nicotine.
- Hormonal changes: Menopausal women equate their apnea-hypopnea index with that of men because estrogen and progesterone maintain proper muscle tone in the premenopausal period.

19.5 Clinical Picture of Obstructive Sleep Apnea

From a clinical point of view, this sleep disorder is manifested by a noisy vibration of the airways called snoring, but also by suffocation, morning headache, daytime sleepiness, and decreased ability to concentrate [23]. The most important symptoms and the common clinical findings are presented in Table 19.1.

19.6 Diagnosis of Obstructive Sleep Apnea

The diagnosis of OSAS is made through polysomnography, which is the gold standard diagnostic test being performed during the night and allows the monitoring of different physiological and pathological parameters, such as the apnea and hypopnea index, oxyhemoglobin saturation, excitations and microexcitations, postural changes, distribution of sleep stages, electrocardiographic recording, and intensity and frequency of snoring [16]. OSAS is confirmed if one of the following two conditions exists: (1) an AHI $\geq$15 events per hour in a relatively asymptomatic patient and (2) an AHI $\geq$5 events per hour in a patient with more than two clinical features

Table 19.1 Common symptoms and findings in OSAS

Symptoms of OSAS	Examination findings in OSAS
Snoring	Body mass index $\geq$30 kg/m^2
Choking or gasping at night	Enlarged neck circumference $\geq$43 cm
Excessive daytime sleepiness	Systolic blood pressure $\geq$140 mmHg
Morning headaches	Crowded upper airway
Insomnia with frequent awakenings	Dysrhythmias (e.g., atrial fibrillation)
Lack of concentration	Lower extremity edema (heart failure)
Cognitive deficits	Accentuated P2 heart sounds (pulmonary HTN)
Changes in mood	Nasal obstruction
Nocturia	Decreased oxygen saturation

[24]. A negative result does not exclude the diagnosis of OSAS particularly in high-risk patients, and polysomnography should be repeated. Also, other conditions should be suspected in such cases for differential diagnosis including moderate or severe pulmonary pathologies, neuromuscular dysfunctions, congestive heart failure, movement disorders, parasomnias, or sleep seizures [25]. At the same time, it should be remembered that when snoring is an isolated finding, with a normal apnea-hypopnea index, snoring can be considered primary or benign snoring [16].

19.7 Associated Conditions of OSAS

19.7.1 Neuropsychiatric Dysfunction

OSAS is related to neurological dysfunctions such as impaired attention, lack of memory, and cognitive deficits, which, together, can result in disability of performance and increased risk of motor vehicle crashes compared with the general population of drivers [26]. Charles et al. found that fatigue induced by OSAS is a contributing factor in 12% of all crashes and in 10% of all near-crashes causing 800,000 collisions per year [27]. Moreover, psychiatric manifestations including moodiness and irritability as well as depression, psychosis, and sexual dysfunction were related to OSAS. Wheaton et al. found in a national survey in the US population that OSAS was associated with probable major depression, and the results are higher among female sex (OR = 5.2; 95% CI: 2.7, 9.9 among women) [28].

19.7.2 Cardiovascular and Cerebrovascular Morbidity

OSAS is associated with an increased risk of cardiovascular morbidity and mortality such as hypertension (with a prevalence between 35 and 80% of the patients), coronary artery disease, stroke, and arrhythmias. There are several mechanisms involved in the development of cardiovascular events like endothelial dysfunction accompanied by a proinflammatory and prooxidant status, hypercoagulability, and imbalance between matrix metalloproteases and their inhibitors [15]. A meta-analysis conducted by Wang et al. showed that severe OSA significantly increases the cardiovascular risk, stroke, and all-cause mortality (relative risk 1.79 for cardiovascular disease, 1.21 for coronary artery disease, 2.15 for stroke, 1.92 for death) [29].

19.7.3 Pulmonary Hypertension or Right-Heart Failure

OSAS is classically associated with pulmonary hypertension (PAH), affecting approximately 10% of patients with OSA [29]. A recent study by Minic et al. found that sleep apnea disturbances were found in 71% of the patients with PAH, and OSA is the most frequent breathing disorder, affecting 56% of them. Also, the authors suggest about the importance of screening for OSAS in patients with PAH [30]. Moreover, Javaheri et al. found that effective treatment of OSA in patients with heart failure is associated with improved survival, while treatment of OSA in patients with PAH is typically associated with modest hemodynamic improvement [31].

19.7.4 Type 2 Diabetes Mellitus

Patients with OSAS have an increased prevalence of insulin resistance as well as type 2 diabetes (T2DM) and diabetes complications [32]. While this association can be manifested through shared same risk factors such as older age, increased waist circumference, higher BMI ≥ 30 kg/m^2, and reduced levels of high-density lipoprotein cholesterol (HDL cholesterol), an independent association between OSA severity, insulin resistance, and type 2 diabetes has been reported in several studies [33, 34]. In one study conducted by Kenderzka et al. about 12% of patients with OSA developed T2DM over a follow-up of 67 months. Moreover, patients with severe OSA (AHI ≥ 30 events per hour) had an approximately 30% higher risk of incident diabetes compared with patients without OSA (AHI <5 events per hour) [34].

19.7.5 Nonalcoholic Fatty Liver Disease

Several studies have found that OSAS is highly prevalent in patients diagnosed with nonalcoholic fatty liver compared to the normal population and could be considered an important risk factor for the development of nonalcoholic steatohepatitis and advanced fibrosis [35, 36]. A recent meta-analysis, by Musso et al. that included 18 cross-sectional studies and 2183 participants, found that patients diagnosed with OSA were at high risk of developing and progressing FGNA, NASH, and advanced fibrosis, regardless of age, sex, and body mass index [37]. Agrawal et al. showed that the severity of OSAS is correlated with the degree of liver fibrosis independent of the presence of metabolic syndrome or obesity [38]. Moreover, a recent study by Krolow et al. which included participants with metabolic conditions, found that moderate and severe degrees of OSA were correlated with increased liver fibrosis [39]. Several studies have found an association between NAFLD and OSAS in the pediatric and adult population [40, 41]. A study published by Nobili et al. showed that the presence and severity of OSA in children are correlated with the severity of liver disease, independent of the presence of abdominal obesity, metabolic syndrome, and insulin resistance [40]. Moreover, Aron-Wisnewsky et al. in a study that included 101 morbidly obese patients who underwent bariatric surgery and liver biopsy, found that chronic intermittent hypoxia remained independently associated with liver fibrosis, fibroinflammation, and NAFLD activity score. However, CIH does not seem to impact adipocyte morphology or adipose tissue macrophage accumulation [41]. There are no guideline recommendations regarding treatment strategy for patients with OSAS and NAFLD [42]. In general, the best approach is the lifestyle modifications, which include physical activity, cessation of smoking and alcohol intake, and weight loss, because it will improve OSA severity and reduce upper airway collapsibility, and it should be strongly recommended to patients with NAFLD and OSA [43]. A recent study by Mersarwi et al. suggests that patients with NAFLD must be screened for OSA due to the fact that a majority of them are asymptomatic [1]. However, there is a necessity for future studies to evaluate the cost-effectiveness impact for screening patients with NAFLD or OSAS.

19.8 Association Between Treatment of OSAS and NAFLD

There are sufficient data to argue that there is an intricate and bidirectional relationship between NAFLD and OSA. The current knowledge showed an increased prevalence of NAFLD in patients with diagnosis of OSA. As previously reported, hypoxia is considered to have a determinant role in NAFLD pathogenesis, and NAFLD represents an additional risk for systemic inflammation in patients with OSA [44]. Jullian-Desayes et al. in a recent meta-analysis, showed that there is a strong association between steatosis and OSA severity, with 85% of severe OSA patients (>30 events/h) having steatosis, while 26% of severe OSA patients having fibrosis [11]. Treatment options for OSA are diverse, but the gold standard for the clinical management of OSA is continuous CPAP treatment [44]. All treatment options for OSA are listed in Table 19.2.

The subtle pathological dynamics between NAFLD and OSA become visible when treatment is initiated. Chen et al. reported that OSA severity was independently associated with liver steatosis and elevation of serum aminotransferases.

Table 19.2 Available treatment options for patients with OSA

Procedure type	Available
Positive airway pressure (PAP)	Continuous PAP (CPAP)
	Bi-level PAP (backup rate, average volume assured pressure support)
Autotitrating PAP	CPAP or bi-level PAP
Surgical treatment	Adenotonsillectomy, nasal surgeries, palatal surgeries, tongue-based surgeries, genioglossus advancement with hyoid suspension, multilevel surgeries (a combination of nasal, palatal, and tongue surgeries)
Maxillomandibular advancement	Enlarges the velo-orohypopharyngeal airway via advancement of anterior pharyngeal tissues attached to the mandible
Oral appliances	Tongue-retaining devices and mandibular advancement devices
Hypoglossal nerve stimulation	Pacemaker-like device connected to a wire attached to a small cuff to the hypoglossal nerve
Weight loss	Obesity should be counseled on long-term weight management. A BMI lower than 25 kg/m^2 through dietary or surgical weight loss is the goal
Positional therapy	Was developed to keep patients in a nonsupine position
Nasal expiratory PAP	The device valve rests in the nose and acts as a one-way resistor, permitting unobstructed inspiration [4]

Three months of CPAP therapy were associated with a significant improvement in liver injury in OSA patients [45]. Similar results were seen in a study by Kim et al. The authors found a favorable dose-response association between the severity of OSA and the improvement in serum aminotransferase levels and the regression of hepatic fibrosis after 6 months of CPAP treatment. Interestingly, these findings were independent from the severity of obesity [46]. In cases of morbid obesity, OSA is associated with liver damage. The role of noninvasive techniques to monitor liver changes during OSA treatment with CPAP remains to be explored in future trials, but Buttacavoli et al. found a positive outcome for using ultrasound liver assessment and CPAP treatment in OSA patients with improvement of liver steatosis [47]. However, a randomized clinical study by Ng et al. reported that CPAP alone did not improve hepatic steatosis and fibrosis [48]. Patients with NAFLD and OSA were randomized equally into two groups.

There were significant correlations between controlled attenuation parameter (CAP), respiratory event index, and oxygen desaturation index. It was noted that weight change over 6 months correlated with changes in both intrahepatic triglyceride and CAP. The additional role of weight reduction through lifestyle modification deserves further investigation [48].

Excess adipose tissue surrounding the upper airway can cause airway narrowing and increase the propensity for collapse during sleep [49]. Therefore, weight loss is mandatory, and several surgical and nonsurgical treatment options are currently available, such as exercise, diet, pharmacological interventions, and bariatric surgery, as a more permanent remedy. There are limited data regarding the efficiency of different weight-loss drugs on OSA patients. Currently, phentermine, topiramate, orlistat, liraglutide, and empagliflozin have been studied in OSA patients with promising results [49, 50]. Bariatric surgery has been extensively used as a more permanent solution for obese patients, and OSA remission can be obtained in the majority (59.2%) of patients with obesity as reported by Currie et al. in a recent paper [51].

In conclusion, recognition of OSA patients among at-risk NAFLD patients and vice versa will not only allow early diagnosis but most importantly institute appropriate therapy that should reduce the burden of OSA-related symptoms with the intent of decreasing adverse cardiovascular and metabolic risk. Individualized therapy should be based on four essential traits such as upper airway obstruction, responsiveness of the upper airway muscles, arousability, and breathing regulation [49]. CPAP is the treatment of choice, but patient compliance is suboptimal. Therefore, the role and efficiency of non-CPAP therapies should be assessed in different at-risk patient categories. Future studies for this novel field of interest are required.

References

1. Mesarwi OA, Loomba R, Malhotra A. Obstructive sleep apnea, hypoxia, and nonalcoholic fatty liver disease. Am J Respir Crit Care Med. 2019;199(7):830–41.
2. Li M, Li X, Lu Y. Obstructive sleep apnea syndrome and metabolic diseases. Endocrinology. 2018;159(7):2670–5. https://doi.org/10.1210/en.2018-00248.

3. Rosato V, Masarone M, Dallio M, et al. NAFLD and extra-hepatic comorbidities: current evidence on a multi-organ metabolic syndrome. Int J Environ Res Public Health. 2019;16(18):3415. https://doi.org/10.3390/ijerph16183415.
4. Boutari C, Mantzoros CS. A 2022 update on the epidemiology of obesity and a call to action: as its twin COVID-19 pandemic appears to be receding, the obesity and dysmetabolism pandemic continues to rage on. Metabolism. 2022;133:155217.
5. https://www.worldobesity.org/about/about-obesity/prevalence-of-obesity. Accessed 18 Sept 2022.
6. https://www.idf.org/news/259:one-billion-people-globally-estimated-to-be-living-with-obesity-by-2030.html. Accessed 26 Sept 2022.
7. Sinn DH, Kang D, Choi SC, Hong YS, Zhao D, Guallar E, Park Y, Cho J, Gwak GY. Nonalcoholic fatty liver disease without metabolic associated fatty liver disease and the risk of metabolic syndrome. Clin Gastroenterol Hepatol. 2022;2022:14.
8. Riazi K, Azhari H, Charette JH, Underwood FE, King JA, Afshar EE, Swain MG, Congly SE, Kaplan GG, Shaheen AA. The prevalence and incidence of NAFLD worldwide: a systematic review and meta-analysis. Lancet Gastroenterol Hepatol. 2022;7(9):851–61. https://doi.org/10.1016/S2468-1253(22)00165-0.
9. Kluge HHP. Weltgesundheitsorganisation Regionalbüro für Europa. WHO European regional obesity report. Geneva: World Health Organization; 2022.
10. Tufik S, Santos-Silva R, Taddei JA, Bittencourt LR. Obstructive sleep apnea syndrome in the Sao Paulo Epidemiologic Sleep Study. Sleep Med. 2010;11(5):441–6.
11. Jullian-Desayes I, Trzepizur W, Boursier J, Joyeux-Faure M, Bailly S, Benmerad M, Le Vaillant M, Jaffre S, Pigeanne T, Bizieux-Thaminy A, Humeau MP, Alizon C, Goupil F, Costentin C, Gaucher J, Tamisier R, Gagnadoux F, Pépin JL. Obstructive sleep apnea, chronic obstructive pulmonary disease and NAFLD: an individual participant data meta-analysis. Sleep Med. 2021;77:357–64.
12. Pouwels S, Sakran N, Graham Y, et al. Non-alcoholic fatty liver disease (NAFLD): a review of pathophysiology, clinical management and effects of weight loss. BMC Endocr Disord. 2022;22:63.
13. Benjafield AV, Ayas NT, Eastwood PR, Heinzer R, Ip MSM, Morrell MJ, Nunez CM, Patel SR, Penzel T, Pépin JL, Peppard PE, Sinha S, Tufik S, Valentine K, Malhotra A. Estimation of the global prevalence and burden of obstructive sleep apnoea: a literature-based analysis. Lancet Respir Med. 2019;7(8):687–98.
14. Faber J, Faber C, Faber AP. Obstructive sleep apnea in adults. Dental Press J Orthod. 2019;24(3):99–109.
15. Hopps E, Caimi G. Obstructive sleep apnea syndrome: links between pathophysiology and cardiovascular complications. Clin Invest Med. 2015;38(6):E362–70.
16. Dempsey JA, Veasey SC, Morgan BJ, O'Donnell CP. Pathophysiology of sleep apnea. Physiol Rev. 2010;90(1):47–112.
17. Schwab RJ, Gefter WB, Pack AI, Hoffman EA. Dynamic imaging of the upper airway during respiration in normal subjects. J Appl Physiol. 1993;74:1504–14.
18. Schwartz AR, Schneider H, Smith PL. Upper airway surface tension: is it a significant cause of airflow obstruction during sleep? J Appl Physiol. 2003;95:1759–60.
19. Phipps PR, Starritt E, Caterson I, Grunstein RR. Association of serum leptin with hypoventilation in human obesity. Thorax. 2002;57:75–6.
20. Yokoe T, Minoguchi K, Matsuo H, Oda N, Minoguchi H, Yoshino G, Hirano T, Adachi M. Elevated levels of C-reactive protein and interleukin-6 in patients with obstructive sleep apnea syndrome are decreased by nasal continuous positive airway pressure. Circulation. 2003;107:1129–34.
21. Paschetta E, Belci P, Alisi A, et al. OSAS-related inflammatory mechanisms of liver injury in nonalcoholic fatty liver disease. Mediat Inflamm. 2015;2015:815721.
22. Lavie L. Obstructive sleep apnoea syndrome—an oxidative stress disorder. Sleep Med Rev. 2003;7(1):35–51.

23. Stansbury RC, Strollo PJ. Clinical manifestations of sleep apnea. J Thorac Dis. 2015;7(9):E298–310.
24. Foroughi M, Razavi H, Malekmohammad M, Adimi Naghan P, Jamaati H. Diagnosis of obstructive sleep apnea syndrome in adults: a brief review of existing data for practice in Iran. Tanaffos. 2016;15(2):70–4.
25. Levendowski DJ, Zack N, Rao S, Wong K, Gendreau M, Kranzler J, Zavora T, Westbrook PR. Assessment of the test-retest reliability of laboratory polysomnography. Sleep Breath. 2009;13(2):163–7.
26. Olaithe M, Bucks RS. Executive dysfunction in OSA before and after treatment: a meta-analysis. Sleep. 2013;36(9):1297–305.
27. George CF. Sleep apnea, alertness, and motor vehicle crashes. Am J Respir Crit Care Med. 2007;176(10):954–6.
28. Wheaton AG, Perry GS, Chapman DP, Croft JB. Sleep disordered breathing and depression among U.S. adults: National Health and Nutrition Examination Survey, 2005–2008. Sleep. 2012;35(4):461–7.
29. Wang X, Ouyang Y, Wang Z, Zhao G, Liu L, Bi Y. Obstructive sleep apnea and risk of cardiovascular disease and all-cause mortality: a meta-analysis of prospective cohort studies. Int J Cardiol. 2013;169(3):207–14.
30. Minic M, Granton JT, Ryan CM. Sleep disordered breathing in group 1 pulmonary arterial hypertension. J Clin Sleep Med. 2014;10:277–83.
31. Javaheri S, Javaheri S, Javaheri A. Sleep apnea, heart failure, and pulmonary hypertension. Curr Heart Fail Rep. 2013;10(4):315–20.
32. Botros N, Concato J, Mohsenin V, Selim B, Doctor K, Yaggi HK. Obstructive sleep apnea as a risk factor for type 2 diabetes. Am J Med. 2009;122(12):1122–7.
33. Punjabi NM, Shahar E, Redline S, Gottlieb DJ, Givelber R, Resnick HE, Sleep Heart Health Study Investigators. Sleep-disordered breathing, glucose intolerance, and insulin resistance: the sleep heart health study. Am J Epidemiol. 2004;160(6):521–30.
34. Kendzerska T, Gershon AS, Hawker G, Tomlinson G, Leung RS. Obstructive sleep apnea and incident diabetes. A historical cohort study. Am J Respir Crit Care Med. 2014;190(2):218–25.
35. Cakmak E, Duksal F, Altinkaya E, Acibucu F, Dogan OT, Yonem O, Yilmaz A. Association between the severity of nocturnal hypoxia in obstructive sleep apnea and non-alcoholic fatty liver damage. Hepat Mon. 2015;15(11):e32655.
36. Corey KE, Misdraji J, Gelrud L, et al. Obstructive sleep apnea is associated with nonalcoholic steatohepatitis and advanced liver histology. Dig Dis Sci. 2015;60(8):2523–8.
37. Musso G, Cassader M, Olivetti C, et al. Association of obstructive sleep apnoea with the presence and severity of non-alcoholic fatty liver disease. A systematic review and meta-analysis. Obes Rev. 2013;14(5):417–31.
38. Agrawal S, Duseja A, Aggarwal A, et al. Obstructive sleep apnea is an important predictor of hepatic fibrosis in patients with nonalcoholic fatty liver disease in a tertiary care center. Hepatol Int. 2015;9(2):283–91.
39. Krolow GK, Garcia E, Schoor F, Araujo FBS, Coral GP. Obstructive sleep apnea and severity of nonalcoholic fatty liver disease. Eur J Gastroenterol Hepatol. 2021;33(8):1104–9.
40. Nobili V, Cutrera R, Liccardo D, et al. Obstructive sleep apnea syndrome affects liver histology and inflammatory cell activation in pediatric nonalcoholic fatty liver disease, regardless of obesity/insulin resistance. Am J Respir Crit Care Med. 2014;189(1):66–76.
41. Aron-Wisnewsky J, Minville C, Tordjman J, Lévy P, Bouillot JL, Basdevant A, Bedossa P, Clément K, Pépin JL. Chronic intermittent hypoxia is a major trigger for non-alcoholic fatty liver disease in morbid obese. J Hepatol. 2012;56(1):225–33.
42. Wijarnpreecha K, Aby ES, Ahmed A, Kim D. Evaluation and management of extrahepatic manifestations of nonalcoholic fatty liver disease. Clin Mol Hepatol. 2021;27(2):221–35.
43. Melaku YA, Reynolds AC, Appleton S, Sweetman A, Shi Z, Vakulin A, Catcheside P, Eckert DJ, Adams R. High-quality and anti-inflammatory diets and a healthy lifestyle are associated with lower sleep apnea risk. J Clin Sleep Med. 2022;18(6):1667–79.

44. Umbro I, Fabiani V, Fabiani M, Angelico F, Del Ben M. Association between non-alcoholic fatty liver disease and obstructive sleep apnea. World J Gastroenterol. 2020;26(20):2669–81.
45. Chen X, Lin X, Chen LD, Lin QC, Chen GP, Yu YH, Huang JC, Zhao JM. Obstructive sleep apnea is associated with fatty liver index, the index of nonalcoholic fatty liver disease. Eur J Gastroenterol Hepatol. 2016;28:650–5.
46. Kim D, Ahmed A, Kushida C. Continuous positive airway pressure therapy on nonalcoholic fatty liver disease in patients with obstructive sleep apnea. J Clin Sleep Med. 2018;14:1315–22.
47. Buttacavoli M, Gruttad'Auria CI, Olivo M, Virdone R, Castrogiovanni A, Mazzuca E, Marotta AM, Marrone O, Madonia S, Bonsignore MR. Liver steatosis and fibrosis in OSA patients after long-term CPAP treatment: a preliminary ultrasound study. Ultrasound Med Biol. 2016;42:104–9.
48. Ng SSS, Wong VWS, Wong GLH, Chu WCW, Chan TO, To KW, Ko FWS, Chan KP, Hui DS. Continuous positive airway pressure does not improve nonalcoholic fatty liver disease in patients with obstructive sleep apnea. A randomized clinical trial. Am J Respir Crit Care Med. 2021;203(4):493–501.
49. Randerath W, de Lange J, Hedner J, Ho JPTF, Marklund M, Schiza S, Steier J, Verbraecken J. Current and novel treatment options for obstructive sleep apnoea. ERJ Open Res. 2022;8(2):00126–2022.
50. Blackman A, Foster GD, Zammit G, Rosenberg R, Aronne L, Wadden T, et al. Effect of liraglutide 3.0 mg in individuals with obesity and moderate or severe obstructive sleep apnea: the SCALE sleep apnea randomized clinical trial. Int J Obes. 2016;40(8):1310–9.
51. Currie AC, Kaur V, Carey I, Al-Rubaye H, Mahawar K, Madhok B, Small P, McGlone ER, Khan OA. Obstructive sleep apnea remission following bariatric surgery: a national registry cohort study. Surg Obes Relat Dis. 2021;17(9):1576–82.

Nonalcoholic Fatty Liver Disease and Psoriasis

20

Laura Huiban, Anca Trifan, and Carol Stanciu

20.1 Introduction

Nonalcoholic fatty liver disease (NAFLD) is a complex and multifactorial syndrome with a broad range of hepatic manifestations, from simple hepatic steatosis to the more severe steatohepatitis which could lead to liver fibrosis and cirrhosis [1, 2]. The main pathogenic route that determines the suitable premises for NAFLD development includes visceral obesity, metabolic syndrome, systemic inflammation, and insulin resistance, all of which were also identified as significant risk factors to exacerbate psoriasis [3, 4]. Moreover, the prevalence of NAFLD in psoriatic patients and of psoriasis in NAFLD patients previously reported by numerous studies suggested a bidirectional relationship between these two pathological conditions [5–9].

20.2 Definitions, Epidemiology, and Clinical Presentation of NAFLD in Psoriasis

NAFLD is currently defined as the excessive triglyceride accumulation in the hepatocytes that is not mediated by alcohol consumption or other specific factors (heredity, acquired metabolic imbalance, steatosis-facilitating medication) [10]. NAFLD is a chronic progressive pathological condition characterized by different stages, from simple hepatic steatosis to inflammatory-mediated steatohepatitis (NASH), and that could further worsen to liver fibrosis, cirrhotic processes, liver failure, and

L. Huiban (✉) · A. Trifan · C. Stanciu
Gastroenterology Department, Grigore T. Popa University of Medicine and Pharmacy, Iasi, Romania

Institute of Gastroenterology and Hepatology, St. Spiridon Emergency Hospital, Iasi, Romania

© The Author(s), under exclusive license to Springer Nature Switzerland AG 2023
A. Trifan et al. (eds.), *Essentials of Non-Alcoholic Fatty Liver Disease*,
https://doi.org/10.1007/978-3-031-33548-8_20

hepatocellular carcinoma, as the vicious cycle within the metabolic and inflammatory interaction gains magnitude and complexity [11–13].

The more recent studies considered that NAFLD could be the hepatic manifestation of metabolic syndrome [14–16]. However, the emerging obesity-independent factors leading to NAFLD also associating it with several new pathological conditions (such as psoriasis, osteoporosis, endocrinopathies, sleep apnea, and colorectal cancer) suggested that NAFLD could be the result of a much more complex interaction between pathological causes and favorable premises [17–19] (Fig. 20.1). One particular pathological mechanism was reported to trigger the development of NAFLD–psoriasis-mediated inflammation.

The prevalence of NAFLD is that high in the general population that some consider it a modern epidemic [20–23]. Recent epidemiological studies reported that up to 37% of adults and 10% of children of the general population are affected by NAFLD despite that the diagnosis rate remains lower due to the asymptomatic clinical presentation of the stages not characterized by hepatic inflammation [24, 25]. Also, NAFLD increases the mortality rates in general population by adding 5–7 deaths per 1000 person-years [4]. Approximately 3–10% of the NAFLD adult and rarely children cases progress to NASH and cirrhosis, but most of the deaths are associated with major cardiovascular events [10]. Similar to cardiovascular risk, the risk associated with the progression from NAFLD to NASH is often seen in one-third of the obese patients and in one-twentieth of the lean patients [25]. It was showed that the prevalence and severity of NAFLD significantly increase by direct correlation to obesity prevalence and severity [25]. However, NAFLD prevalence was showed to vary by relation to age, sex, and ethnicity. A recent report summarized that male sex, older age, and Latin American ethnicity seem to increase NAFLD prevalence [26, 27]. Despite the lesser prevalence in Caucasian population (39%, as compared to 83% in Latin Americans, as presented by van der Voort [26]), Klujszo et al. [27] and Bellinato et al. [28] commented that NAFLD is the most frequent liver pathology in the Western countries affecting up to 46% of the population. According to recent reports, up to 70% of type 2 diabetic patients [28],

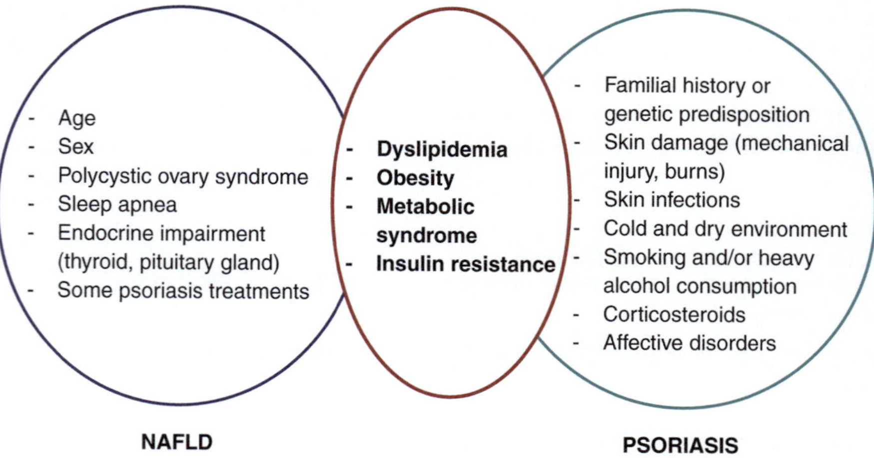

Fig. 20.1 Independent and shared risk factors of NAFLD and psoriasis

up to 65% of obese patients affected by metabolic syndrome, and up to 50% of dyslipidemic patients are also diagnosed with NAFLD [29]. Moreover, due to their partly shared pathophysiology, NAFLD was found to affect more than 40% of the young psoriatic patients and up to 70% of the older ones, as two strong predictors of NAFLD were psoriasis and metabolic syndrome, according to a prospective population-based cohort study conducted in Rotterdam [30].

Psoriasis was originally defined as an inflammatory skin condition characterized by epidermal hyperproliferation, aberrant keratinocyte differentiation, and angiogenesis, in an autoimmune mediation context [31]. However, the more recent studies that focused on psoriatic comorbidities suggested that psoriasis could be a complex multisystemic disease that is mainly affecting keratinocyte functions and of which abnormal inflammatory modulation leads to low-grade chronic systemic inflammation easily transferred to the other organs [32–34]. It was showed that keratinocyte-mediated inflammation could lead to arthropathy, uveitis, inflammatory bowel diseases, and metabolic syndrome, all of which were previously documented as frequent psoriatic comorbid conditions [35, 36]. Interestingly, a similar potentiating effect was showed for the steatohepatitis-mediated inflammation that could determine keratinocyte proliferation, often observed in psoriasis [35].

Just as in NAFLD case, obesity, diabetes, and stress are thought to contribute to the risk of developing psoriasis, while the latter is thought to increase the risk for autoimmune and inflammatory conditions, such as cardiovascular diseases [37]. Also, the prevalence correlational studies showed that NAFLD could increase the severity and duration of skin psoriatic outbreaks and predispose to diabetes, severe liver conditions, and multiple sclerosis [38], despite that psoriasis prevalence in general population is relatively low (up to 2–3% of the world population), as compared to NAFLD prevalence. Of all, the most relevant association was established between psoriasis and NAFLD, as Gandha et al. confirmed that they are directly associated, as suggested by the significant correlation between liver steatosis stage and psoriatic skin surface area and severity [39]. Moreover, Roberts et al. showed that psoriatic patients with NAFLD seem to progress to more severe hepatic damage [3].

20.3 Diagnosis of NAFLD in Psoriasis

Psoriasis is clinically presented as clearly edged variable areas of skin surfaces covered by erythematous plaques and silvery-white scales that are identified mostly on the scalp, elbows, knees, and umbilical and lumbar areas [35]. Despite the apparent pure dermatological picture, psoriasis was described as a multisystemic disease of inflammatory etiology. The biochemical assessment of the psoriatic patients' serum could reveal altered lipid and glucose metabolism, increase of transaminases, and sustained inflammatory state [35]. These profiles are usually the ones that notify the dermatologist of possible NAFLD comorbidity in psoriatic patients, as some of the mentioned changes were also reported in NAFLD.

The sustained yet low-magnitude inflammatory state promoted by pro-inflammatory cytokines' presence was confirmed in both NAFLD and psoriatic patients. However, psoriasis was found to cause significantly more severe hepatic manifestations of NAFLD, while the risk for severe liver fibrosis could be higher in patients affected by both psoriasis and NAFLD [40], while more severe psoriatic skin lesions were reported in NAFLD patients [41]. All these observations led to the psoriasis–NAFLD pathophysiological interaction hypothesis based on the hepato-dermal axis [42].

NAFLD is often asymptomatic unless the hepatic damage causes significant clinical manifestation or abdominal tenderness upon palpation. Some of the NAFLD patients may exhibit nonspecific clinical manifestations, such as fatigue and abdominal pain [43]. Most of the asymptomatic NAFLD cases are initially diagnosed during routine blood work or imaging screening. Routine liver function test results could be mildly modified and that is often the NAFLD diagnosis initiation. Aspartate aminotransferase (AST) and alanine aminotransferase (ALT) serum levels are occasionally increased, without exceeding 3–5 normal values, while AST/ALT ratio remains greater than 1. γ-Glutamyl transferase (GGT) serum concentrations are increased in most cases. High alkaline phosphatase serum concentrations, dyslipidemic profiles, elevated serum total bilirubin, and decreased serum albumin levels are also reported in NAFLD [29], but the biochemical assessment is not decisive since it could not be modified in up to two-thirds of the NAFLD patients [43].

Despite that liver imaging (ultrasonography, computerized tomography, or magnetic resonance imaging) is not able to differentiate between steatosis and inflammation or indicate the presence of fibrosis, it reveals that 5–30% of the hepatic tissues are steatotic [44, 45]. Fibrosis presence—usually indicating NASH—requires liver assessment through vibration-controlled transient elastography or magnetic resonance elastography and liver biopsy, the gold standard in diagnosis, but extremely invasive and potentially damaging [29, 46]. Thus, the lesser harmful method of the NAFLD fibrosis scores is preferred [29, 47, 48] (Table 20.1).

Table 20.1 Diagnosis chart of NAFLD [27, 29, 35, 40]

Component	Characteristics
Associated risks	Type 2 diabetes, metabolic syndrome, obesity, psoriasis
Clinical symptoms	Mainly asymptomatic Rarely abdominal tenderness upon palpation (in severe cases) Nonspecific symptoms, such as fatigue and abdominal pain
Blood	↑ AST, ALT (<3–5 × normal ranges); AST/ALT >1 ↑ ALP, GGT; ↑ total bilirubin; ↑ serum albumin Dyslipidemic profiles, elevated serum total bilirubin, and decreased serum albumin levels
Imaging	5–30% of the liver tissues affected by steatosis
Liver elastography	Liver fibrosis (indicating progression to NASH)
Liver biopsy	Gold standard in diagnosis; confirmation of NAFLD for all stages and complications
Fibrosis-4 index	= Age (year) × AST (U/L)/[PLT (109/L) × ALT ½ (U/L)]
NAFLD fibrosis score	= −1.675 + 0.037 × age (year) + 0.094 × BMI (kg/m^2) + 1.13 × glucose intolerance (yes = 1, no = 0) + 0.99 × AST/ALT − 0.013 × platelet count (10^9/L) − 0.66 × albumin (g/dL)

20.4 Pathophysiology of NAFLD in Psoriasis

The pathophysiological mechanisms underlying NAFLD development and progression have long been discussed and debated. Though NAFLD is currently considered a multilayered, multifactorial, and possibly multisystemic disease, the latest advance in this domain supported the previous description of this disease as being the hepatic manifestation of metabolic syndrome [49–53]. Aresse et al. discussed the increased heterogeneity of NAFLD-affected population and concluded that a multitude of factors including genetic predisposition, physiologic, and environmental factors could variably contribute to NAFLD development and progression, thus determining many clinically different phenotypical variants [52]. Many of the NAFLD patients are affected by different stages of obesity. However, a particular NAFLD patient group, namely "lean NAFLD" patients, has normal body index, but increased systemic inflammation suggesting that the adipokine-mediated pathway could not be the sole player in NAFLD progression to NASH [9, 53]. These pathophysiological aspects are mainly contributing to treatment options and to understanding how NAFLD pathophysiology is associated with other chronic conditions in a comorbid way.

Despite that some disagreements and gaps regarding the NAFLD pathophysiology remain, it is generally accepted that the multicomponent pathomechanisms include the unbalance in metabolic homeostasis and subsequent adipose tissue-mediated inflammation. As previously stated, the development and progression of metabolic syndrome with its different phenotypes (diabetes, dyslipidemia, obesity, or other comorbid conditions) lead to abdominal fat tissue accumulation, which could provide sufficient background for hepatic steatosis. Insulin resistance, promoting hepatic inflammation by increased pro-inflammatory cytokine release, leads to significant adipose lipolysis that generates free fatty acid efflux mediating macrophage recruitment and hepatic de novo lipogenesis, both of which are demonstrated to promote interconnected liver steatosis and inflammation [8, 54]. Additionally, the steatotic liver is furthermore vulnerable to oxidative stress (lipid peroxidation) and inflammation-mediated hepatic injury (apoptosis, necrosis, fibrosis, and ultimately cirrhosis) mediated by mitochondrial dysfunction, profibrogenic pathway, and hepatic stellate cell activation [25, 40]. Notwithstanding, recent studies on the pathogenesis of NAFLD suggested that it could be a much complex mechanism than previously thought and acknowledged by the previously described "two-hit" hypothesis [31]. At least, a multiple-component NAFLD pathogenesis could explain the complex interactions between NAFLD and other pathological states with which it shares significant pathogenic factors.

Psoriasis is mainly developing based on altered skin immunity leading to sustained, self-amplifying inflammatory signaling that promotes aberrant keratinocyte proliferation and differentiation. The main inflammatory response pathways that are impaired in psoriatic skin are associated with IL-17/IL-23-, IL-22-, and TNF-α-mediated T-helper lymphocyte activity [9]. It is believed that alongside keratinocyte stimulation, the pro-inflammatory state promoted by adipocyte accumulation could trigger and sustain chronic systemic inflammation mediated by IL-17 via keratinocyte activation [3, 35]. Consequently, a molecular cascade triggered by dendritic cell, T lymphocyte, macrophage, and neutrophil activation leads to IL-17 secretion.

Similar inflammatory mediation was also observed in NAFLD due to the visceral adipose tissues' potential to modulate interleukin-mediated inflammatory response. It was previously shown that pro-inflammatory T-helper 17 axis could be implicated in both NAFLD and psoriasis pathomechanisms, as well as in obesity, diabetes, and atherosclerosis. In liver, Th-17 was tied to NAFLD progression to NASH, as IL-17 mediates hepatic stellate cell activation and collagen production [55]. Other cytokines implicated in inflammation modulation in both NAFLD and psoriasis are IL-1, IL-2, and IL-6 [56].

Hepatic inflammation, hepatocyte apoptosis, and necrosis are also mediated by adipokines and their imbalanced secretion. Adipokines are cytokines mainly secreted by the white adipose tissues and control adipose tissue formation and local and hepatic lipid metabolism. In this way, psoriatic skin-derived TNF-α and IL-17 could induce hepatic inflammation and trigger insulin resistance and fibrogenesis, while pro-inflammatory signals originating in the inflamed liver could worsen the psoriatic skin manifestations [42].

In contrast to keratinocyte-mediated immune cell activation, the secretory functions of adipocytes produce abnormally elevated levels of TNF-α and leptin, often in response to increased hepatic free saturated fatty acid content, which causes hepatocyte necrosis and apoptosis. The implication of the free fatty acids released from the abnormal adipocytes was previously tied to psoriasis development and severity. Additionally, it was showed that both NAFLD and psoriatic patients exhibit decreased adiponectin levels, suggesting that not only the adipose tissue promotes inflammatory response, but also the balance between inflammatory and anti-inflammatory cytokines is not maintained [35].

The interplay between psoriatic skin and steatotic liver in terms of immune mediation was previously described as the hepato-dermal axis and partly explains the direct two-way communication between these two pathological conditions and their shared pathogenesis [42] (Fig. 20.2). This could also explain why several biological agents against NAFLD offer positive response in psoriatic patients (IL-17 and IL-23 antagonists).

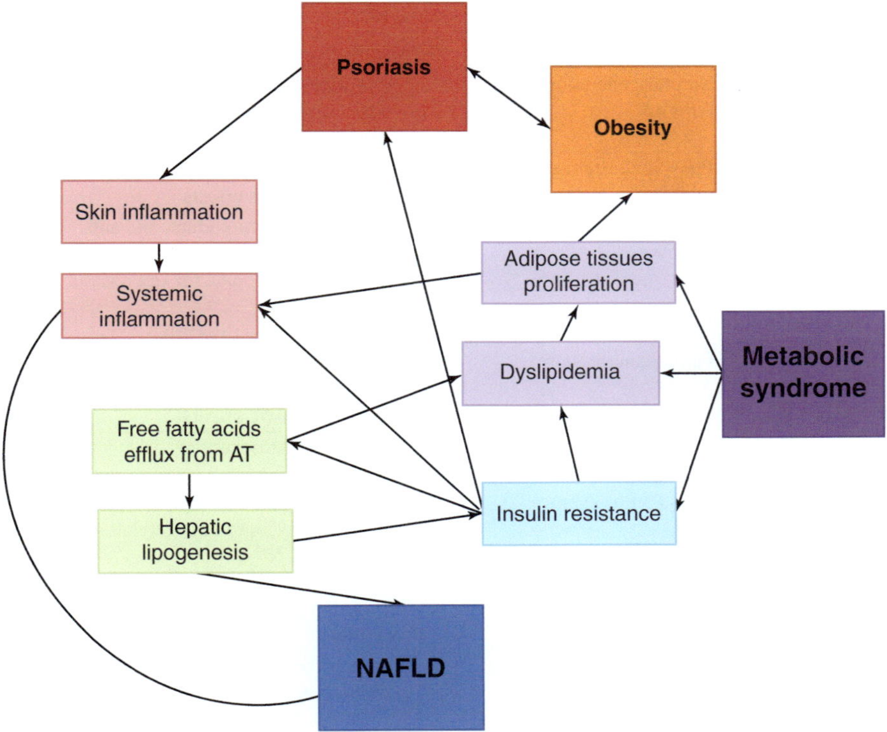

Fig. 20.2 Shared pathophysiology mechanisms of NAFLD and psoriasis

20.5   Management of NAFLD in Psoriasis

In general, NAFLD treatment narrows down to changes in lifestyle and diet, as no current drug can provide complete remission (Table 20.2). Liver fat accumulation limitation, weight loss, and specifically treating metabolic syndrome-associated comorbidities are the main solutions for NAFLD management. Also, the measures to reduce oxidative stress, mitochondrial dysfunction, and insulin resistance could slow down NAFLD progression to NASH. Physical exercise was demonstrated to show significant potential in decreasing hepatic lipid accumulation, systemic and local oxidative stress, and hepatic inflammation. While fructose was previously reported as an important promoter of hepatic fat accumulation by disrupting the intestinal barrier, it must be avoided in NAFLD. On the contrary, vitamin D, vitamin E, and omega-3 fatty acid supplementation could bring significant benefits in NAFLD patient management [20, 57].

Table 20.2 Hepatic effects of drugs used in psoriasis treatment [9, 27, 28]

Drug	Anti-psoriatic effects	Hepatic effects
Acitretin	Second-generation retinoid	– Improves insulin resistance – Rare, altered liver enzyme activity – Hyperlipidemia
Apremilast	Phosphodiesterase-4 inhibitor	– Improves glucose and lipid metabolism – No hepatotoxic effects
Cyclosporine	Polypeptide calcineurin inhibitor	– Antifibrotic, antioxidant, and anti-inflammatory effects – Potentiates adiponectin and resistin activities – Potentially hyperlipidemia
Dimethyl fumarate	Fumaric acid ester	– Antifibrotic, antioxidant, and anti-inflammatory effects – No hepatotoxic effects
Methotrexate	Dihydrofolate reductase inhibitor	– Highly hepatotoxic
Adalimumab	Anti-TNF-α agent	– Improves GGT activity – Reduces glycoprotein acetylation, CRP, IL-6, and TNF-α – No hepatotoxic effects – Protective against liver fibrosis development
Etanercept	Anti-TNF-α agent	– Antioxidant and anti-inflammatory properties – Hepatoprotective (normalizes transaminase levels) – Glucose metabolism improvement – Pro-inflammatory adipokine inhibition – Protective against liver fibrosis development
Infliximab	Anti-TNF-α agent	– Adiponectin and IL-6 activities' potentiation – Could cause autoimmune hepatitis responsive to steroid treatment – Increases BMI and body weight
Secukinumab	Anti-IL-17	– Systemic inflammation reduction – Antioxidant effects – No hepatotoxic effects
Ustekinumab	Anti-IL-12/23	– Alters liver function (increased transaminase serum levels) – Potent inhibitor of TNF-α, IL-1b, IL-17a, and IL-6

In psoriatic patients, NAFLD must be treated according to the general guidelines, while some specific medication for psoriasis must be used with extreme caution due to hepatotoxic potential. Apremilast, acitretin, dimethyl fumarate, and most of the biological agents are well tolerated due to their decreased hepatotoxicity, while methotrexate, cyclosporin, and acitretin must be avoided in NAFLD and psoriasis patients or in psoriasis patients that exhibit increased risk for NAFLD development due to their potential to trigger or worsen NAFLD-dependent or -independent liver injury [3, 9, 58–63]. However, at least cyclosporine and dimethyl fumarate hepatotoxic effects were demonstrated as being transitory and reversible and only mildly affecting liver enzyme activity. On the other hand, cyclosporin and acitretin could induce hyperlipidemia, thus facilitating hepatic steatosis. Etanercept, infliximab, and adalimumab were reported to increase body weight and body mass index and should be used with caution in psoriasis patients predisposed to or affected by NAFLD [64].

Recently, several psoriasis-specific treatments were showed to address the shared pathophysiological mechanisms, and current efforts are made to evaluate their potential benefits against hepatic steatosis and in preventing the progression to NASH. The non-biological agents used in psoriasis treatment were showed to potentially modulate insulin resistance (acitretin) and glucose and lipid metabolism (apremilast) and to exhibit antifibrotic, antioxidant, and anti-inflammatory effects (cyclosporin and dimethyl fumarate) [65–68]. Nevertheless, some of the biological agents (TNF-α inhibitors) could be used to prevent liver fibrosis. Of all, ustekinumab was reported to exhibit considerable anti-inflammatory effects acting as a potent inhibitor of TNF-α, IL-1b, IL-17a, and IL-6 [9].

20.6 Conclusions

NAFLD and psoriasis are two apparently very distinct pathological conditions that are related to metabolic syndrome, insulin resistance, and chronic low-grade systemic inflammation. However, the link between them seems not entirely understood and could be the result of a multifactorial interaction involving the hepato-dermal axis. The management of NAFLD and psoriasis is rather complex, especially when they co-occur. The treatment for psoriasis should be carefully administered to NAFLD-diagnosed or -predisposed patients, while it was demonstrated that some of the common biological agents used in psoriasis treatment could be useful in NAFLD cases with promising results.

References

1. Watanabe S, Hashimoto E, Ikejima K, et al. Evidence-based clinical practice guidelines for nonalcoholic fatty liver disease/nonalcoholic steatohepatitis. J Gastroenterol. 2015;50:364–77. https://doi.org/10.1007/s00535-015-1050-7.
2. Huby T, Gautier EL. Immune cell-mediated features of non-alcoholic steatohepatitis. Nat Rev Immunol. 2022;22:429–43. https://doi.org/10.1038/s41577-021-00639-3.
3. Belinchón-Romero I, Bellot P, Romero-Pérez D, et al. Non-alcoholic fatty liver disease is associated with bacterial translocation and a higher inflammation response in psoriatic patients. Sci Rep. 2021;11:8593. https://doi.org/10.1038/s41598-021-88043-8.
4. Gau SY, Huang KH, Lee CH, Kuan YH, Tsai TH, Lee CY. Bidirectional association between psoriasis and nonalcoholic fatty liver disease: real-world evidence from two longitudinal cohort studies. Front Immunol. 2022;13:840106.

5. Roberts KK, Cochet AE, Lamb PB, Brown PJ, Battafarano DF, Brunt EM, Harrison SA. The prevalence of NAFLD and NASH among patients with psoriasis in a tertiary care dermatology and rheumatology clinic. Aliment Pharmacol Ther. 2015;41(3):293–300. https://doi.org/10.1111/apt.13042.

6. Gaspari C, Carvalho G, Anjos L, et al. FRI0453 the increased prevalence of NAFLD is worrisome among patients with psoriatic arthritis. Ann Rheum Dis. 2016;75:600.

7. Li AA, Ahmed A, Kim D. Extrahepatic manifestations of nonalcoholic fatty liver disease. Gut and Liver. 2020;14:168–78. https://doi.org/10.5009/gnl19069.

8. Soto-Angona Ó, Anmella G, Valdés-Florido MJ, et al. Non-alcoholic fatty liver disease (NAFLD) as a neglected metabolic companion of psychiatric disorders: common pathways and future approaches. BMC Med. 2020;18:261. https://doi.org/10.1186/s12916-020-01713-8.

9. Balak DMW, Piaserico S, Kasujee I. Non-alcoholic fatty liver disease (NAFLD) in patients with psoriasis: a review of the hepatic effects of systemic therapies. Psoriasis (Auckl). 2021;7(11):151–68. https://doi.org/10.2147/PTT.S342911.

10. Smith BW, Adams LA. Non-alcoholic fatty liver disease. Crit Rev Clin Lab Sci. 2011;48(3):97–113.

11. Carr RM, Oranu A, Khungar V. Nonalcoholic fatty liver disease: pathophysiology and management. Gastroenterol Clin N Am. 2016;45(4):639–52. https://doi.org/10.1016/j.gtc.2016.07.003.

12. Kořínková L, Pražienková V, Černá L, Karnošová A, Železná B, Kuneš J, Maletínská L. Pathophysiology of NAFLD and NASH in experimental models: the role of food intake regulating peptides. Front Endocrinol. 2020;11:597583. https://doi.org/10.3389/fendo.2020.597583.

13. Pouwels S, Sakran N, Graham Y, et al. Non-alcoholic fatty liver disease (NAFLD): a review of pathophysiology, clinical management and effects of weight loss. BMC Endocr Disord. 2022;22:63. https://doi.org/10.1186/s12902-022-00980-1.

14. Kim CH, Younossi ZM. Nonalcoholic fatty liver disease: a manifestation of the metabolic syndrome. Cleve Clin J Med. 2008;75(10):721–8. https://doi.org/10.3949/ccjm.75.10.721.

15. Paschos P, Paletas K. Nonalcoholic fatty liver disease and metabolic syndrome. Hippokratia. 2009;13(1):9–19.

16. Godoy-Matos AF, Silva Júnior WS, Valerio CM. NAFLD as a continuum: from obesity to metabolic syndrome and diabetes. Diabetol Metab Syndr. 2020;12:60. https://doi.org/10.1186/s13098-020-00570-y.

17. Della PG, Vetrani C, Brancato V, et al. Effects of a multifactorial ecosustainable isocaloric diet on liver fat in patients with type 2 diabetes: randomized clinical trial. BMJ Open Diabetes Res Care. 2020;8:e001342. https://doi.org/10.1136/bmjdrc-2020-001342.

18. Aamir B, Ajay D, Arka D, Manu M, Pramil T. Non-alcoholic fatty liver disease development: a multifactorial pathogenic phenomena. Liver Res. 2022;6(2):72–83. https://doi.org/10.1016/j.livres.2022.05.002.

19. Sharma D, Mandal P. NAFLD: genetics and its clinical implications. Clin Res Hepatol Gastroenterol. 2022;46(9):102003. https://doi.org/10.1016/j.clinre.2022.102003.

20. Hassen G, Singh A, Belete G, Jain N, De la Hoz I, Camacho-Leon GP, Dargie NK, Carrera KG, Alemu T, Jhaveri S, Solomon N. Nonalcoholic fatty liver disease: an emerging modern-day risk factor for cardiovascular disease. Cureus. 2022;14(5):e25495. https://doi.org/10.7759/cureus.25495.

21. Perumpail BJ, Khan MA, Yoo ER, Cholankeril G, Kim D, Ahmed A. Clinical epidemiology and disease burden of nonalcoholic fatty liver disease. World J Gastroenterol. 2017;23(47):8263–76. https://doi.org/10.3748/wjg.v23.i47.8263.

22. Sherif ZA. The rise in the prevalence of nonalcoholic fatty liver disease and hepatocellular carcinoma. In: Nonalcoholic fatty liver disease—an update. London: IntechOpen; 2019. https://doi.org/10.5772/intechopen.85780.

23. Vernon G, Baranova A, Younossi ZM. Systematic review: the epidemiology and natural history of non-alcoholic fatty liver disease and non-alcoholic steatohepatitis in adults. Aliment Pharmacol Ther. 2011;34:274–85. https://doi.org/10.1111/j.1365-2036.2011.04724.x.

24. Li J, Zou B, Yeo YH, Feng Y, Xie X, Lee DH, et al. Prevalence, incidence, and outcome of non-alcoholic fatty liver disease in Asia, 1999–2019: a systematic review and meta-analysis. Lancet Gastroenterol Hepatol. 2019;4(5):389–98. https://doi.org/10.1016/S2468-1253(19)30039-1.
25. Prussick R, Prussick C, Nussbaum A. Nonalcoholic fatty liver disease and psoriasis what a dermatologist needs to know. J Clin Aesthet Dermatol. 2015;8(3):43–5.
26. Van der Voort EA, Koehler EM, Dowlatshahi EA, Hofman A, Stricker BH, Janssen HL, et al. Psoriasis is independently associated with nonalcoholic fatty liver disease in patients 55 years old or older: results from a population-based study. J Am Acad Dermatol. 2014;70:517–24.
27. Klujszo E, Parcheta A, Witkowska AB, Krecisz B. Non-alcoholic fatty liver disease in patients with psoriasis: therapeutic implications. Adv Dermatol Allergol. 2020;37(4):468–74. https://doi.org/10.5114/ada.2019.83983.
28. Bellinato F, Gisondi F, Mantovani A, Girolomoni G, Targher G. Risk of non-alcoholic fatty liver disease in patients with chronic plaque psoriasis: an updated systematic review and meta-analysis of observational studies. J Endocrinol Investig. 2022;45:1277–88. https://doi.org/10.1007/s40618-022-01755-0.
29. Carrascosa JM, Bonanad C, Dauden E, Botella R, Olveira-Martín A. en nombre del Grupo de Trabajo en Inflamación Sistémica en Psoriasis. Psoriasis e hígado graso no alcohólico. Actas Dermosifiliogr. 2017;108:506–14.
30. van der Voort EA, Koehler EM, Nijsten T, Stricker BH, Hofman A, Janssen HL, et al. Increased prevalence of advanced liver fibrosis in patients with psoriasis: a cross-sectional analysis from the Rotterdam study. Acta Derm Venereol. 2016;96:213–7.
31. Raharja A, Mahil SK, Barker JN. Psoriasis: a brief overview. Clin Med (Lond). 2021;21(3):170–3. https://doi.org/10.7861/clinmed.2021-0257.
32. Oliveira Mde F, Rocha Bde O, Duarte GV. Psoriasis: classical and emerging comorbidities. An Bras Dermatol. 2015;90(1):9–20. https://doi.org/10.1590/abd1806-4841.20153038.
33. Yamamoto T. Psoriasis and connective tissue diseases. Int J Mol Sci. 2020;21(16):5803. https://doi.org/10.3390/ijms21165803.
34. Tashiro T, Sawada Y. Psoriasis and systemic inflammatory disorders. Int J Mol Sci. 2022;23(8):4457. https://doi.org/10.3390/ijms23084457.
35. Ganzetti G, Campanati A, Offidani A. Non-alcoholic fatty liver disease and psoriasis: so far, so near. World J Hepatol. 2015;7(3):315–26. https://doi.org/10.4254/wjh.v7.i3.315.
36. Boehncke WH, Boehncke S. More than skin-deep: the many dimensions of the psoriatic disease. Swiss Med Wkly. 2014;144:w13968. https://doi.org/10.4414/smw.2014.13968.
37. Torres T, Bettencourt N. Psoriasis: the visible killer. Rev Port Cardiol. 2014;33:95–9.
38. Madanagobalane S, Anandan S. The increased prevalence of non-alcoholic fatty liver disease in psoriatic patients: a study from South India. Australas J Dermatol. 2012;53(3):190–7. https://doi.org/10.1111/j.1440-0960.2012.00905.x.
39. Gandha N, Wibawa LP, Jacoeb TNA, Sulaiman AS. Correlation between psoriasis severity and nonalcoholic fatty liver disease degree measured using controlled attenuation parameter. Psoriasis (Auckl). 2020;20(10):39–44. https://doi.org/10.2147/PTT.S272286.
40. Prussick RB, Miele L. Nonalcoholic fatty liver disease in patients with psoriasis: a consequence of systemic inflammatory burden? Br J Dermatol. 2018;179:16–29. https://doi.org/10.1111/bjd.16239.
41. Heitmann J, Frings VG, Geier A, Goebeler M, Kerstan A. Non-alcoholic fatty liver disease and psoriasis—is there a shared proinflammatory network? JDDG J Dtsch Dermatol Ges. 2021;19:517–28. https://doi.org/10.1111/ddg.14425.
42. Mantovani A, Gisondi P, Lonardo A, Targher G. Relationship between non-alcoholic fatty liver disease and psoriasis: a novel hepato-dermal axis? Int J Mol Sci. 2016;17:217.
43. Dowman JK, Tomlinson JW, Newsome PN. Systematic review: the diagnosis and staging of non-alcoholic fatty liver disease and non-alcoholic steatohepatitis. Ailment Pharmacol Ther. 2011;33(5):525–40.
44. Cobbold JFL, Patel D, Taylor-Robinson SD. Assessment of inflammation and fibrosis in non-alcoholic fatty liver disease by imaging-based techniques. J Gastroenterol Hepatol. 2012;27:1281–92. https://doi.org/10.1111/j.1440-1746.2012.07127.x.

45. Adori C, Daraio T, Kuiper R, Barde S, Horvathova L, Yoshitake T, Ihnatko R, Valladolid-Acebes I, Vercruysse P, Wellendorf AM, Gramignoli R, Bozoky B, Kehr J, Theodorsson E, Cancelas JA, Mravec B, Jorns C, Ellis E, Mulder J, Uhlén M, Bark C, Hökfelt T. Disorganization and degeneration of liver sympathetic innervations in nonalcoholic fatty liver disease revealed by 3D imaging. Sci Adv. 2021;7(30):eabg5733. https://doi.org/10.1126/sciadv.

46. Rockey DC, Caldwell SH, Goodman ZD, Nelson RC, Smith AD. Liver biopsy. Hepatology. 2009;49:1017–44.

47. Treeprasertsuk S, Björnsson E, Enders F, Suwanwalaikorn S, Lindor KD. NAFLD fibrosis score: a prognostic predictor for mortality and liver complications among NAFLD patients. World J Gastroenterol. 2013;19(8):1219–29. https://doi.org/10.3748/wjg.v19.i8.1219.

48. Angulo P, Hui JM, Marchesini G, Bugianesi E, George J, Farrell GC, et al. The NAFLD fibrosis score: a noninvasive system that identifies liver fibrosis in patients with NAFLD. Hepatology. 2007;45:846–54.

49. Kotronen A, Yki-Järvinen H. Fatty liver: a novel component of the metabolic syndrome. Arterioscler Thromb Vasc Biol. 2008;28:27–38.

50. Targher G, Tilg H, Byrne CD. Non-alcoholic fatty liver disease: a multisystem disease requiring a multidisciplinary and holistic approach. Lancet Gastroenterol Hepatol. 2021;6(7):578–88. https://doi.org/10.1016/S2468-1253(21)00020-0.

51. Byrne CD, Targher G. NAFLD: a multisystem disease. J Hepatol. 2015;62(1 Suppl):S47–64. https://doi.org/10.1016/j.jhep.2014.12.012.

52. Arrese M, Arab JP, Barrera F, Kaufmann B, Valenti L, Feldstein AE. Insights into nonalcoholic fatty-liver disease heterogeneity. Semin Liver Dis. 2021;41(4):421–34. https://doi.org/10.1055/s-0041-1730927.

53. Young S, Tariq R, Provenza J, et al. Prevalence and profile of nonalcoholic fatty liver disease in lean adults: systematic review and meta-analysis. Hepatol Commun. 2020;4(7):953–72. https://doi.org/10.1002/hep4.1519.

54. Wenk KS, Arrington KC, Ehrlich A. Psoriasis and nonalcoholic fatty liver disease. J Eur Acad Dermatol Venereol. 2011;25:383–91.

55. Takaki A, Kawai D, Yamamoto K. Multiple hits, including oxidative stress, as pathogenesis and treatment target in non-holic steatohepatitis (NASH). Int J Mol Sci. 2013;14(10):20704–28. https://doi.org/10.3390/ijms141020704422.

56. Marra M, Campanati A, Testa R, Sirolla C, Bonfigli AR, Franceschi C, Marchegiani F, Offidani A. Effect of etanercept on insulin sensitivity in nine patients with psoriasis. Int J Immunopathol Pharmacol. 2007;20:731–6.

57. Gallego-Durán R, Cerro-Salido P, Gomez-Gonzalez E, Pareja MJ, Ampuero J, Rico MC, Aznar R, Vilar-Gomez E, Bugianesi E, Crespo J, González-Sánchez FJ, Aparcero R, Moreno I, Soto S, Arias-Loste MT, Abad J, Ranchal I, Andrade RJ, Calleja JL, Pastrana M, Iacono OL, Romero-Gómez M. Imaging biomarkers for steatohepatitis and fibrosis detection in nonalcoholic fatty liver disease. Sci Rep. 2016;6:31421. https://doi.org/10.1038/srep31421.

58. Mazzilli S, Lanna C, Chiaramonte C, et al. Real-life experience of apremilast in psoriasis and arthritis psoriatic patients: preliminary results on metabolic biomarkers. J Dermatol. 2020;47(6):578–82. https://doi.org/10.1111/1346-8138.15293.

59. Roenigk HH, Callen JP, Guzzo CA, et al. Effects of Acitretin on the liver. J Am Acad Dermatol. 1999;41(4):584–8.

60. Michalska-Bańkowska A, Grabarek B, Wcisło-Dziadecka D, et al. The impact of diabetes and metabolic syndromes to the effectiveness of cyclosporine a pharmacotherapy in psoriatic patients. Dermatol Ther. 2019;32(3):e12881. https://doi.org/10.1111/dth.12881.

61. Bacchetti T, Campanati A, Ferretti G, Simonetti O, Liberati G, Offidani AM. Oxidative stress and psoriasis: the effect of antitumour necrosis factor-α inhibitor treatment. Br J Dermatol. 2013;168(5):984–9. https://doi.org/10.1111/bjd.12144.

62. Cooper KD, Voorhees JJ, Fisher GJ, Chan LC, Gupta AK, Baadsgaard O. Effects of cyclosporine on immunologic mechanisms in psoriasis. J Am Acad Dermatol. 1990;23(6–2):1318–28.

63. Nedelcu RI, Balaban M, Turcu G, Brinzea A, Ion DA, Antohe M, Hodorogea A, Calinescu A, Badarau AI, Popp CG, Popp CG, et al. Efficacy of methotrexate as anti-inflammatory and anti-proliferative drug in dermatology: three case reports. Exp Ther Med. 2019;18:905–10.
64. Wu MY, Yu CL, Yang SJ, et al. Change in body weight and body mass index in psoriasis patients receiving biologics: a systematic review and network meta-analysis. J Am Acad Dermatol. 2020;82(1):101–9. https://doi.org/10.1016/j.jaad.2019.07.103.
65. Lanna C, Cesaroni GM, Mazzilli S, et al. Small molecules, big promises: improvement of psoriasis severity and glucidic markers with apremilast: a case report. Diabetes Metab Syndr Obes. 2019;12:2685–8. https://doi.org/10.2147/DMSO.S229549.
66. Lee CS, Li K. A review of acitretin for the treatment of psoriasis. Expert Opin Drug Saf. 2019;8(6):769–79. https://doi.org/10.1517/14740330903393732.
67. Afra TP, Razmi TM, Dogra S. Apremilast in psoriasis and beyond: big hopes on a small molecule. Indian Dermatol Online J. 2019;10(1):1–12. https://doi.org/10.4103/idoj.IDOJ_437_18.
68. Corazza M, Odorici G, Conti A, et al. Dimethyl fumarate treatment for psoriasis in a real-life setting: a multicentric retrospective study. Dermatol Ther. 2021;34(5):e15066. https://doi.org/10.1111/dth.15066.

Current Management and Pipeline Treatment Approaches in NAFLD: Summary of Ongoing RCTs and Future Directions

Cristina Muzica, Anca Trifan, Sebastian Zenovia, Irina Girleanu, Camelia Cojocariu, and Carol Stanciu

21.1 Introduction

Nonalcoholic fatty liver disease (NAFLD) physiopathology relies on the "two-hit theory," which includes liver steatosis as the first "hit," followed by a second "hit" consisting of oxidative stress, abnormal lipid metabolism, and an improper immune response, which induce further injury to hepatocytes, resulting in nonalcoholic steatohepatitis (NASH) [1, 2]. There are several signaling pathways through which NAFLD and NASH occur. Lipid synthesis and lipotoxicity determine an inflammatory response followed by cell death and fibrosis, this process resulting from increased lipid synthesis and uptake in the liver that outpaces lipid oxidation and elimination. In addition to the liver, insulin-sensitive organs like adipose tissue and muscle create adipokines and myokines, which support oxidative stress and inflammation in the liver, respectively. Through the metabolism of pathogen-associated molecular patterns (PAMPs), bile acids, and other compounds, the gut microbiota controls the inflammatory response and hepatic fat buildup. Kupffer cells that are already present in the liver are activated, and leukocytes (such as neutrophils and monocytes) are drawn to the liver as part of innate immune responses related to NAFL/NASH. Another element causing liver inflammation is lymphocyte-mediated adaptive immunity. Extracellular vesicles stimulate immunological cells and hepatic stellate cells, driving inflammation in NAFL/NASH. Lipotoxicity-induced hepatocyte death, which includes apoptosis, necroptosis, pyroptosis, and ferroptosis, is a significant driver in the evolution of NAFL/NASH [3].

C. Muzica (✉) · A. Trifan · S. Zenovia · I. Girleanu · C. Cojocariu · C. Stanciu
Gastroenterology Department, Grigore T. Popa University of Medicine and Pharmacy, Iasi, Romania

Institute of Gastroenterology and Hepatology, St. Spiridon Emergency Hospital, Iasi, Romania

© The Author(s), under exclusive license to Springer Nature Switzerland AG 2023
A. Trifan et al. (eds.), *Essentials of Non-Alcoholic Fatty Liver Disease*,
https://doi.org/10.1007/978-3-031-33548-8_21

Considering the fact that nowadays the treatment of most diseases follows the concept of precision medicine, the treatment of NAFLD and NASH must have therapeutic targets aimed at the interruption of these pathways. The main goal in the management of NAFLD patients is to identify patients at risk for progression to fibrosis and liver cirrhosis and to offer therapeutic intervention. Treatment in NAFLD includes lifestyle changes, pharmacotherapy, and surgery. The sequence of implementation of these treatment methods is established according to the stage of the disease and takes into consideration the patient's preferences, the concept of "empowering the patient" being all the more important in the case of patients with NAFLD since they associate, in most cases, with diabetes mellitus and obesity, with this cluster of diseases being able to significantly affect the quality of life. Hence, the key therapeutic objectives in NAFLD are the lowering of metabolic risk factors and the management of the metabolic syndrome. In NAFLD patients, losing weight and changing one's lifestyle can significantly improve histology outcomes. These therapies are sufficiently beneficial in just 10–20% of patients, and there are several difficulties in adopting them in daily practice [4].

21.2 Lifestyle Changes

In NAFLD patients without fibrosis development, it is generally recommended to start with lifestyle changes which consist of dietary changes, exercise, and weight loss [5]. Thus, lifestyle modifications represent the first-line treatment option. According to several studies, weight loss significantly improves the histological characteristics of NASH, and there is a distinct dose-response relationship. Hepatic steatosis might be improved with weight loss of at least 3–5%, while reducing inflammatory activity requires a 5–7% weight loss; furthermore, it seems that a weight drop of over 10% is associated with the regression of fibrosis [6].

21.2.1 Calorie-Restricted Diet

Based on the results from numerous studies which demonstrated significant benefits in adopting a calorie-restricted diet in NAFLD patients, current guidelines state the importance of introducing a diet-based strategy in the management of these patients [7]. Thus, consuming a diet with fewer calories per day than what is needed for survival, such as the Mediterranean diet, can lower body weight, hepatic lipid accumulation, and insulin resistance as well as increase serum levels of monounsaturated and n-3 polyunsaturated fatty acids and decrease serum levels of saturated fatty acids [8].

The benefits of weight loss and calorie-restricted diets in patients with NAFLD are well demonstrated by robust data. For example, Holmer et al. recently published an open-label randomized controlled trial which included 74 NAFLD patients who were randomly assigned in a 1:1:1 ratio to a 12-week treatment with either a 5:2 diet with intermittent calorie restriction (500 kcal/day for women and 600 kcal/day for men) for two nonconsecutive days per week or a low-carb high-fat diet with an average daily calorie intake of 1600 kcal/day for women and 1900 kcal/day for men. The authors found that findings showed that low-carb high-fat diet and 5:2 diet are both superior to general lifestyle change in terms of reducing hepatic steatosis and body weight [9].

The general recommendations regarding diet in patients with NAFLD which can improve body weight are the following [10]

- To reduce the quantity of sugar by avoiding sweets, processed foods, sugared dairy products, and sugar-sweetened beverages.
- To consume low-fat meat and low-fat dairy products, which will reduce saturated fat and cholesterol.
- To increase n-3 fatty acids by eating fish, walnuts, and olive oil.
- To avoid ultra-processed food.

Another advantage regarding dietary intervention is that it can modify gut microbiota components and enhance the health of NAFLD patients including body weight loss and improved insulin sensitivity [11].

21.2.2 Physical Activity

Recent research has found a link between health-enhancing physical activity and a lower risk of both NAFLD and lean NAFLD in the general population [12]. Health-enhancing physical activity is defined as either vigorous activity at least 3 days per week or seven or more days per week of any combination of walking, moderate, or vigorous activities [12].

By enhancing the phagocytic ability of liver-resident Kupffer cells (KCs) and lowering hepatic inflammation and fibrogenesis, long-term exercise can prevent the development of NASH [13]. Through the activation of the AMP-activated protein kinase (AMPK) and PPARg-coactivator-1 (PGC-1a) signaling pathways, a mouse study found that maternal exercise can reduce Western-style diet (WSD)-induced obesity and enhance hepatic lipid metabolism [14]. In obese adults, exercise-training interventions can also lower blood pressure, insulin resistance, and intrahepatic fat deposition [15]. However, the stress of the workplace and fast meals make changing one's lifestyle extremely difficult or lead to most individuals giving up in the process.

Even though research on the benefits of exercise on NAFLD is still relatively new, experimental and clinical evidence emphasizes the value of exercise, particularly vigorous intensity exercise that significantly lowers intrahepatic lipid content and delays the development of NASH.

21.3 Bariatric Surgery

By limiting food intake, regulating gut hormone release, and correcting metabolic malfunction, bariatric surgery (BS), also known as weight-loss surgery, is thought to be the most effective technique to treat obesity and diabetes [16]. In comparison to standard obesity care, BS can dramatically lower mortality and lengthen life span in persons with obesity, according to a meta-analysis [17]. The change in liver function tests (LFTs) 1 year after surgery shows that the bariatric surgeries sleeve gastrectomy (SG) and Roux-en-Y gastric bypass (RYGB) on NAFLD and NASH are comparably effective [18].

There may be some discrepancies brought on by BS methods, according to other investigations [19, 20]. For instance, a 5-year follow-up study demonstrated that Roux-en-Y gastric bypass has a higher efficacy compared to sleeve gastrectomy in terms of improving weight loss and reducing hypertension, but that there was no difference in the remission of T2DM, obstructive sleep apnea syndrome, or improvement in quality of life [21].

21.4 Pharmacotherapy

According to recent guidelines in NAFLD, pharmacotherapy is considered in patients presenting with progressive forms of NASH, those with early-stage NASH who have associated risk factors for fibrosis development, and those with active NASH with evidence of high necroinflammatory activity [7]. The therapeutic goal is to reduce NASH-related mortality and progression to cirrhosis, liver failure, and hepatocellular carcinoma (HCC), and a surrogate endpoint is represented by the resolution of NASH-defining lesions. Currently, numerous randomized clinical trials (RCTs) are underway to evaluate the effects of therapeutic agents with promising results.

21.4.1 Therapeutic Agents for T2DM and Obesity

Particularly in patients with a higher BMI, the occurrence of NAFLD is highly correlated with T2DM and obesity [22, 23]. In contrast, NAFLD is less common in T2DM patients who are treated with insulin, sodium glucose cotransporter-2 (SGLT2) inhibitors, and GLP-1 receptor antagonists [24].

As a potential treatment for NAFLD/NASH, the reprogramming of anti-obesity or antidiabetic medications like pioglitazone and saroglitazar is being investigated. In a mouse NASH model, saroglitazar, a combined PPAR-a/g agonist, can reduce hepatic lipid accumulation, lobular inflammation, hepatocyte ballooning, and liver fibrosis [25]. In patients with NAFLD or NASH, 4 mg of saroglitazar significantly reduced ALT and liver fat content, improved insulin resistance, and improved dyslipidemia, according to a phase II clinical trial research [26].

Farnesoid X receptor (FXR) is activated by bile acids, and evidence from the current literature showed that it is crucial for maintaining glucose homeostasis and hepatic lipid buildup and has a major impact on insulin sensitivity [27, 28]. The nonsteroidal FXR agonist cilofexor possesses anti-inflammatory and antifibrotic properties. In a phase II trial investigation, it was discovered that cilofexor significantly reduced blood levels of C4, primary bile acids, and serum-glutamyl transferase in NASH patients, but not liver fibrosis and stiffness [29].

By inhibiting de novo lipogenesis, reducing liver inflammation and cell death, and boosting fatty acid oxidation, SGLT2 inhibitors such as canagliflozin, dapagliflozin, and empagliflozin have pleiotropic effects to treat NAFLD and T2DM [30].

Metformin and insulin-based therapies have been shown to reduce hepatic fat storage when GLP-1 receptor agonists are used [31]. They can also somewhat lessen liver fibrosis.

Patients with T2DM should use metformin as their first line of treatment because it lowers triglycerides, total cholesterol, and LDL while lowering blood sugar levels [32]. However, there is still controversy around the effects of metformin and dipeptidyl peptidase-4 (DPP-4) inhibitors in the management of NAFLD [33].

21.4.2 Vitamin E

Vitamin E is a fat-soluble vitamin presenting under several forms of which α-tocopherol is the most important, being the only one with pharmacological features which allow to be used by the human body. Considering that the changes in NAFLD are promoted by an increase in oxidative stress, vitamin E is one of many antioxidants that has been extensively studied for its potential to treat NAFLD. It stabilizes cell membranes by defending unsaturated fatty acids from lipid peroxidation and the ensuing reactive oxygen species (ROS). Adjuvant vitamin E therapy is more beneficial for adult patients with NAFLD than for pediatric patients, according to a recent meta-analysis of clinical trials [34]. In HIV-infected patients, vitamin E can help alleviate NASH as shown by a decrease in the serum biomarkers ALT and cytokeratin 18 for hepatocyte death [35].

Consumption of meals high in polyphenols also boasts positive effects for NAFLD patients, as polyphenols as anti-inflammatory and antioxidant reagents exhibit a protective effect in liver disease [36]. For instance, NAFLD incidence is decreased by a high consumption of lignans, a significant group of low-molecular-weight polyphenols found in plants like whole grains [37].

However, the therapy with vitamin E needs some precautions as it is associated with some adverse events. Data shows that the mortality rate increases at doses >400 IU/day, and it also increases the risk of hemorrhagic stroke and prostate cancer.

21.4.3 Anti-Cell Death Agents

As NAFLD and NASH advance, lipotoxicity destroys hepatic cells, produces inflammatory cytokines and chemokines, and activates hepatic stellate cells (HSCs). As a result, it is crucial to prevent cellular death when treating chronic liver illness. In patients with NASH and F2–F3 liver fibrosis, for instance, selonsertib, a specific inhibitor of apoptotic signal-regulating kinase 1, had an antifibrotic effect [38]. However, selonsertib monotherapy did not lessen liver fibrosis in individuals with NASH and bridging fibrosis (F3) or compensated cirrhosis (F4) when compared to placebo control treatment, according to two phase III clinical trials [39]. Therefore, selonsertib does not meet the criteria to be recommended yet in the management of NAFLD.

21.4.4 Antifibrotics

The development of liver fibrosis and NAFLD into fibrotic NASH can be stopped by antifibrotic drugs. Activated HSCs are the primary cells that produce extracellular matrix proteins during liver fibrosis [40]. The basic strategies for combating liver fibrosis involve preventing HSC activation and expansion and using medications to reduce inflammation and cell death. The treatments for NAFLD or NASH outlined above are also available for treating liver fibrosis. Some organic materials have a variety of outcomes. For instance, in mice with diet-induced NASH, scoparone, a bioactive component from a Chinese herb, can reduce hepatic steatosis, inflammation, cell death, and fibrosis [41].

Treatments for NAFLD and NASH also have some alternative targets, including G protein-coupled receptors (GPCRs), estrogen-related receptor alpha (ERR), bone morphogenetic proteins (BMPs), and KLFs [42].

21.5   Pipeline Treatments

21.5.1 Beyond Phase II Therapeutic Agents

Current therapeutic agents that have passed phase II, are illustrated in Table 21.1.

As previously mentioned, FXR has a positive impact on glucose homeostasis and hepatic lipid production and may even modify liver fibrosis [43]. Considering the potential beneficial role of FXR in NAFLD, OCA, an FXR agonist, has been extensively studied and proposed as a novel medicine for possible approval after phase II and III RCTs in patients with NASH and severe fibrosis consistently demonstrated its efficacy on fibrosis regression [44, 45]. The results from phase III REGENERATE trial showed that OCA at a dose of 25 mg was able to improve fibrosis and resolute NASH-associated changes when compared to placebo; taken together, it appears that up to five individuals must be treated for one patient's fibrosis to either improve or not worsen [46]. Regarding adverse events, it seems that OCA at 25 mg/day was linked to pruritus in 50% of patients, with severe intensity in 28% [46]. Considering that pruritus could severely decrease the quality of life, it is possible that some patients will stop the therapy because of it. Another adverse event that could occur is an elevation of LDL cholesterol, which could be managed by using a statin [46].

Peroxisome proliferator-activated receptor α (PPAR) and PPARδ control a number of metabolic processes, the most important being the decrease of cholesterol levels and the activation of genes that control fatty acid oxidation and lipid transport [47, 48], and are highly expressed in hepatocytes. Elafibranor is a dual agonist for these receptors and has been studied for the treatment of NAFLD. Preclinical models and early human studies revealed that elafibranor functions as an insulin sensitizer, potentially improving hepatic steatosis, inflammation, and fibrosis. Although in the phase II GOLDEN-505 study the primary outcome was not achieved as there

Table 21.1 Current therapeutic agents that have passed phase II

Phase III randomized controlled trial	Therapeutic agent	Mechanism of action	Dosage (per 24 h) (mg)	Duration (weeks)	Outcome
REGENERATE [45]	Obeticholic acid	FXR agonist	25	72	Interim analysis data submitted to the FDA and received a CRL for additional post-interim data
RESOLVE-IT [50]	Elafibranor	PPARα and PPARδ agonist	120	72	Interim analysis failed to show any treatment effect; the program has been terminated
ARMOR [52]	Aramchol	SCD1 inhibitor	600	52	Ongoing
AURORA	Cenicriviroc	CCR2–CCR5 antagonist	150	52	Terminated due to lack of efficacy
MAESTRO [51]	Resmetirom	THRβ agonist	80–100	52	Ongoing

CCR CC-chemokine receptor, *CRL* complete response letter, *FXR* farnesoid X receptor, *PPAR* peroxisome proliferator-activated receptor, *SCD1* stearoyl-CoA desaturase 1, *THRβ* thyroid hormone receptor-β

was no difference between elafibranor and placebo, a dose of 120 mg per day for 52 weeks in patients with fibrosis stage F2 or F3 resulted in noticeably higher rates of NASH resolution than those observed in the placebo group in the post hoc analysis [49]. Following these results, a phase III trial (RESOLVE IT) continued to investigate the effects elafibranor (120 mg daily or placebo) for 72 weeks on liver histology in patients with F2 and F3 NASH, but unfortunately the trial did not meet the primary endpoint, achieving a response rate of 19.2% compared to 14.7% in the placebo arm [50].

Another two therapeutic agents which are currently undergoing evaluation through phase III RCTs are resmetirom and aramchol. Resmetirom is a thyroid hormone receptor (THR) agonist with oral activity that targets the liver and has a far higher selectivity for THR than triiodothyronine (T3) [51]. According to a phase II study, resmetirom showed a relative decrease in liver fat compared to those who received a placebo and, more importantly, was linked to greater rates of NASH resolution (27.4% resmetirom versus 6.5% placebo; $P = 0.02$) [51]. The other agent is aramchol, a bile acid-to-fatty acid conjugate which inhibits the stearoyl-CoA desaturase 1 (SCD1) enzyme, which has an important role in the process of liver steatosis development. The phase IIb ARREST study demonstrated that aramchol at 600 mg per day was linked to a tendency for greater rates of NASH remission without fibrosis worsening [52].

21.5.2 Phase II Therapeutic Agents

21.5.2.1 GLP-1 Receptor Agonists

Liraglutide and semaglutide are glucagon-like peptide 1 (GLP1) receptor agonists, which have received FDA approval for the treatment of T2DM and are investigated in clinical trials for the treatment of NASH. Liraglutide showed a significant improvement in the liver histology in NASH patients (in 39% of liraglutide-treated patients versus 9% of placebo) [53]. In a phase II study, semaglutide demonstrated a dose-response relationship, with a 59% resolution of NASH in the group receiving 0.4 mg compared to 17% in the placebo group ($P = 0.001$, semaglutide 0.4 mg versus placebo) [54]. Semaglutide taken once weekly is now being studied as a treatment for people with compensated cirrhosis and NASH who do not have varices or ascites as a sign of portal hypertension [55].

21.5.2.2 Galectin 3 Inhibitors

Belapectin is an inhibitor of galectin 3 that has a positive impact on liver fibrosis and portal hypertension that is currently under evaluation in NAFLD and NASH patients. A phase IIb trial demonstrated that after a year of belapectin 2 mg/kg and 8 mg/kg, it did not achieve the desired outcome of significant reduction in HVPG or fibrosis [56]. However, 2 mg/kg of belapectin was linked to a decrease in HVPG at 52 weeks compared with baseline and a decreased development of new varices in the subset of 81 individuals without esophageal varices at baseline [56]. Thus, belapectin is now studied in a two-stage phase IIb/III trial where the primary outcome is to evaluate the proportion of patients in the belapectin treatment groups who develop new esophageal varices at 18 months of treatment compared to the proportion in the placebo group in patients with NASH-cirrhosis without esophageal varices (NCT04365868).

21.5.2.3 FXR Agonists

Cilofexor, a selective nonsteroidal FXR agonist, has shown improved markers of cholestasis and decreased liver enzymes in individuals with primary sclerosing cholangitis and is now being evaluated in a phase III trial [57]. Furthermore, in a phase II randomized, placebo-controlled trial in patients with NASH without cirrhosis, cilofexor determined a significant reduction in hepatic fat (30% in 39% of patients) after therapy for 24 weeks at a dose of 100 mg daily [58].

21.5.2.4 ACC Inhibitors

The liver acetyl-CoA carboxylase (ACC) direct inhibitor *firsocostat* decreased de novo lipogenesis and liver fat in a randomized, placebo-controlled study, which included patients without cirrhosis but with one or more of the following criteria: (1) hepatic steatosis of at least 8% based on MRI examination and liver stiffness of at least 2.5 kPa and (2) histology-proven NASH with F2 or F3 fibrosis [59]. By 12 weeks, 48% of patients receiving firsocostat at a dose of 20 mg showed at least a 30% reduction in MRI from baseline, compared to 15% of those receiving placebo ($P = 0.004$) [59].

21.5.2.5 Fibroblast Growth Factor 21 Analogues

A pegylated homologue of fibroblast growth factor (FGF21) is **pegbelfermin**, which demonstrated a significant reduction in absolute hepatic fat fraction compared to placebo in a phase IIa, which included patients with NASH150 who were examined (NCT02413372). Patients received 20 mg weekly (5.2% at 20 mg versus 1.3% in those with placebo, respectively; $P = 0.008$) [60]. Adults with NASH and liver fibrosis stage F3 or F4 are being treated with pegbelfermin in phase IIb trials (FALCON1 and FALCON2; NCT03486899 and NCT03486912, respectively).

A phase IIa trial with once-weekly dosage has examined **efruxifermin**, an FGF21 analogue designed to match the biological activity profile of native FGF21. In the BALANCED research, efruxifermin was administered subcutaneously for 16 weeks to 80 patients with biopsy-proven NASH (NCT03976401) at three different daily dose levels (28 mg, 50 mg, and 70 mg) or a placebo [61]. Efruxifermin determined absolute liver fat reductions at 12 weeks considerably higher compared to placebo (12%, 13%, and 14% versus 0.3%) [61]. Furthermore, it achieved a 28% improvement in fibrosis by at least two stages across all dose groups, with a 38% response rate in the 50 mg daily dose group, and 48% NASH resolution without worsening of fibrosis across all dose groups, with a 54% response rate in the 50 mg daily dose group [61]. In light of the rapid resolution of NASH and regression of fibrosis, these outcomes are encouraging. We anticipate the replication of these findings in a larger cohort with favorable safety and tolerability characteristics for prolonged medication usage.

21.6 Conclusions

The eagerness for the approval of medications for patients with NAFLD is justified, but it should not take away the importance of the currently existing, easily accessible, and less expensive options. In addition to weight loss of 10% or more in a year, these solutions also involve the best management of comorbidities. The new and emerging therapies for NAFLD are promising, but further evidence to endorse their efficacy in improving the outcome in these patients is still needed.

References

1. Day CP, James OF. Steatohepatitis: a tale of two "hits"? Gastroenterology. 1998;114:842–5.
2. Loomba R, Friedman SL, Shulman GI. Mechanisms and disease consequences of nonalcoholic fatty liver disease. Cell. 2021;184:2537–64.
3. Xiaohan X, Poulsen KL, Lijuan W, Liu S, Miyata T, Song Q, Wei Q, Zhao C, Lin C, Yang J. Targeted therapeutics and novel signaling pathways in non-alcohol-associated fatty liver/steatohepatitis (NAFL/NASH). Signal Transduct Target Ther. 2022;7:287.
4. Vilar-Gomez E, Martinez-Perez Y, Calzadilla-Bertot L, et al. Weight loss through lifestyle modification significantly reduces features of nonalcoholic steatohepatitis. Gastroenterology. 2015;149(2):367–78.e5.
5. Vachliotis I, Goulas A, Papaioannidou P, Polyzos SA. Nonalcoholic fatty liver disease: lifestyle and quality of life. Hormones (Athens). 2022;21:41–9.
6. Hannah WN Jr, Harrison SA. Effect of weight loss, diet, exercise, and bariatric surgery on nonalcoholic fatty liver disease. Clin Liver Dis. 2016;20:339–50.

7. European Association for the Study of the Liver (EASL); European Association for the Study of Diabetes (EASD); European Association for the Study of Obesity (EASO). EASL–EASD–EASO clinical practice guidelines for the management of non-alcoholic fatty liver disease. J Hepatol. 2016;64:1388–402.

8. Ristic-Medic D, Kovacic M, Takic M, Arsic A, Petrovic S, Paunovic M, Jovicic M, Vucic V. Calorie-restricted Mediterranean and low-fat diets affect fatty acid status in individuals with nonalcoholic fatty liver disease. Nutrients. 2020;13:15.

9. Holmer M, Lindqvist C, Petersson S, Moshtaghi-Svensson J, Tillander V, Brismar TB, Hagström H, Stål P. Treatment of NAFLD with intermittent calorie restriction or low-carb high-fat diet—a randomised controlled trial. JHEP Rep. 2021;3:100256.

10. Francque SM, et al. Non-alcoholic fatty liver disease: a patient guideline. JHEP Rep. 2021;3(5):100322.

11. Ghetti FDF, De Oliveira DG, De Oliveira JM, Ferreira LEVVDC, Cesar DE, Moreira APB. Effects of dietary intervention on gut microbiota and metabolic-nutritional profile of outpatients with non-alcoholic steatohepatitis: a randomized clinical trial. J Gastrointest Liver Dis. 2019;28:279–87.

12. Jang DK, Lee JS, Lee JK, Kim YH. Independent association of physical activity with nonalcoholic fatty liver disease and alanine aminotransferase levels. J Clin Med. 2019;8:1013. https://doi.org/10.3390/jcm8071013.

13. Miura I, Komine S, Okada K, Wada S, Warabi E, Uchida F, Oh S, Suzuki H, Mizokami Y, Shoda J. Prevention of non-alcoholic steatohepatitis by long-term exercise via the induction of phenotypic changes in Kupffer cells of hyperphagic obese mice. Physiol Rep. 2021;9:e14859.

14. Kasper P, Breuer S, Hoffmann T, Vohlen C, Janoschek R, Schmitz L, Appel S, Fink G, Hünseler C, Quaas A, et al. Maternal exercise mediates hepatic metabolic programming via activation of AMPK-PGC1a axis in the offspring of obese mothers. Cell. 2021;10:1247.

15. Battista F, Ermolao A, van Baak MA, Beaulieu K, Blundell JE, Busetto L, Carraça EV, Encantado J, Dicker D, Farpour-Lambert N, et al. Effect of exercise on cardiometabolic health of adults with overweight or obesity: focus on blood pressure, insulin resistance, and intrahepatic fat—a systematic review and meta-analysis. Obes Rev. 2021;22:e13269.

16. Cornejo-Pareja I, Clemente-Postigo M, Tinahones FJ. Metabolic and endocrine consequences of bariatric surgery. Front Endocrinol. 2019;10:626.

17. Syn NL, Cummings DE, Wang LZ, Lin DJ, Zhao JJ, Loh M, Koh ZJ, Chew CA, Loo YE, Tai BC, et al. Association of metabolic–bariatric surgery with long-term survival in adults with and without diabetes: a one-stage meta-analysis of matched cohort and prospective controlled studies with 174,772 participants. Lancet. 2021;397:1830–41.

18. Cherla DV, Rodriguez NA, Vangoitsenhoven R, Singh T, Mehta N, McCullough AJ, Brethauer SA, Schauer PR, Aminian A. Impact of sleeve gastrectomy and Roux-en-Y gastric bypass on biopsy-proven non-alcoholic fatty liver disease. Surg Endosc. 2019;34:2266–72.

19. Kalinowski P, Paluszkiewicz R, Ziarkiewicz-Wróblewska B, Wróblewski T, Remiszewski P, Grodzicki M, Krawczyk M. Liver function in patients with nonalcoholic fatty liver disease randomized to Roux-en-Y gastric bypass versus sleeve gastrectomy. Ann Surg. 2017;266:738–45.

20. Wölnerhanssen BK, Peterli R, Hurme S, Bueter M, Helmiö M, Juuti A, Meyer-Gerspach AC, Slawik M, Peromaa-Haavisto P, Nuutila P, et al. Laparoscopic Roux-en-Y gastric bypass versus laparoscopic sleeve gastrectomy: 5-year outcomes of merged data from two randomized clinical trials (SLEEVEPASS and SM-BOSS). BJS. 2021;108:49–57.

21. Pajecki D, Dantas ACB, Tustumi F, Kanaji AL, de Cleva R, Santo MA. Sleeve gastrectomy versus Roux-en-Y gastric bypass in the elderly: 1-year preliminary outcomes in a randomized trial (BASE trial). Obes Surg. 2021;31:2359–63.

22. Loosen SH, Demir M, Kunstein A, Jördens M, Qvarskhava N, Luedde M, Luedde T, Roderburg C, Kostev K. Variables associated with increased incidence of non-alcoholic fatty liver disease (NAFLD) in patients with type 2 diabetes. BMJ Open Diabetes Res Care. 2021;9:e002243.

23. Ganjooei NA, Jamialahmadi T, Nematy M, Jangjoo A, Goshayeshi L, Khadem-Rezaiyan M, Reiner Ž, Alidadi M, Markin AM, Sahebkar A. The role of lipid profile as an independent

predictor of non-alcoholic steatosis and steatohepatitis in morbidly obese patients. Front Cardiovasc Med. 2021;8:682352.

24. Kumar DP, Caffrey R, Marioneaux J, Santhekadur PK, Bhat M, Alonso C, Koduru SV, Philip B, Jain MR, Giri SR, et al. The PPAR α/γ agonist saroglitazar improves insulin resistance and steatohepatitis in a diet induced animal model of nonalcoholic fatty liver disease. Sci Rep. 2020;10:1–14.

25. Gawrieh S, Noureddin M, Loo N, Mohseni R, Awasty V, Cusi K, Kowdley KV, Lai M, Schiff E, Parmar D, et al. Saroglitazar, a PPAR-α/γ agonist, for treatment of nonalcoholic fatty liver disease: a randomized controlled double-blind phase 2 trial. Hepatology. 2021;74(4):1809–24.

26. Schmitt J, Kong B, Stieger B, Tschopp O, Schultze SM, Rau M, Weber A, Mullhaupt B, Guo GL, Geier A. Protective effects of farnesoid X receptor (FXR) on hepatic lipid accumulation are mediated by hepatic FXR and independent of intestinal FGF15 signal. Liver Int. 2015;35:1133–44.

27. Liu M, Zhang G, Wu S, Song M, Wang J, Cai W, Mi S, Liu C. Schaftoside alleviates HFD-induced hepatic lipid accumulation in mice via upregulating farnesoid X receptor. J Ethnopharmacol. 2020;255:112776.

28. Amano Y, Shimada M, Miura S, Adachi R, Tozawa R. Effects of a farnesoid X receptor antagonist on hepatic lipid metabolism in primates. Eur J Pharmacol. 2014;723:108–15.

29. Zhang E, Zhao Y, Hu H. Impact of sodium glucose cotransporter 2 inhibitors on nonalcoholic fatty liver disease complicated by diabetes mellitus. Hepatol Commun. 2021;5:736–48.

30. Wong C, Lee MH, Yaow CYL, Chin YH, Goh XL, Ng CH, Lim AYL, Muthiah MD, Khoo CM. Glucagon-like peptide-1 receptor agonists for non-alcoholic fatty liver disease in type 2 diabetes: a meta-analysis. Front Endocrinol. 2021;12:609110.

31. Sivitz WI, Phillips LS, Wexler DJ, Fortmann SP, Camp AW, Tiktin M, Perez M, Craig J, Hollander PA, Cherrington A, et al. Optimization of metformin in the GRADE cohort: effect on glycemia and body weight. Diabetes Care. 2020;43:940–7.

32. Gillani SW, Ghayedi N, Roosta P, Seddigh P, Nasiri O. Effect of metformin on lipid profiles of type 2 diabetes mellitus: a meta-analysis of randomized controlled trials. J Pharm Bioallied Sci. 2021;13:76–82.

33. Lamos EM, Kristan M, Siamashvili M, Davis SN. Effects of anti-diabetic treatments in type 2 diabetes and fatty liver disease. Expert Rev Clin Pharmacol. 2021;10:1–16.

34. Amanullah I, Khan YH, Anwar I, Gulzar A, Mallhi TH, Raja AA. Effect of vitamin E in non-alcoholic fatty liver disease: a systematic review and meta-analysis of randomised controlled trials. Postgrad Med J. 2019;95:601–11.

35. Sebastiani G, Saeed S, Lebouche B, De Pokomandy A, Szabo J, Haraoui L-P, Routy J-P, Wong P, Deschenes M, Ghali P, et al. Vitamin E is an effective treatment for nonalcoholic steatohepatitis in HIV mono-infected patients. AIDS. 2020;34:237–44.

36. Abenavoli L, Larussa T, Corea A, Procopio A, Boccuto L, Dallio M, Federico A, Luzza F. Dietary polyphenols and non-alcoholic fatty liver disease. Nutrients. 2021;13:494.

37. Salehi-Sahlabadi A, Teymoori F, Jabbari M, Momeni A, Mokari-Yamchi A, Sohouli M, Hekmatdoost A. Dietary polyphenols and the odds of non-alcoholic fatty liver disease: a case-control study. Clin Nutr ESPEN. 2021;41:429–35.

38. Loomba R, Lawitz E, Mantry PS, Jayakumar S, Caldwell SH, Arnold H, Diehl AM, Djedjos CS, Han L, Myers RP, et al. The ASK1 inhibitor selonsertib in patients with nonalcoholic steatohepatitis: a randomized, phase 2 trial. Hepatology. 2018;67:549–59.

39. Harrison SA, Wong V, Okanoue T, Bzowej N, Vuppalanchi R, Younes Z, Kohli A, Sarin S, Caldwell SH, Alkhouri N, et al. Selonsertib for patients with bridging fibrosis or compensated cirrhosis due to NASH: results from randomized phase III STELLAR trials. J Hepatol. 2020;73:26–39.

40. Kisseleva T. The origin of fibrogenic myofibroblasts in fibrotic liver. Hepatology. 2017;65:1039–43.

41. Liu B, Deng X, Jiang Q, Li G, Zhang J, Zhang N, Xin S, Xu K. Scoparone alleviates inflammation, apoptosis and fibrosis of non-alcoholic steatohepatitis by suppressing the TLR4/NF-κB signaling pathway in mice. Int Immunopharmacol. 2019;75:105797.

42. Sun N, Shen C, Zhang L, Wu X, Yu Y, Yang X, Yang C, Zhong C, Gao Z, Miao W, et al. Hepatic Krüppel-like factor 16 (KLF16) targets PPARα to improve steatohepatitis and insulin resistance. Gut. 2020;10:1136.

43. Carr RM, Reid AE. FXR agonists as therapeutic agents for non-alcoholic fatty liver disease. Curr Atheroscler Rep. 2015;17:16.

44. Neuschwander-Tetri BA, et al. Farnesoid X nuclear receptor ligand obeticholic acid for non-cirrhotic, non-alcoholic steatohepatitis (FLINT): a multicentre, randomised, placebo-controlled trial. Lancet. 2015;385:956–65.

45. Younossi Z, et al. Positive results from REGENERATE: a phase 3 international, randomized, placebo-controlled study evaluating obeticholic acid treatment for NASH [abstract GS-06]. J Hepatol. 2019;70:E5.

46. Younossi ZM, et al. Obeticholic acid for the treatment of non-alcoholic steatohepatitis: interim analysis from a multicentre, randomised, placebo-controlled phase 3 trial. Lancet. 2019;394:2184–96.

47. Grygiel-Górniak B. Peroxisome proliferator-activated receptors and their ligands: nutritional and clinical implications—a review. Nutr J. 2014;13:17.

48. Rotman Y, Sanyal AJ. Current and upcoming pharmacotherapy for non-alcoholic fatty liver disease. Gut. 2017;66:180–90.

49. Ratziu V, et al. Elafibranor, an agonist of the peroxisome proliferator-activated receptor-α and -δ, induces resolution of nonalcoholic steatohepatitis without fibrosis worsening. Gastroenterology. 2016;150:1147–1159.e5.

50. Harrison SA, et al. RESOLVE-IT® phase 3 trial of elafibranor in NASH: final results of the week 72 interim surrogate efficacy analysis (Poster). Hepatology. 2020;72:162.

51. Harrison SA, et al. Resmetirom (MGL-3196) for the treatment of non-alcoholic steatohepatitis: a multicentre, randomised, double-blind, placebo-controlled, phase 2 trial. Lancet. 2019;394:2012–24.

52. Ratziu V, et al. One-year results of the global phase 2b randomized placebo-controlled ARREST trial of aramchol, a stearoyl CoA desaturase inhibitor, in patients with NASH [abstract]. Hepatology. 2018;68:LB-5.

53. Armstrong MJ, et al. Liraglutide efficacy and action in non-alcoholic steatohepatitis (LEAN): study protocol for a phase II multicentre, double-blinded, randomised, controlled trial. BMJ Open. 2013;3:e003995.

54. Newsome PN, et al. A placebo-controlled trial of subcutaneous semaglutide in nonalcoholic steatohepatitis. N Engl J Med. 2020;384(12):1113–24. https://doi.org/10.1056/NEJMoa2028395.

55. Harrison SA, et al. Semaglutide for the treatment of non-alcoholic steatohepatitis: trial design and comparison of non-invasive biomarkers. Contemp Clin Trials. 2020;97:106174.

56. Chalasani N, et al. Effects of belapectin, an inhibitor of galectin-3, in patients with non-alcoholic steatohepatitis with cirrhosis and portal hypertension. Gastroenterology. 2019;158:1334–1345.e5.

57. Trauner M, et al. The nonsteroidal farnesoid X receptor agonist cilofexor (GS-9674) improves markers of cholestasis and liver injury in patients with primary sclerosing cholangitis. Hepatology. 2019;70:788–801.

58. Patel K, et al. Cilofexor, a nonsteroidal FXR agonist, in patients with noncirrhotic NASH: a phase 2 randomized controlled trial. Hepatology. 2020;72:58–71.

59. Loomba R, et al. GS-0976 reduces hepatic steatosis and fibrosis markers in patients with non-alcoholic fatty liver disease. Gastroenterology. 2018;155:1463–1473.e6.

60. Sanyal A, et al. Pegbelfermin (BMS-986036), a PEGylated fibroblast growth factor 21 analogue, in patients with non-alcoholic steatohepatitis: a randomised, double-blind, placebo-controlled, phase 2a trial. Lancet. 2019;392:2705–17.

61. Harrison SA, et al. Efruxifermin (EFX), a long-acting Fc-FGF21 fusion protein, administered for 16 weeks to patients with NASH substantially reduces liver fat and ALT, and improves liver histology: analysis of a randomized, placebo-controlled, phase 2a study (balanced) [abstract]. Hepatology. 2020;72:6A–7A.

Practical Clinical Cases in Nonalcoholic Fatty Liver Disease

Ermina Stratina, Adrian Rotaru, Remus Stafie, and Horia Minea

22.1 First Case Report

A 41-year-old male patient was referred to our gastroenterology outpatient clinic because of elevated liver enzymes, identified at a routine checkup, and fatigue. Prior to admission, he had a history of appendectomy and was diagnosed with grade 1 hypertension, with no drug treatment being initiated. Regarding his family medical history, it was discovered that his father suffered from cardiovascular diseases, but the patient was unable to provide further and more accurate information. After further evaluation, we concluded that the patient was a smoker (7 pack years) and had no history of alcohol abuse (<30 g/day) [1]. In what concerns the physical examination, there were no notable findings. On presentation, the patient had a height of 1.79 m with a body mass index (BMI) of 24.2 kg/m^2.

Blood samples revealed normal white cell count (9.400/μL), platelet count (212.000/μL), and hemoglobin (14.2 g/dL) also being within normal limits. The biochemical test showed a slightly high C-reactive protein (1.8 mg/dL) and an alanine aminotransferase (ALT) of 103 U/L (reference range 9–52 U/L) and aspartate aminotransferase (AST) of 88 U/L (reference range 15–36 U/L). Fasting plasma glucose was within normal limits. In what concerns the lipid profile, there were notable modifications: total cholesterol 247 mg/dL, high-density lipoprotein (HDL) 41 mg/dL, low-density lipoprotein (LDL) 169 mg/dL, and triglycerides 184 mg/dL. Total bilirubin, alkaline phosphatase, gamma-glutamyl transferase (GGT), and albumin had normal values. Immunoglobulins, including IgA, IgG, and IgG, were within normal limits. Serum ferritin and ceruloplasmin were within normal ranges.

E. Stratina (✉) · A. Rotaru · R. Stafie · H. Minea
Gastroenterology Department, Grigore T. Popa University of Medicine and Pharmacy, Iasi, Romania

Institute of Gastroenterology and Hepatology, St. Spiridon Emergency Hospital, Iasi, Romania

A. Trifan et al. (eds.), *Essentials of Non-Alcoholic Fatty Liver Disease*, https://doi.org/10.1007/978-3-031-33548-8_22

Hepatitis B surface antigen, hepatitis B virus core antibody, and hepatitis C virus antibody were all negative. All coagulation tests presented normal values.

An abdominal ultrasonography examination was performed. We identified bright hepatic echoes and increased hepatorenal echogenicity, suggesting the presence of liver steatosis. According to the American Gastroenterology Association Clinical Practice Update on the diagnosis and management of nonalcoholic liver disease in lean individuals [1], fibrosis-4 (FIB4) index was calculated according to the following formula: FIB4 = age (year) × AST (IU/L)/{platelet count (109/L) × [ALT (U/L)]1/2} [2]. The result was an increased value of FIB4, namely 2.13.

Taking into consideration these results, we decided to further perform a second noninvasive test, namely, vibration-controlled transient elastography (VCTE) with controlled attenuation parameter (CAP), which revealed an increased liver stiffness measurement (LSM) and CAP values of 8.1 kPa and 298 dB/m, respectively, corresponding to mild fibrosis (F1) and moderate steatosis (S2) [3].

Considering the results mentioned above, the patient was diagnosed with nonalcoholic steatohepatitis (NASH). According to current guidelines [1], the patient was advised to make several lifestyle changes, including daily exercise and weight loss (3–5% from the current weight). Moreover, we suggested that the patient should monitor his blood pressure frequently and contact his general practitioner if any changes will occur.

At 6-month follow-up, the patient presented a decrease in body weight of around 2.5 kg. Blood tests were collected, and liver enzymes were in the normal range, while total cholesterol and triglycerides, even if a descending trend was observed, still maintained a higher value than the normal range. At the VCTE with CAP examination, there was a slight improvement of the LSM and CAP values, namely 7.9 kPa and 281 dB/m, respectively. In what concerns the eating habits of our patients, he declared that he made some changes by ruling out food rich in saturated fats and adopting a more balanced diet similar to the Mediterranean one.

22.2 Discussions

NAFLD is closely linked to the obesity epidemic and being overweight, but it can also affect those who are slim and have a BMI under 25 kg/m^2 without having any identified risk factors [4, 5]. Vos et al. first used the term "lean NAFLD" in 2011, and since then, new noninvasive diagnostic techniques have been widely accessible and available, raising concerns about the disorder's prevalence. Consequently, early diagnosis is essential for better care [6, 7]. Lean NAFLD is considered to be a serious clinical and diagnostic issue because, in the absence of obesity, which is a clinical marker for steatosis, the diagnosis of liver steatosis or liver damage is usually made too late or not at all. As a result, it is likely too late to begin the essential medical intervention and therapy. The metabolic profiles of lean NAFLD and overweight/obese NAFLD patients are similar and closely linked to those of the metabolic syndrome (MetS), which includes hypertension, low HDLc, hypertriglyceridemia, type 2 diabetes mellitus (T2DM), or increased fasting plasma glucose and increased waist circumference [8, 9].

According to EASL/EASD/EASO NAFLD standards, food and exercise are the recommended treatments for hepatic steatosis. A specific training program is not, however, mentioned. Similar findings from studies looking at how exercise affects NAFLD imply that both strength and aerobic training diminish hepatic steatosis [10, 11]. This evidence was recently supported by a meta-analysis, which found that regardless of the type of exercise program used (aerobic vs. resistance), the degree of steatosis is significantly reduced when a plan involving at least three weekly sessions lasting 40–45 min for 12 weeks is followed [12, 13]. According to research, resistance training is the most beneficial for women, while aerobic exercise appears to be more beneficial for men in terms of reducing hepatic fat [12]. High exercise compliance is obviously necessary; however, a sizeable portion of NAFLD patients may struggle to maintain aerobic exercise training due to coexisting cardiovascular comorbidities or physical impairment brought on by obesity.

22.3 Second Case Report

A 34-year-old male was admitted to our hospital because of fatigue, malaise, and pain below the right costal margin. Prior to admission, he had no important medical history. Concerning his family history, we noted that his mother had T2DM and his brother had cirrhosis but he could not specify the cause. The patient had no history of alcohol abuse, and he did not take any medications at home. On physical examination, the patient had pain on palpation in the right hypochondrium and hepatomegaly. Other clinical findings were not remarkable. One year before admission, his height was 181 cm, his body weight was 125 kg, and his BMI was 38.22 kg/m². On admission, his body weight was 118 kg and his BMI was 36.08 kg/m².

White blood cell count was increased (12,000/μL), platelet count was within normal limits (170,000/μL), and hemoglobin was 13.4 g/dL. C-reactive protein was mildly elevated (1.1 mg/dL). The biochemical test showed a fasting plasma glucose of 180 mg/dL (10 mmol/L) and a glycated hemoglobin A1c (HbA1c) of 9.1%. Also, he had a random glucose level of 272 mg/dL. LFTs showed an ALT of 206 U/L (reference range 9–52 U/L), an AST of 144 U/L (reference range 15–36 U/L), and an ALP of 133 U/L (reference range 40–105 U/L). Also, lipid profile was modified: total cholesterol 282 mg/dL, high-density lipoprotein (HDL) 36 mg/dL, low-density lipoprotein (LDL) 177 mg/dL, and triglycerides 201 mg/dL. Bilirubin, international normalized ratio, and albumin were normal values. Aspartate aminotransferase-to-platelet ratio index (APRI) and FIB4 index were elevated (APRI = 2.1 and FIB4 index = 2.01, respectively). APRI and FIB4 were calculated according to the following formula: APRI = AST level (IU/L)/upper limit of normal AST × 100/platelet count (109/L), and FIB4 = age (year) × AST (IU/L)/{platelet count (109/L) × [ALT (U/L)]1/2} [2, 14]. Serum ferritin and ceruloplasmin were within normal ranges. The hepatitis B surface antigen, hepatitis B virus core antibody, and hepatitis C virus antibody were all negative. Immunoglobulins, including IgA, IgG, and IgG, were within normal limits. Coagulation tests showed a decrease in the percentage of prothrombin time (67.6%). Homeostatic model of assessment of insulin resistance

(HOMA-IR) was 7.9. The HOMA-IR was calculated based on fasting values of plasma glucose and insulin according to the HOMA model formula: HOMA-IR = IRI (μU/mL) × FPG (mg/dL)/405 [15].

Abdominal ultrasonography examination identified bright hepatic echoes, increased hepatorenal echogenicity, and vascular blurring of the portal and hepatic veins, suggestive for diffuse hepatic steatosis. The BARD score was 2 points, which suggested advanced fibrosis [16]. We evaluated the patient by VCTE with CAP. The results showed us an increased CAP and LSM value (342 dB/m and 10.7 kPa, respectively). The cutoffs used for CAP were 285 dB/m for S1, 340 dB/m for S2, and 355 dB/m for S3, respectively. LSM cutoff staging values were as follows: F1 (mild), F2 (significant), F3 (advanced) fibrosis, and F4 (cirrhosis): 5.6–7.1, 7.2–9.4, 9.5–12.4, and ≥12.5 kPa [17, 18].

Based on these findings, the patient was diagnosed with nonalcoholic steato-hepatitis (NASH). He was also diagnosed, for the first time, with T2DM based on the following findings: fasting plasma glucose over 126 mg/dL, random glucose level over 200 mg/dL, and hemoglobin A1c over 6.5% [19]. The patient started insulin therapy because hyperglycemia persisted after admission. After starting insulin treatment, hyperglycemia rapidly improved.

According to the indications of the diabetologist, treatment with subcutaneous injections of the GLP-1R agonist liraglutide was initiated. The patient tolerated liraglutide with no side effects such as nausea or vomiting. Insulin was gradually discontinued after 5 weeks because glycemic control was improved.

After 50 weeks of treatment with liraglutide, the patient's weight loss was 18 kg, LFTs were in the lower normal range (AST 30 U/L, ALT 22 U/L, ALP 58 U/L), glycemic control was improved (HbA1c 5.8%), and lipid profile was normalized without specific treatment. We performed an abdominal ultrasound which objectivated a diminished echogenicity, suggesting an overall reduction in steatosis. Also, CAP and LSM values improved (302 dB/m and 8.4 kPa, respectively).

22.4 Discussion

NAFLD is usually linked to insulin resistance and is regarded as the hepatic manifestation of the metabolic syndrome. T2DM, obesity, hypertension, and dyslipidemia are examples of the conditions that are directly related to the advancement of NAFLD. T2DM has been shown to be one of the major risk factors for [2] the occurrence of cirrhosis, advanced fibrosis, NASH, and hepatocellular cancer [20].

The relationship between NAFLD and T2DM is bidirectional, and it is associated with high rates of mortality. The presence of NAFLD in patients with T2DM promotes the development of severe outcomes, and T2DM enhances the NAFLD-associated complications [21].

The pathophysiology of NASH is with multiple pathways and is closely related to insulin resistance, which is associated with metabolic syndrome, excessive intracellular fatty acids, oxidant stress, and mitochondrial dysfunction. These factors promote systemic and liver inflammation, which leads to hepatic fibrosis [22].

In the modern world, nearly a third of the population suffers from obesity. Obesity is an intricate, multifaceted, and mostly avoidable pathology. The presence and degree of hepatic fibrosis have been linked to one of the most significant risk factors for NAFLD [23]. Obesity and weight increase were found to be independent predictors of liver fibrosis in recent research that included 40,700 participants with NAFLD [24].

The American Diabetes Association highlights the important link between diabetes and obesity and recommends testing and assessing the risk for developing T2DM in asymptomatic patients $\geq$45 years old with excess weight and regardless of age if they have BMI $\geq$40 kg/m^2 [25].

Liver biopsy remains the current gold standard for the diagnosis of NASH. Also, it is the only investigation that can make the difference between NAFL and NASH. The essential criteria to put the diagnosis of NASH are the joint presence of steatosis, ballooning, and lobular inflammation [26]. Despite the advantages, LB is costly, uncomfortable, and with life-threatening risks for patients [27].

Alternative, noninvasive diagnostic methods include imaging-based techniques. US is the first-line investigation used for assessing liver steatosis but is better for evaluating mild and severe steatosis [28]. VCTE with CAP represents an important tool for detecting liver fibrosis and steatosis. When imaging-based techniques are not available, the guidelines recommend using serum biomarkers (AST, ALT, platelets). One of the most crucial prognostic indicators for NAFLD is fibrosis, and individuals who have it are more likely to experience serious outcomes. Regarding the scores for fibrosis, NFS and FIB4 have been validated in ethnically different NAFLD populations, with reliable results [29, 30].

Our patient had obesity for at least 2 years. Also, HOMA-IR, an important parameter for insulin resistance, was increased in this patient at admission. Therefore, hyperinsulinemia due to severe insulin resistance had been present, being involved in the progression of liver fibrosis. Initially, we started the administration of insulin to improve hyperglycemia. Weight loss and glycemic control are effective measures for NASH.

Liraglutide is an analog of glucagon-like peptide-1 (GLP-1), which is linked to adenylate cyclase. The increase in cyclic AMP-induced glucose-dependent release of insulin inhibits the glucose-dependent release of glucagon and slows gastric emptying to increase the control of blood sugar. Liraglutide is widely used in the treatment of diabetic patients [31]. Recent papers demonstrated the pleiotropic effects of liraglutide: reduce intrahepatic fat, ALT, and TG in T2DM patients with NAFLD. Also, it has been approved that liraglutide has the effect of decreasing liver lipid content and then treating NAFLD in animal studies [32].

The patient showed notable results after 50 weeks of treatment with a GLP-1R agonist. He lost 18 kg of body weight (from a baseline of 118 kg), and LFT and lipid profile have been normalized. The patient was not evaluated by LB before and after treatment, and this represents one limitation of our study.

In conclusion, the clinical presentation of NAFLD/NASH cases can be in various forms. Considering the increased prevalence of NAFLD in obese and diabetic patients and the emergence of new drugs, it is important to develop screening strategies for these categories. Also, further studies will be needed for the assessment of the efficacy of GLP-1 on NASH.

22.5   Third Case Report

A 53-year-old female patient was referred to our gastroenterology outpatient clinic because of abdominal pain located in the right hypochondrium associated with nausea without vomiting. Prior to admission, she had a history of grade 2 hypertension in treatment, grade 1 obesity, extrauterine pregnancy for which she underwent surgery at 29 years old, and gallbladder lithiasis discovered 3 years prior to admission. Regarding her family medical history, we have discovered that her mother suffers from type 2 diabetes mellitus (T2DM) and her brother is currently under treatment for psoriasis. After further evaluation, we concluded that the patient was not smoking and had no history of alcohol abuse (<30 g/day). In what concerns the physical examination, the patient had a blood pressure of 145/80 mmHg and pain in the right hypochondrium, without other notable changes. On presentation, the patient had a height of 1.58 m, a BMI of 32.1 kg/m^2, and a waist circumference of 118 cm.

Blood samples revealed normal white cell count (6100/µL), platelet count (311,000/µL), and hemoglobin (13.9 g/dL) also being within normal limits. Regarding the lipid profile, important modifications were discovered, namely a total cholesterol of 287 mg/dL, low HDLc levels (32 mg/dL), high low-density lipoprotein (LDLc) levels (177 mg/dL), and a high value of triglycerides (203 mg/dL). Biochemical test showed a normal C-reactive protein and an alanine aminotransferase (ALT) of 39 U/L (reference range 9–52 U/L) and an aspartate aminotransferase (AST) of 27 U/L (reference range 15–36 U/L). Fasting plasma glucose was within normal limits. Total bilirubin, alkaline phosphatase, gamma-glutamyl transferase (GGT), and albumin had normal values. Immunoglobulins, including IgA, IgG, and IgG, were within normal limits. Serum ferritin and ceruloplasmin were within normal ranges. Hepatitis B surface antigen, hepatitis B virus core antibody, and hepatitis C virus antibody were all negative, and all coagulation tests presented normal values.

Abdominal ultrasonography examination was performed. We identified an increased liver echogenicity suggesting the presence of hepatic steatosis and hepatomegaly. The portal vein was normal in size. Moreover, the diagnosis of gallbladder lithiasis was confirmed, but no signs of inflammation were discovered. No other important changes were identified.

According to the current guidelines on the management of NAFLD, FIB4 index was calculated according to the following formula: FIB4 = age (year) × AST (IU/L)/ {platelet count (109/L) × [ALT (U/L)]1/2} [1, 28]. The result was an increased value of FIB4, namely 1.87.

Taking into consideration these results, we decided to further perform a second noninvasive test, namely, VCTE with CAP, which revealed increased LSM and CAP values: 6.9 kPa and 354 dB/m, respectively, corresponding to mild fibrosis (F1) and severe steatosis (S3) [3].

Finally, the patient was diagnosed with nonalcoholic fatty liver disease. Moreover, our patient presented 3 out of 5 components of the MetS (high blood pressure, dyslipidemia, and increased waist circumference), and the diagnosis was established accordingly [33].

According to current recommendations, the patient was encouraged to adopt a number of lifestyle adjustments, including regular exercise and weight loss. In addition to suggesting aerobic and resistance training, a general recommendation was given to minimize the consumption of simple sugars, industrial fructose, and saturated fats. The patient was advised to monitor her blood pressure periodically and notify her primary care physician of any changes. Furthermore, treatment with rosuvastatin 20 mg daily was initiated for dyslipidemia.

At the 6-month follow-up, the patient's body weight had decreased by around 5 kilograms. Blood tests revealed that liver enzymes remained within the normal range, while total cholesterol and triglycerides, despite a decreasing trend, nonetheless remained over the normal range. At the VCTE with CAP examination, there was a slight improvement of the LSM and CAP values, namely 6.6 kPa and 322 dB/m, respectively. Regarding dietary and lifestyle modifications, she stated that she finds it challenging to adopt new eating and living habits and this is why the patient was referred to a nutrition specialist in order to provide a more holistic care.

22.6 Discussions

NAFLD is nevertheless closely linked to the obesity epidemic and being overweight [34]. NAFLD is one of the most significant causes of liver pathology globally, and it is likely to overtake other causes as the primary cause of end-stage liver disease in the next decades, as evidenced by prior studies [4]. Based on current knowledge, the pathogenesis of NAFLD is a multifactorial and multistep process [35]. Among the established clinical conditions closely associated with NAFLD, abdominal obesity and other characteristics of MetS, such as disturbed glucose metabolism with insulin resistance, dyslipidemia, hypertension, and other metabolic disorders linked to increased cardiovascular risk, are given special consideration [36, 37]. As a result, the current understanding of the intimate and reciprocal association between NAFLD and MetS has evolved, and the bidirectional relationship between the two disorders is now widely recognized [38, 39].

As NAFLD has steadily risen in importance on a global scale, it has become increasingly apparent that the phrase "nonalcoholic" contains fundamental flaws. This description overemphasizes the absence of alcohol consumption and underemphasizes the metabolic danger [40]. As a result, a new terminology has been designed to better illustrate the close connection between NAFLD and metabolic diseases, specifically metabolic associated fatty liver disease (MAFLD) [41].

Increases in the prevalence of both MetS and NAFLD are mostly attributable to changes in nutrition and lifestyle in industrialized and developing nations, respectively. This tendency increases mortality and morbidity related to metabolic, hepatic, and cardiovascular conditions [42, 43].

22.7 Fourth Case Report

A 23-year-old woman was emergently admitted to the hospital because of upper gastrointestinal bleeding. Endoscopically, gastric ulcer Forrest III class was discovered. Prior to admission, she daily used nonsteroidal anti-inflammatory drugs for 1 year due to back pain and biliary colic. During anamnesis, we noticed an irregular menstrual cycle at 2 months and the impossibility of getting pregnant for 1 year. The patient had no history of alcohol consumption or drug use. During the physical examination, hirsutism, acne, and obesity were noticed, with an abdominal circumference of 105 cm and a BMI of 33 kg/m². Moreover, the patient had pain on palpation in the right hypochondrium and hepatomegaly.

Laboratory tests showed a mild level of hemoglobin of 9.4 g/dL. White blood cell count and platelet count were within normal limits. C-reactive protein was elevated (2.0 mg/dL). The coagulation profile was in normal limits. LFT showed an alanine aminotransferase (ALT) of 155 U/L (reference range 15–36 U/L) and an alkaline phosphatase (ALP) of 110 (reference range 40–105 U/L). The lipid profile was modified with total cholesterol of 300 mg/dL, high-density lipoprotein (HDL) of 39 mg/dL, low-density lipoprotein (LDL) of 221 mg/dL, and triglycerides of 200 mg/dL. Bilirubin and albumin had normal values. Hepatitis B surface antigen, hepatitis B virus core antibody, and hepatitis C virus antibody were all negative. Ceruloplasmin was within normal limits, while ferritin was lower than the normal value. The fasting plasma glucose level was 120 mg/dL. After stabilization of the upper gastrointestinal bleeding, a glucose tolerance test was performed, with a level of glucose of 153 mg/dL after 2 h, resulting in decreased glucose tolerance.

Abdominal ultrasound identified increased homogeneous echogenicity of the liver compared to the kidney and difficult identification of the hepatic veins and multiple hyperreflective images on the topography of the cholecyst. The structure of the ovaries was modified, each one having an increased volume (12 cm³). The evaluation of the liver using VCTE with CAP showed an increased LSM and CAP (9.5 kPa and 310 dB/m). The cutoffs used for CAP were 285 dB/m for S1, 340 dB/m for S2, and 355 dB/m for S3, respectively. LSM cutoff staging values were as follows: F1 (mild), F2 (significant), F3 (advanced) fibrosis, and F4 (cirrhosis): 5.6–7.1, 7.2–9.4, 9.5–12.4, and ≥12.5 kPa.

Through a multidisciplinary collaboration, an endovaginal ultrasound was performed, each ovary having dimensions of 12 cm³ and at least 30 small cysts. According to the anamnesis, clinical, and ultrasound investigation, the supposition of polycystic ovary syndrome was set. The patient had all three Rotterdam criteria: clinical manifestation of hyperandrogenism, sporadic ovulation, and polycystic ovarian changes. HOMA-IR was 3.6. The HOMA-IR was calculated based on fasting values of plasma glucose and insulin according to the HOMA model formula: HOMA-IR = IRI (µU/mL) × FPG (mg/dL)/405. Therefore, the laboratory tests focused on the hormone profile in order to exclude other etiologies. The levels of prolactin, thyroid hormones, cortisol, and ACTH were within physiological limits. The ratio of LH/FSH was 3 (above the normal level of 2), while the increased level of testosterone and estradiol and the low level of progesterone supported the diagnostic assumption.

Besides the reason for hospitalization (upper gastrointestinal bleeding, iron deficiency anemia for which she received martial therapy and proton pump inhibitors), the patient was diagnosed with polycystic ovary syndrome, nonalcoholic steatohepatitis (NASH), decreased glucose tolerance, and high blood pressure grade 1 with very high additional risk. In a setting of a multidisciplinary team, including a gastroenterologist, endocrinologist, diabetologist, and dietitian, besides the diet control and exercise for weight lost, the patient started oral administration with metformin for the reduction of insulin resistance. Moreover, due to the fact that the patient denied the intention of pregnancy, she received combined oral contraception with an antiandrogenic effect.

After a 6-month period of treatment, the patient lost 20 kg, with an improvement in the physical appearance (hirsutism) and menstrual cycle every 30 days. LFTs reached a normal range (ALT 40 U/L, AST 34 U/L), and the glycemic control was improved to 98 mg/dL. The abdominal ultrasound proved a diminished echogenicity of the liver. Moreover, the values for CAP and LSM reduced significantly (270 dB/m, 8.6 kPa).

22.8 Discussions

NAFLD represents a common cause of chronic liver disease worldwide, with a constantly increasing prevalence. Being a diagnostic of exclusion, common etiologies such as alcohol consumption and viral infections must be ruled out. Besides having a strong connection with obesity, unhealthy lifestyle, and metabolic syndrome, NAFLD is also linked with endocrinological disorders such as growth hormone deficiency, glucocorticoid excess, reduced level of thyroid hormones, and polycystic ovary syndrome (PCOS) [44, 45].

PCOS is a pathology diagnosed among young women during the childbearing period. The prevalence varies between 4 and 21% worldwide, depending on the diagnostic criteria. In order to establish the endocrine pathology, Rotterdam standards are mostly used, with at least two criteria being necessary in order to confirm the disease: clinical manifestations of hyperandrogenism, sporadic ovulation or absence of ovulation, and imagistic confirmations of the polycystic ovarian changes. Moreover, other endocrine disorders must be ruled out: hyperprolactinemia, thyroid, and adrenal disorder, or androgen-secreting tumors [46, 47]. The simultaneous hepatic and ovarian dysfunctions were described for the first time by Brown et al. (2005) when a liver biopsy performed on a 24-year-old patient with PCOS and elevated transaminase confirmed the NASH diagnosis [48]. Insulin resistance and obesity are indicated as the main risk factors for the progression of NAFLD in PCOS. However, hyperandrogenemia also influences evolution, although the exact mechanism is not fully understood [49].

As in the majority of NAFLD cases, the patient does not present specific symptoms related to liver injury, with fatigue, malaise, and discomfort in the right hypochondrium being the most frequent. A similar situation was described in our case, where the patient presented at the hospital due to upper gastrointestinal bleeding.

Standard management of NAFLD in PCOS does not exist, and current approach focused on lifestyle changes, pharmacological treatment, and bariatric surgery [50, 51].

Designing a diet that allows sustained weight loss and physical exercises are the first lines of treatment for overweight or obese patients. Moreover, it decreases the level of androgens and contributes to the normalization of menstrual cycles and the improvement of cardio-metabolic markers. In the case of the presented patient, the modification of the lifestyle had an important impact on the liver parameters by normalizing the enzymes of hepatocytolysis and decreasing the degree of fat loading [52]. In a study that included 293 patients who followed a hypocaloric diet and moderate physical activity for 52 weeks, of those who managed to lose at least 10% of their body weight, in the case of 90%, the resolution was confirmed NASH, while at 45%, the level of fibrosis decreased significantly [53].

Used in clinical practice for over 60 years, as a first-line treatment for type 2 diabetes, metformin is frequently used in PCOS to counteract insulin resistance. In the case of the presented patient, in addition to the significant decrease in body mass index and the reduction of the parameters evaluated by elastometry, the normalization of the menstrual cycle and the improvement of hirsutism represent additional benefits of metformin [54]. An alternative to metformin is the GLP-1 receptor agonist, liraglutide, whose effect of reducing insulin resistance, weight loss, and implicitly the fat load of the liver has been confirmed in various randomized studies such as Frøssing et al. whose 26 weeks' trial with liraglutide proved a reduced liver fat content of 44% and decrease in visceral adipose tissue by 18% [55].

In conclusion, PCOS represents a complex pathology with silent damage to the liver parenchyma, without having a standardized approach. However, by identifying one of the specific manifestations, including NAFLD, the implementation of a therapeutic strategy improves the quality of life.

References

1. Long MT, Noureddin M, Lim JK. AGA clinical practice update: diagnosis and management of nonalcoholic fatty liver disease in lean individuals: expert review. Gastroenterology. 2022;163(3):764–774.e1.
2. Kim BK, Kim DY, Park JY, Ahn SH, Chon CY, Kim JK, Paik YH, Lee KS, Park YN, Han KH. Validation of FIB-4 and comparison with other simple noninvasive indices for predicting liver fibrosis and cirrhosis in hepatitis B virus-infected patients. Liver Int. 2010;30(4):546–53.
3. Eddowes PJ, Sasso M, Allison M, Tsochatzis E, Anstee QM, Sheridan D, Guha IN, Cobbold JF, Deeks JJ, Paradis V, Bedossa P, Newsome PN. Accuracy of FibroScan controlled attenuation parameter and liver stiffness measurement in assessing steatosis and fibrosis in patients with nonalcoholic fatty liver disease. Gastroenterology. 2019;156(6):1717–30.
4. Feldman A, Eder SK, Felder TK, Kedenko L, Paulweber B, Stadlmayr A, Huber-Schönauer U, Niederseer D, Stickel F, Auer S, Haschke-Becher E, Patsch W, Datz C, Aigner E. Clinical and metabolic characterization of lean Caucasian subjects with non-alcoholic fatty liver. Am J Gastroenterol. 2017;112(1):102–10.
5. Wattacheril J, Sanyal AJ. Lean NAFLD: an underrecognized outlier. Curr Hepatol Rep. 2016;15(2):134–9.

6. Tilg H, Effenberger M. From NAFLD to MAFLD: when pathophysiology succeeds. Nat Rev Gastroenterol Hepatol. 2020;17(7):387–8.

7. Vos B, Moreno C, Nagy N, Féry F, Cnop M, Vereerstraeten P, Devière J, Adler M. Lean non-alcoholic fatty liver disease (Lean-NAFLD): a major cause of cryptogenic liver disease. Acta Gastroenterol Belg. 2011;74(3):389–94.

8. Fracanzani AL, Petta S, Lombardi R, Pisano G, Russello M, Consonni D, Di Marco V, Cammà C, Mensi L, Dongiovanni P, Valenti L, Craxì A, Fargion S. Liver and cardiovascular damage in patients with lean nonalcoholic fatty liver disease, and association with visceral obesity. Clin Gastroenterol Hepatol. 2017;15(10):1604–1611.e1.

9. Sookoian S, Pirola CJ. Systematic review with meta-analysis: risk factors for non-alcoholic fatty liver disease suggest a shared altered metabolic and cardiovascular profile between lean and obese patients. Aliment Pharmacol Ther. 2017;46(2):85–95.

10. Keating SE, Hackett DA, Parker HM, O'Connor HT, Gerofi JA, Sainsbury A, Baker MK, Chuter VH, Caterson ID, George J, Johnson NA. Effect of aerobic exercise training dose on liver fat and visceral adiposity. J Hepatol. 2015;63(1):174–82.

11. Sung KC, Ryu S, Lee JY, Kim JY, Wild SH, Byrne CD. Effect of exercise on the development of new fatty liver and the resolution of existing fatty liver. J Hepatol. 2016;65(4):791–7.

12. Hashida R, Kawaguchi T, Bekki M, Omoto M, Matsuse H, Nago T, Takano Y, Ueno T, Koga H, George J, Shiba N, Torimura T. Aerobic vs. resistance exercise in non-alcoholic fatty liver disease: a systematic review. J Hepatol. 2017;66(1):142–52.

13. Takahashi H, Kotani K, Tanaka K, Egucih Y, Anzai K. Therapeutic approaches to nonalcoholic fatty liver disease: exercise intervention and related mechanisms. Front Endocrinol (Lausanne). 2018;15(9):588.

14. Lin Z-H, Xin Y-N, Dong Q-J, Wang Q, Jiang X-J, Zhan S-H, Sun Y, Xuan S-Y. Performance of the aspartate aminotransferase-to-platelet ratio index for the staging of hepatitis C-related fibrosis: an updated meta-analysis. Hepatology. 2011;53:726–36.

15. Tohidi M, Ghasemi A, Hadaegh F, Derakhshan A, Chary A, Azizi F. Age- and sex-specific reference values for fasting serum insulin levels and insulin resistance/sensitivity indices in healthy Iranian adults: Tehran Lipid and Glucose Study. Clin Biochem. 2014;47(6):432–8.

16. Cichoż-Lach H, Celiński K, Prozorow-Król B, Swatek J, Słomka M, Lach T. The BARD score and the NAFLD fibrosis score in the assessment of advanced liver fibrosis in nonalcoholic fatty liver disease. Med Sci Monit. 2012;18(12):CR735–40.

17. Sasso M, Beaugrand M, et al. Controlled attenuation parameter (CAP): a novel VCTE™ guided ultrasonic attenuation measurement for the evaluation of hepatic steatosis: preliminary study and validation in a cohort of patients with chronic liver disease from various causes. Ultrasound Med Biol. 2010;36(11):1825–35.

18. Ferraioli G. Quantitative assessment of liver steatosis using ultrasound controlled attenuation parameter (Echosens). J Med Ultrasonics. 2021;48:489–95.

19. American Diabetes Association Professional Practice Committee. 2. Classification and diagnosis of diabetes: standards of Medical Care in Diabetes-2022. Diabetes Care. 2022;45(Suppl 1):S17–38.

20. Vieira Barbosa J, Lai M. Nonalcoholic fatty liver disease screening in type 2 diabetes mellitus patients in the primary care setting. Hepatol Commun. 2021;5:158–67.

21. Younossi Z, Tacke F, Arrese M, Chander Sharma B, Mostafa I, Bugianesi E, et al. Global perspectives on nonalcoholic fatty liver disease and nonalcoholic steatohepatitis. Hepatology. 2019;69:2672–82.

22. Younossi ZM. The epidemiology of nonalcoholic steatohepatitis. Clin Liver Dis (Hoboken). 2018;11:92–4.

23. Hruby A, Hu FB. The epidemiology of obesity: a big picture. PharmacoEconomics. 2015;33(7):673–89.

24. Kim Y, Chang Y, Cho YK, Ahn J, Shin H, Ryu S. Obesity and weight gain are associated with progression of fibrosis in patients with nonalcoholic fatty liver disease. Clin Gastroenterol Hepatol. 2019;17:543–550.e542.

25. American Diabetes Association. Standards of medical care in diabetes—2012. Diabetes Care. 2012;35(Supplement 1):S11–63.
26. Ratziu V, Charlotte F, Heurtier A, Gombert S, Giral P, Bruckert E, Grimaldi A, Capron F, Poynard T. Sampling variability of liver biopsy in nonalcoholic fatty liver disease. Gastroenterology. 2005;128(7):1898–906.
27. Copel L, Sosna J, Kruskal JB, Kane RA. Ultrasound-guided percutaneous liver biopsy: indications, risks, and technique. Surg Technol Int. 2003;11:154–60.
28. European Association for the Study of the Liver (EASL); European Association for the Study of Diabetes (EASD); European Association for the Study of Obesity (EASO). EASL–EASD–EASO clinical practice guidelines for the management of non-alcoholic fatty liver disease. J Hepatol. 2016;64(6):1388–402.
29. Siddiqui MS, Vuppalanchi R, Van Natta ML, Hallinan E, Kowdley KV, Abdelmalek M, Neuschwander-Tetri BA, Loomba R, Dasarathy S, Brandman D, Doo E, Tonascia JA, Kleiner DE, Chalasani N, Sanyal AJ, NASH Clinical Research Network. Vibration-controlled transient elastography to assess fibrosis and steatosis in patients with nonalcoholic fatty liver disease. Clin Gastroenterol Hepatol. 2019;17(1):156–163.e2.
30. Petta S, Vanni E, Bugianesi E, Di Marco V, Cammà C, Cabibi D, Mezzabotta L, Craxì A. The combination of liver stiffness measurement and NAFLD fibrosis score improves the noninvasive diagnostic accuracy for severe liver fibrosis in patients with nonalcoholic fatty liver disease. Liver Int. 2015;35(5):1566–73.
31. Feng W, Gao C, Bi Y, Wu M, Li P, Shen S, et al. Randomized trial comparing the effects of gliclazide, liraglutide, and metformin on diabetes with non-alcoholic fatty liver disease. J Diabetes. 2017;9:800–9.
32. Moreira GV, Azevedo FF, Ribeiro LM, Santos A, Guadagnini D, Gama P, et al. Liraglutide modulates gut microbiota and reduces NAFLD in obese mice. J Nutr Biochem. 2018;62:143–54.
33. Chalasani N, Younossi Z, Lavine JE, Charlton M, Cusi K, Rinella M, Harrison SA, Brunt EM, Sanyal AJ. The diagnosis and management of nonalcoholic fatty liver disease: practice guidance from the American Association for the Study of Liver Diseases. Hepatology. 2018;67(1):328–57.
34. Marchesini G, Bugianesi E, Forlani G, Cerrelli F, Lenzi M, Manini R, Natale S, Vanni E, Villanova N, Melchionda N, Rizzetto M. Nonalcoholic fatty liver, steatohepatitis, and the metabolic syndrome. Hepatology. 2003;37(4):917–23.
35. Paik JM, Golabi P, Younossi Y, Mishra A, Younossi ZM. Changes in the global burden of chronic liver diseases from 2012 to 2017: the growing impact of NAFLD. Hepatology. 2020;72(5):1605–16.
36. Hardy T, Oakley F, Anstee QM, Day CP. Nonalcoholic fatty liver disease: pathogenesis and disease spectrum. Annu Rev Pathol. 2016;23(11):451–96.
37. Polyzos SA, Kountouras J, Mantzoros CS. Obesity and nonalcoholic fatty liver disease: from pathophysiology to therapeutics. Metabolism. 2019;92:82–97.
38. Kim D, Chung GE, Kwak MS, Seo HB, Kang JH, Kim W, Kim YJ, Yoon JH, Lee HS, Kim CY. Body fat distribution and risk of incident and regressed nonalcoholic fatty liver disease. Clin Gastroenterol Hepatol. 2016;14(1):132–8.e4.
39. Yki-Järvinen H. Non-alcoholic fatty liver disease as a cause and a consequence of metabolic syndrome. Lancet Diabetes Endocrinol. 2014;2(11):901–10.
40. Ma J, Hwang SJ, Pedley A, Massaro JM, Hoffmann U, Chung RT, Benjamin EJ, Levy D, Fox CS, Long MT. Bi-directional analysis between fatty liver and cardiovascular disease risk factors. J Hepatol. 2017;66(2):390–7.
41. Younossi ZM, Rinella ME, Sanyal AJ, Harrison SA, Brunt EM, Goodman Z, Cohen DE, Loomba R. From NAFLD to MAFLD: implications of a premature change in terminology. Hepatology. 2021;73(3):1194–8.
42. Eslam M, Sanyal AJ, George J, International Consensus Panel. MAFLD: a consensus-driven proposed nomenclature for metabolic associated fatty liver disease. Gastroenterology. 2020;158(7):1999–2014.e1.

43. Rinaldi L, Pafundi PC, Galiero R, Caturano A, Morone MV, Silvestri C, Giordano M, Salvatore T, Sasso FC. Mechanisms of non-alcoholic fatty liver disease in the metabolic syndrome. A narrative review. Antioxidants (Basel). 2021;10(2):270.

44. Legro RS, Arslanian SA, Ehrmann DA, Hoeger KM, Murad MH, Pasquali R, Welt CK, Endocrine Society. Diagnosis and treatment of polycystic ovary syndrome: an Endocrine Society clinical practice guideline. J Clin Endocrinol Metab. 2013;98:4565–92.

45. Younossi Z, Anstee QM, Marietti M, Hardy T, Henry L, Eslam M, George J, Bugianesi E. Global burden of NAFLD and NASH: trends, predictions, risk factors and prevention. Nat Rev Gastroenterol Hepatol. 2018;15(1):11–20.

46. Bozdag G, Mumusoglu S, Zengin D, Karabulut E, Yildiz BO. The prevalence and phenotypic features of polycystic ovary syndrome: a systematic review and meta-analysis. Hum Reprod. 2016;31:2841–55.

47. Lizneva D, Suturina L, Walker W, et al. Criteria, prevalence, and phenotypes of polycystic ovary syndrome. Fertil Steril. 2016;106(1):6–15.

48. Brown AJ, Tendler DA, McMurray RG, Setji TL. Polycystic ovary syndrome and severe non-alcoholic steatohepatitis: beneficial effect of modest weight loss and exercise on liver biopsy findings. Endocr Pract. 2005;11(5):319–24.

49. Pasquali R, Oriolo C. Obesity and androgens in women. Hyperandrog Women. 2019;53:120–34.

50. Falzarano C, et al. Nonalcoholic fatty liver disease in women and girls with polycystic ovary syndrome. J Clin Endocrinol Metabol. 2022;107(1):258–72.

51. Sarkar M, Terrault N, Chan W, Cedars MI, Huddleston HG, Duwaerts CC, Balitzer D, Gill RM. Polycystic ovary syndrome (PCOS) is associated with NASH severity and advanced fibrosis. Liver Int. 2020;40(2):355–9.

52. Vilar-Gomez E, Martinez-Perez Y, Calzadilla-Bertot L, et al. Weight loss through lifestyle modification significantly reduces features of nonalcoholic steatohepatitis. Gastroenterology. 2015;149(2):367–378.e5.

53. Bordewijk EM, Nahuis M, Costello MF, et al. Metformin during ovulation induction with gonadotrophins followed by timed intercourse or intrauterine insemination for subfertility associated with polycystic ovary syndrome. Cochrane Database Syst Rev. 2017;1(1):CD009090.

54. Shamim H, Jean M, Umair M, Muddaloor P, Farinango M, Ansary A, Dakka A, Nazir Z, White CT, Habbal AB, Mohammed L. Role of metformin in the management of polycystic ovarian syndrome-associated acne: a systematic review. Cureus. 2022;14(8):e28462.

55. Frøssing S, Nylander M, Chabanova E, et al. Effect of liraglutide on ectopic fat in polycystic ovary syndrome: a randomized clinical trial. Diabetes Obes Metab. 2018;20(1):215–8.

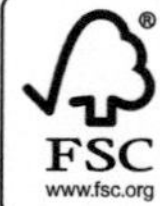